AF618206

Blood Supply of Bone

Springer
London
Berlin
Heidelberg
New York
Barcelona
Budapest
Hong Kong
Milan
Paris
Santa Clara
Singapore
Tokyo

Murray Brookes and William J. Revell

Blood Supply of Bone

Scientific Aspects

With 235 Figures
plus 10 Colour Plates

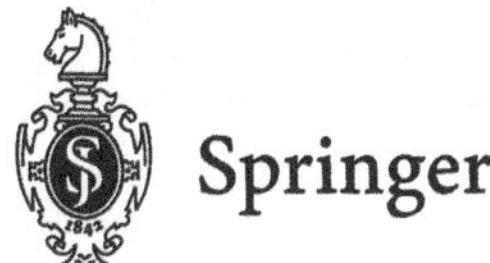

Springer

Murray Brookes, DM (Oxon), MA, DLO (RCS) England
Professor Emeritus, University of London
Academic Department of Orthopaedics,
Rayne Institute, St Thomas's Hospital,
Lambeth Palace Road, London SE1 7EH, UK

William J. Revell, BA, MSc, PhD (Lond)
Academic Department of Orthopaedics, Rayne Institute,
St Thomas's Hospital, Lambeth Palace Road, London SE1 7EH, UK

Cover illustrations: Front cover: Sagittal microangiograph of a human fetal tibia (Chapter 3, Figure 2). Back cover: Cross-sectional microangiograph of a canine femur (Chapter 9, Figure 14).

ISBN-13:978-1-4471-1545-8

British Library Cataloguing in Publication Data
Brookes, Murray
Blood supply of bone: scientific aspects
1. Bones - Blood-vessels
I. Title II. Revell, William J.
612. 7'5
ISBN-13:978-1-4471-1545-8

Library of Congress Cataloging-in-Publication Data
Brookes, Murray.
Blood supply of bone: scientific aspects / Murray Brookes and William J. Revell. - Rev. and updated ed.
p. cm.
Includes bibliographical references and index.
ISBN-13:978-1-4471-1545-8 e-ISBN-13:978-1-4471-1543-4
DOI: 10.1007/978-1-4471-1543-4

1. Bones - Blood-vessels. 2. Bones–Growth. I. Revell, William J., 1946- . II. Title.
[DNLM: 1. Bone and Bones - blood supply. WE 200 B872b 1998]
QP88.2.B76 1998
612.7'5 - dc21
DNLM/DLC 97-31214
for Library of Congress CIP

Softcover reprint of the hardcover 1st edition 1998

This is a revised and updated edition of *The Blood Supply of Bone*, previously published in 1971 by Butterworth Scientific Ltd.

Typeset by EXPO Holdings, Malaysia

28/3830-543210 Printed on acid-free paper

Dedication

To Our Wives and Children

Werkleute sind wir, Knappen, Jünger, Meister,
Und bauen dich, du hohen Mittelschiff.

Das Stundenbuch.
Rainer Maria Rilke.

Preface to the first edition

This book on the blood supply of bone was begun 5 years ago as an introduction to the anatomical study of the vascular architecture of the skeleton. But the central position held by bone vascularization in the growth and mutability of bones and joints fortunately made the book outgrow its original intention: it has not outgrown its limitations. A detailed account of the mechanisms of calcification, collagenogenesis and matrix formation has been put aside. Instead I have chosen to emphasize the controlling role of the osseous circulation in osteogenesis, and the linkage it provides between bone metabolism, bone mechanics and bone pathology.

In the precious hours that I could sequestrate for my researches from a busy teaching curriculum, I have enjoyed the co-operation of many clinicians and academic colleagues. I would like to acknowledge their kindness in making clinical material or scientific equipment accessible to me, and their timely advice and early encouragement. My thanks are due to the Sir Halley Stewart Trust, the Medical Research Council and the Governors of Guy's Hospital Medical School, who have supported my researches financially. It is particularly pleasing for me to record an additional debt that I owe to Professor Roger Warwick, which cannot be repaid by the publication of this book in whose compilation he has shown a continual interest. Among the many who have diligently rendered me technical assistance, none will begrudge my mentioning a special debt of gratitude to my wife, for her part-time labour as a research secretary in the midst of a large and lively household.

Murray Brookes
1971

Preface to the second edition

More than a quarter of a century has gone by since the publication of the *Blood Supply of Bone* in 1971. In this time it has been pleasing to see the intensification of bone mechanical and molecular biological studies, if only because the stated aim in the Preface to the first edition was to emphasize the "vascular linkage between bone metabolism, bone mechanics and bone pathology". That purpose has not changed, and the participation of bone mechanics in the life of bone has never been far from our discussion of the blood supply of bone, the two indivisible aspects of the osteogenic coin. Mechanics affect bone formation; without blood flow there is no osteogenesis.

Unfortunately, our subject itself has outgrown its original capacity to include, in a single volume, significant areas of orthopaedic practice. It has therefore become imperative to reserve a subsequent volume devoted to the vascular control of bone remodelling, and its influence on some of the major features of clinical orthopaedics, such as fracture repair, chronic disorders of bone production, bone prosthetics and skeletal malformation.

It is with great pleasure that this book gives us an opportunity to thank Professor Frederick Heatley, Head of the Academic Orthopaedic Department in St Thomas's Hospital, London, for always supporting us in our endeavours and providing us, by his own initiatives, with space and facilities to carry out bone research for the past 20 years. There can be no question but that without his continual generosity, our collaborative investigations would never have come about, and most certainly this new edition of the *Blood Supply of Bone* would never have been written.

We also thank our postgraduate pupils, who over the years have developed their skills while amplifying our knowledge. We thank, in particular, Mr Richard Brueton, Dr Seba Chandararaj, Mr Mark Churchill, Mr Charles Gallanaugh, Professor Miles Irving, Dr Khin U. May, Mr Mohinder Singh, Mr John Spencer and Professor Darrel Wijeratne, whose thesis work on the skeleton was personally supervised by one of us (M.B.), and who permitted us to make citation of their research. And most happily we wish to thank Esther Brookes for her daily labour in preparing an acceptable text, including the Bibliography, for our publishers Springer Verlag.

Murray Brookes
William Revell
1997

Preface to the second edition

Contents

COLOUR PLATES

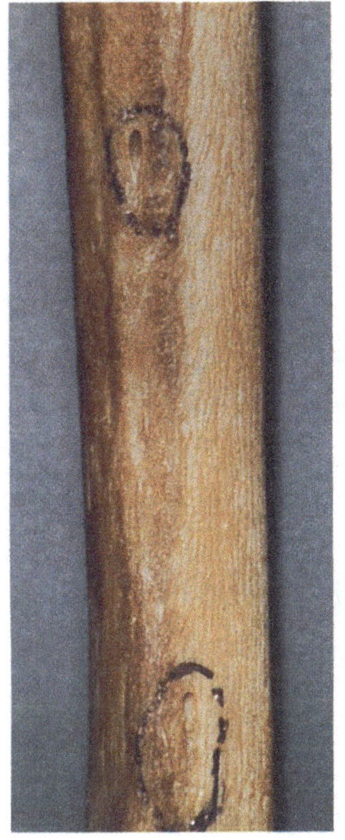

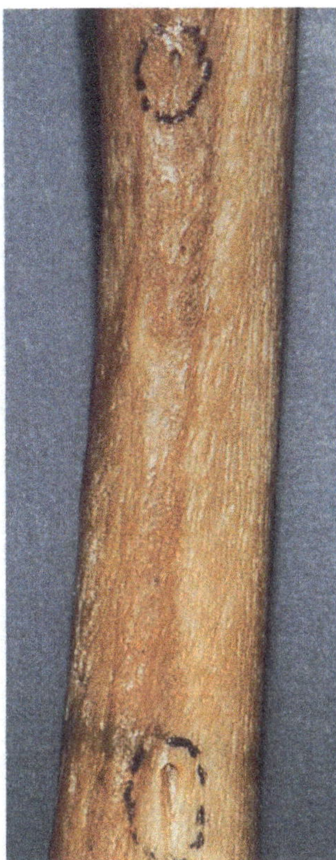

Fig. 2.14. (*far left*) Two femoral nutrient foramina of similar size on the linea aspera. (Original: Natural size).

Fig. 2.15. (*left*) Two femoral nutrient foramina; the upper one is smaller. (Original: Natural size).

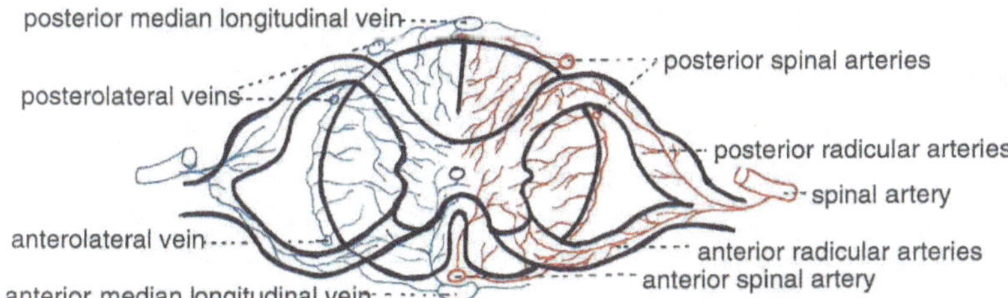

Fig. 5.7. (*above*) Plan of the spinal cord and its intrinsic blood vessels, united by longitudinal arterial and venous columns. (Based on Gray 1989.)

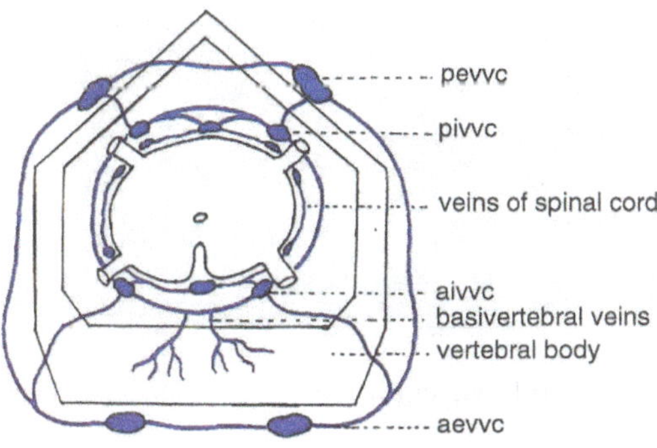

Fig. 5.8. (*left*) Plan of the three great venous circles around each vertebra and the spinal cord, showing **pevvc** and **pivvc**, external and internal vertebral venous columns; **aevvc** and **aivvc**, corresponding anterior columns; and the innermost venous circles of the spinal cord and their longitudinal anastomoses. The caval, azygos, abdominal and pelvic venous systems communicate with the vertebral veins.

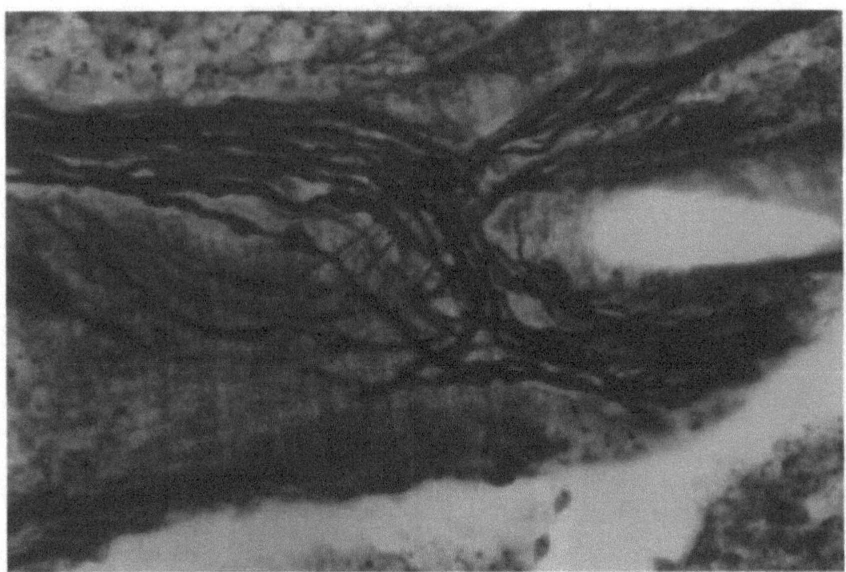

Fig. 8.20. A large nerve bundle dividing at the bifurcation of a medullary artery. (Dog; Linder's silver impregnation; Original magnification ×450)

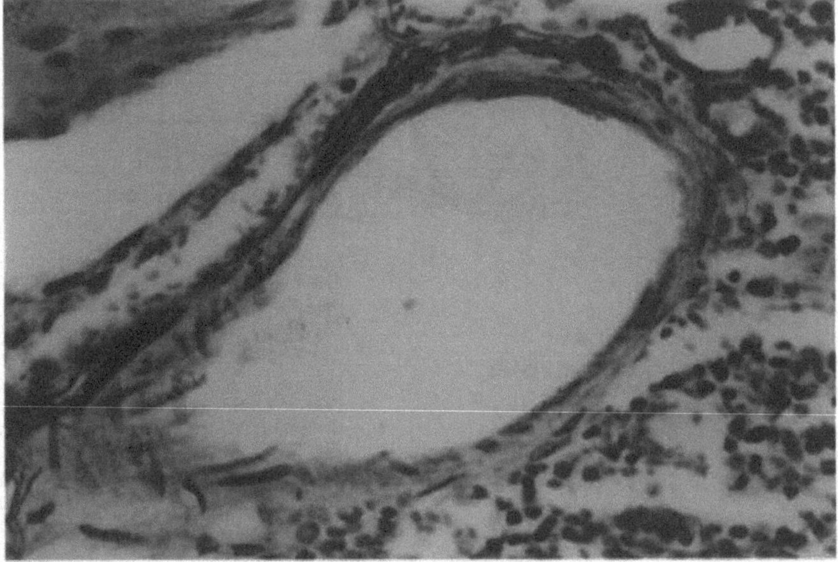

Fig. 8.21. Perivascular fibres in contact with a small epiphyseal artery. (Dog, Linder's silver impregnation; Original magnification ×420)

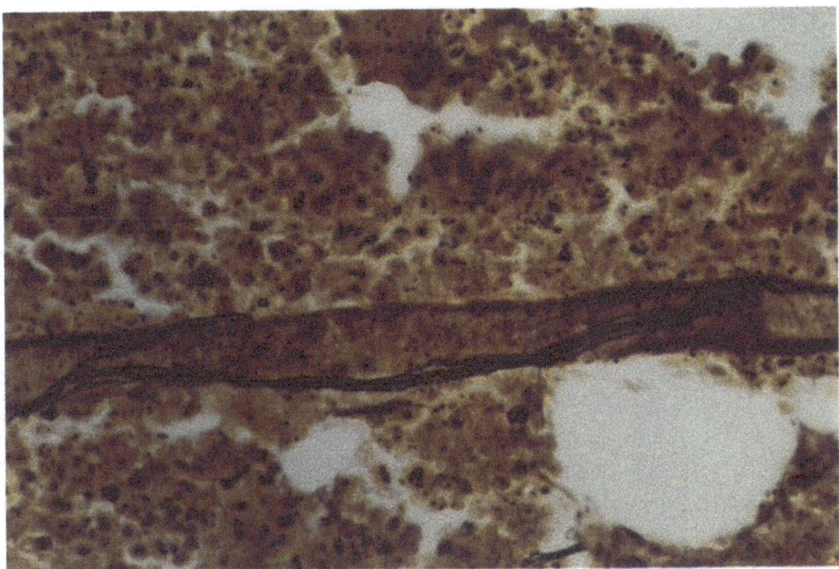

Fig. 8.22. Straight arteriole in bone marrow with its sympathetic fibres. (Dog, Linder's silver impregnation; Original magnification ×420)

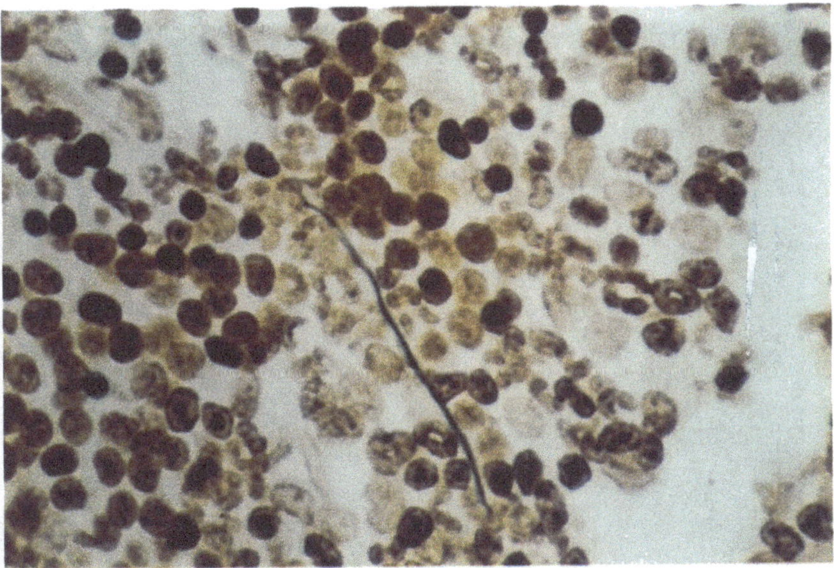

Fig. 8.23. A solitary nerve fibre running between parenchymal cells. (Dog, Linder's silver impregnation; Original magnification ×420)

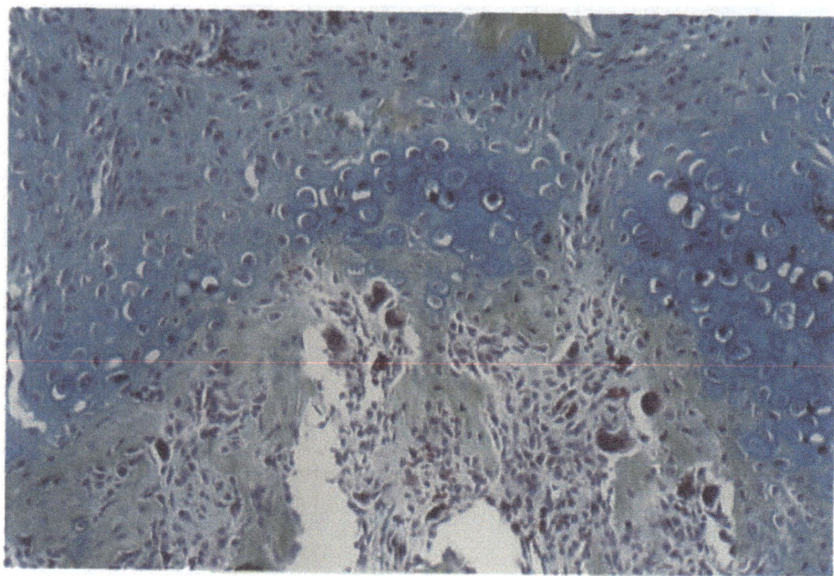

Fig. 8.38. Photomicrograph of a section through the site of a rat fibular fracture (4 days post-operation), stained with Elbadawi's (1976) hexachrome modification of Movat's stain. The purple "giant cells" close to the blue cartilage, are primitive angioblastic islands in the EM.

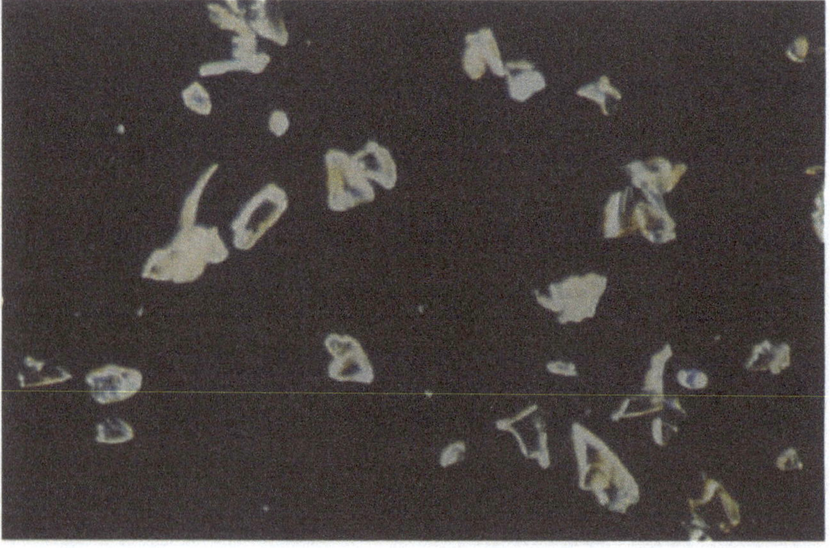

Fig. 19.1. Polarized light view of prepared resin particles. The mean length along the long axis is 32.28 μm.

Chapter 1
Introduction

Historical beginnings

The manner in which bones obtain a blood supply has engaged the attention of anatomists for nearly three centuries. Nevertheless, it must be admitted that progress in the study of the vascular architecture of the skeleton and the significance of its circulation has been unusually slow, and at times refractory. Indeed, it is only in the final decade of the twentieth century that it has become possible to give a brief account of the anatomy of the circulation in long bones, which can rightfully claim general acceptance, and on the basis of scientific demonstration supplicate for freedom from controversy.

Fifty years ago and more, vascular studies on bones were a rarity, in part because adequate techniques for visualizing blood vessels in bone were not available,and suitable microradiographic apparatus had not yet been devised. Furthermore, the microscopic investigation of bones is beset with practical difficulties peculiar to bones alone. Their hardness is an obstacle to dissection and their opaqueness requires modifications to be made in what are routine and well-established histological procedures in other, but soft, tissues. Even today, Araldite embedding of undecalcified bone samples followed by sectioning with powerful microtomes, tends to be confined to specialized and well-endowed laboratories, creating problems of access to the imaginative experimentalist.

But the chief impediment to the spirit of enquiry has doubtless been provided by the very nature of the bones themselves. Their solidity; their provision of a supporting and protecting frame to the soft organs of the body; their manifest function as mechanical levers and fixed points facilitating movement and progression; their apparently enduring quality in life and immutability after death; and their persistence as memorials to extinct species and fossil men: all these are are attributes which do not immediately declare an innate vitality. It is understandable, therefore, that in the past, as in the present, there have always been those who preferred not to study the skeleton as a living component of the body, but to investigate its mechanical and engineering properties, especially in relation to posture and locomotion, and to deal with bones as if they were inert, permanent and dead.

Yet, however vaguely comprehended the manner of their nutrition may have been in the past, the lifeless appearance of bones never beguiled those anatomists who recognized the vitality of the skeleton in its capacity for growth and repair. In the literary monuments recording the patient industry of von Haller (1763),

Hunter (1772), Winslow (1776), Bichat (1801), Mascagni (1819), Cooper (1822) and their learned nineteenth century successors, right up to the present-day flood of texts and papers of recent investigators, a gradually unfolding account may be found of the circulation of the blood in bones and its relation to their structure and function. The account is far from being complete, and improved methods of investigation have raised new problems before offering a final solution to the old. It is appropriate therefore, to make mention of three great men whose original contributions to the study of bone vascularization supplied a starting point for the inquiries of succeeding generations.

In 1674, in a letter to the Royal Society, Antonie van Leeuwenhoek, a citizen of Delft, a draper by trade and the founder of microscopical science, wrote:

> I have several times endeavoured to observe the parts of a Bone, and at first I imagined, I saw on the surface of the Shinbone of a Cow several small veins.... I thought likewise, I saw then also, that that Bone consisted of united Globules. Afterwards I viewed the Shinbone of a Calf, in which I found several little holes, passing from without inwards; and I then imagined, that this Bone had divers small pipes going longwayes.

Fifteen years later, in 1691, Clopton Havers, born in Essex, an undergraduate of Cambridge, but who received his MD from the University of Utrecht, published in London his *Osteologia Nova, or Some New Observations of the Bones, communicated to the Royal Society in several Discourses*. In this book he described how a large nutrient artery pierces the shaft of long bones and enters and ramifies in bone marrow. From the yellow marrow of the femora which he examined microscopically, little bags of fat could be shaken free, each provided with an arterial stalk. This ramified on the surface of the lobule and secreted an oily medullary substance. He surmised that by contraction of the marrow lobules, medullary oil was expelled into a system of "straight channels" – soon referred to everywhere as the Haversian canals – which he found in the bones of both ox and man. The oil provided suppleness to the cortical lamellae of which he was again the first observer. In the Latin of the Leyden edition (1734) Havers wrote, "Pariter eos [poros rectos] in humano osse, non sine summa delectatione, intuitus sum" (I was particularly pleased to observe them [the straight channels] in human bone as well). "Per os medullosum oleum se ipsum diffundit, laminisque immediate providet" (A medullary oil spread through the bone from within, and made direct provision for its laminae). Havers also described groups of arteries which entered the extremities of long bones. In his opinion they formed a vascular mesh in the cortex which gave rise to "vast numbers of veins" leaving the bone at its periosteal surface. This is the earliest observation on the centrifugal nutrition of bone cortex from the marrow outwards, through the compact bone of the shaft, into the veins of the periosteum.

It will be noticed that Havers himself was uncertain whether all the minute canals he had observed in bone cortex actually contained blood vessels, or medullary oil which percolated from the marrow cavity. The doubt was finally resolved by Albinus in 1754 with the publication of his third volume of *Annotationes Academicae*. Albinus in his own lifetime had become an acknowledged master of the vascular injection technique commonplace in halls of dissection for displaying the blood vessels of the human body. He wrote how he was surprised to find that the tiny canals of bone cortex, visible in a hand lens, did not simply contain medullary oil but enclosed fine blood vessels. "Postquam autem vasa implevi, diffractis ossibus per longitudinem, non vacuos, sed impletos canaliculos eorum vidi: et...ut impleti a vasis essent" (However, once I had filled the vessels and split the bones longitudinally, I saw that the canals were not empty but had been filled as if by blood vessels). His findings were not due to extravasation of perfusate, but to its passage along distended vessels in the bone canals. Furthermore, vessels both entered and left the bone at its internal and external surfaces, so that half was supplied from medullary and half from periosteal vessels. "Apparuit igitur, ubi, quasque per vias, quae per ossa penetrare vasa dixi, intrent exeantve: quorum quae ab exteriore parte sunt, ea rami vasorum sunt periostei: quae ab interiore, ad medullam visa sunt pertinere" (It therefore appeared as I have said previously, that whatever the routes by which blood vessels penetrate the bones, whether going in or coming out, those from the outer part of the bone are branches of the periosteal vessels; those which come from the inner aspect of the cortex belong to the medullary system). In this way was introduced the long-lived notion of a combined medullary and periosteal vascularization of the cortex of long bones at all times, which has been accepted for 200 years without qualification by all except those modern investigators who have troubled themselves to reexamine the question (Brookes & Harrison 1957; Rhinelander 1968; Gunst 1980; Dillaman 1984; Montgomery *et al.* 1988; Dillaman *et al.* 1991; Bridgeman & Brookes 1996). Nevertheless we owe a debt of gratitude to Albinus, whose great authority made the concept of bone vascularization acceptable to all his contemporaries and established once and for all the basic function of the Haversian canals of bone, hinted at by Leeuwenhoek but described and made generally known by Havers himself.

Modern vascular studies

By the beginning of the nineteenth century, it was generally accepted that in their internal structure bones are as full of blood as soft tissues, with greater powers of repair than most, and are subject like them to periods of growth and decay and to daily renewal of their substance. It has now become axiomatic that an adequate blood supply is the indispensable basis of the vitality and growth of bones and their mutability in response to environmental changes. Moreover, bone as a tissue is normally formed and broken down in relation to blood vessels, because these are the route by which diffusible ions and molecules pass to bone cells and into the organic matrix and mineral component of bone substance. It follows that the vascular anatomy of bones has an important bearing on their shape and microscopic structure, and profoundly influences these characters in both health and disease. Furthermore, the modern study of the microcirculation and vascular reactivity of bone tissue has allowed workers in various centres to make considerable progress towards an elucidation of the physiology of the osseous circulation and its relationship to the control of bone growth.

Several modern methods have been highly successful in yielding anatomical data bearing on the layout of blood vessels in bones. The most frequently used procedure in anatomical vascular studies is the injection of radiopaque media into the main vessels of a limb. After fixation, the isolated bones are then sectioned into slices about 400 μm thick and X-rayed (Tucker 1949; de Marneffe 1951; Kelly *et al.* 1959; Brookes 1967a; Rhinelander 1968). For microangiography, special apparatus is required that permits continuous exposure (10 min) of specimens to low kilovoltage emissions (12 kV), in order to study vascular details in bone, especially in small laboratory animals. The writer has for many years employed a Hilger and Watts microfocal unit and used it, in later years, as in the projection method (Cunningham 1960) of microradiography. Exposures are made on Kodak maximum resolution film, which after development may be further magnified photographically as desired. By varying the nature of the perfusate (most frequently a barium sulphate suspension), its concentration and its site of injection, the three major parts of the circulation in bones, arteries, capillaries and veins can be delineated.

India ink perfusions (Pinard 1952; Novak 1959; Irving 1965; Brookes & Helal 1968b) are very helpful for filling capillaries, but the necessary celloidin processing and clearing of thick tissue sections for optical microscopy is time-consuming and tedious. Nevertheless, the sharpness of contrast and the possibility of magnification to ×250 cannot be equalled by microradiographic examination of vascular networks.

Vascular perfusion with plastic materials (de Marneffe 1951; Wray & Lynch 1959), especially neoprene, followed by bone corrosion in strong acids and subsequent display of vascular leashes under the light microscope, is a helpful auxiliary technique. The electron microscope (EM) has not yet been fully exploited for bone vascular studies, possibly because of the difficulties in cutting ultra-thin sections of a hard tissue impregnated with calcium salts. EM studies on the vessels of bone marrow have, however, been carried out on marrow cores removed from the bone shaft after fixation (Zamboni & Pease 1961; Skawina *et al.* 1994a,b). Juxta-epiphyseal vessels, because of their situation next to soft cartilage and within a yielding primary spongiosa, are comparatively easy to examine with the EM (Brookes & Landon 1963).

Nevertheless, it cannot be emphasized sufficiently that modern methods have not rendered obsolete the more venerable techniques of dissection and paraffin histology of bone materials. The former is still used to study the fine details of the gross blood supply of bones in clinically important areas (Tucker 1949; Rogers & Gladstone 1950; Howe *et al.* 1950; Stilwell 1959), or with experimental investigation in animals (Kistler 1934; Hughes 1952; Parouti 1962; Torreilles 1962). Paraffin histology is a necessary concomitant of microangiographic studies, in order to establish the nature of the vessels which have been visualized and their relation to cartilage and bone. Especially in cortical vascular studies, it is regrettable that light microscopy has only too frequently been employed in support of conclusions which otherwise are based solely on X-ray or perfusion appearances. It is not surprising, therefore, that the detailed anatomy of the cortical blood vessels is an area still awaiting elucidation, particularly in relation to vascular changes during senescence and disease (Trueta 1968; Bridgeman & Brookes 1996; Crock 1996).

The tubular bones of the skeleton have been an object of vascular study more often than other types. Tubular bones, both long and short, are roughly cylindrical in shape. They possess a shaft of compact bone, the cortex, which encloses a central medullary or marrow cavity. Since Galenic times (AD 130–200), the extremities of a tubular bone have been referred to as their epiphyses. Each is covered by an articular cartilage. The shaft of the bone was for a time referred to as its diaphysis after Heister (1732), a pupil of Albinus, had used this otherwise botanical word in this sense. Nowadays the diaphysis denotes only the major portion of the shaft, continuous with the proximal and distal metaphyses. The metaphysis, a word coined by Kölliker (1873), is that part of the shaft adjacent to an epiphysis and separated from it in growing bones by a growth cartilage. Spongy, or cancellous, bone is found in both epiphysis and metaphysis. They are encased in only a thin shell of compact bone. Bone marrow is found in the marrow cavity of the diaphysis and also in the cancelli or intratrabecular spaces of spongy bone. It can be either fatty or haemopoietic, although the distinction is only one of degree; haemopoietic marrow contains some fat cells, but they do not feature prominently. Several named groups of vessels are usually described as being concerned in the supply of blood to bones. Macroscopic *nutrient* arteries perforate the cortex of the shaft and the bone extremities. The ramifications of these vessels in bone marrow are known as *medullary* arteries. The compact bone of the shaft is irrigated by *cortical* blood vessels whose circulatory features can be treated separately from those of the *periosteal* vascular bed. In a long bone epiphysis, *juxta-articular* and *juxta-epiphyseal* vessels are found in association with articular and growth cartilages respectively.

These several regions of the osseous circulation are discussed in the following pages, but it is emphasized that the blood circulation in the skeleton as a whole is a subunit integrated within the cardiovascular system, the latter containing within itself several specialized circulations, each with its own peculiarities. In the osseous circulation there are three main vascular groupings, namely afferent arteries, an interposed functional vascular lattice and efferent veins. Only the functional vascular lattice is the site of ionic exchange between blood and bone/bone marrow, and it consists of a network of capillaries or sinusoids. The *afferent vessels* are the extra-osseous nutrient arteries and their intra-osseous medullary branches, and the periosteal arteries in the ageing skeleton. The *functional vascular lattice* is a sinusoid network, whether in haemopoietic or fatty marrow or in cancellous bone. Unusually long and wide sinusoids make up the functional vascular lattice in compact bone. The *efferent vessels* comprise on the

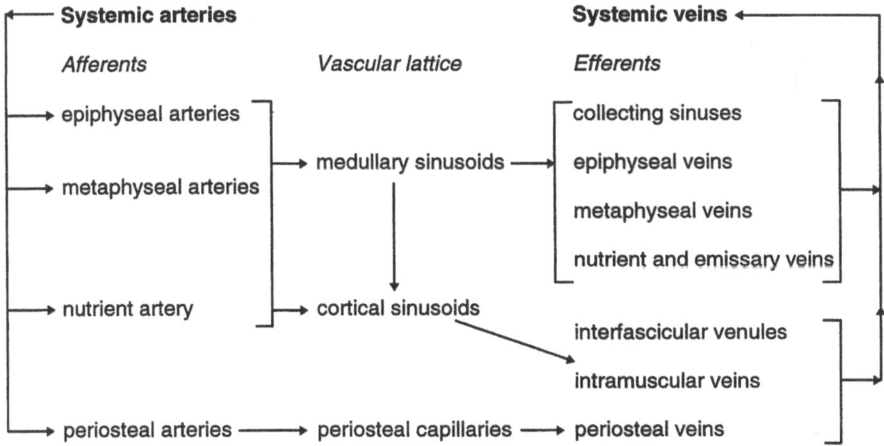

Fig. 1.1. Vascular pathways in a long bone. In senescence both medullary and periosteal blood supplies are present. In youth, periosteal arteries do not supply the cortex. Venous drainage is centrifugal.

one hand veins in the periosteum and attached muscles and large medullary venous sinuses and nutrient veins on the other hand. Through these numerous vessels, the osseous circulation is drained into the systemic veins of the cardiovascular system (Fig. 1.1, *previous page*).

Chapter 2

Nutrient vessels in long bones

Nutrient arteries

In tubular bones generally, a systemic artery usually runs parallel to the long axis of the bone and gives rise to an artery which enters the diaphysis. Myo-periosteal vessels (Barkow 1868) form transverse anastomoses around the shaft and bone extremities, giving origin to numerous nutrient vessels penetrating the bony epiphyses and metaphyses. There are considerable species differences in the systemic origin of afferent vessels to bones (Figs 2.1, 2.5), but in a given species variation is slight. The vessels are easy to demonstrate in man and in other animals (Howe *et al.* 1950; Rogers & Gladstone 1950; Brookes & Harrison 1957; Brookes 1958b; Fitzgerald 1961; Parouti 1962; Torreilles 1962), and dissection reveals the remarkable constancy in pattern of the arteries that supply tubular bones in general (Figs 2.1–2.8). This pattern comprises diaphyseal, epiphyseal and metaphyseal nutrient arterial groups, an arrangement which has long been clearly recognized (Testut 1880; Lexer *et al.* 1904).

Nutrient veins

The various groups are closely accompanied in their extra-osseous course by veins. The venous radicles emerging from the bone are more numerous than the entering arteries. The principal nutrient artery, for example, in its canal is surrounded by a leash of venules coalescing into one or two large nutrient veins. In cancellous bone extremities, many foramina give exit to veins alone, so that the number of nutrient veins draining a bone exceeds that of the nutrient arteries supplying it. In addition, perfused preparations clearly show that the veins are more capacious than the arteries they accompany.

It would seem therefore that if a vascular derangement occurs in a bone, it is more likely to be on account of an arterial inadequacy than a venous impediment.

Arteries of the diaphysis

Even in large mammals, these vessels are generally classified as small arteries. Typically, a principal nutrient artery pierces the diaphysis at the nutrient

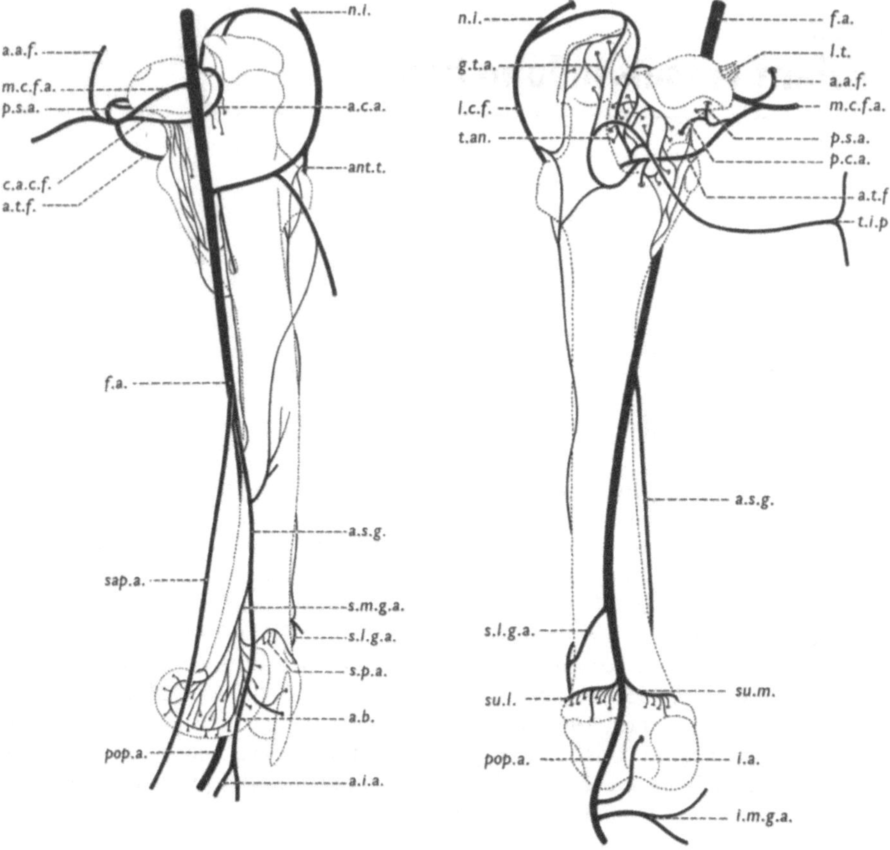

Fig. 2.1. Arterial supply of rabbit femur: anterior aspect.

Fig. 2.2. Arterial supply of rabbit femur: posterior aspect.

Key to Figures 2.1 and 2.2

a.a.f.	artery to acetabular fossa
a.b.	articular branch
a.c.a.	anterior cervical arteries
a.i.a.	anterior intercondylar artery
a.s.g.	anteria suprema genu
a.t.f.	artery to trochanteric fossa
ant.t.	anastomosis around third trochanter
c.a.c.f.	circulus arteriosus capitis femoris
f.a.	femoral artery
g.t.a.	arteries to greater trochanter
i.a.	intercondylar artery
i.m.g.a.	inferior medial genicular artery
l.c.f.	lateral circumflex femoral artery
l.t.	ligamentum teres
m.c.f.a.	medial circumflex femoral artery
n.i.	nutrient to ilum
p.c.a.	posterior cervical arteries
pop.a.	popliteal artery
p.s.a.	posterior subcapital artery
sap.a.	saphenous artery
s.l.g.a.	superior lateral genicular artery
s.m.g.a.	superior medial genicular artery
s.p.a.	suprapatellar arteries
su.l.	lateral supracondylar artery
su.m.	medial supracondylar artery
t.an.	trochanteric anastomosis
t.i.p.a.	trochanteric branch of internal pudendal artery

foramen, passing through the cortex in the nutrient canal to ramify finally in the marrow cavity (Figs 2.9–2.11). This vessel is referred to simply as the nutrient artery almost universally; by some it is called the principal nutrient artery to distinguish it from all the other smaller arteries which perforate the bony epiphyses. However all arteries are nutrient, but the artery to the diaphysis of long bones has been known as *arteria nutricia* (Latin: nutricare, to nourish) for too long for any change in name to be of advantage. It is the largest among the many arteries which perforate a long bone, in particular those at its extremities.

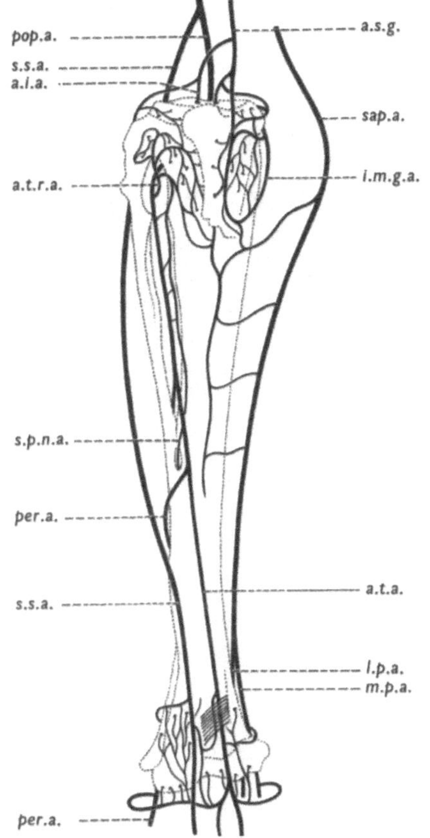

Fig. 2.3. Arterial supply of rabbit tibiofibula: anterior aspect.

Fig. 2.4. Arterial supply of rabbit tibiofibula: posterior aspect.

Key to Figures 2.3 and 2.4

a.i.a.	anterior intercondylar artery
a.s.g.	arteria suprema genu
a.t.a.	anterior tibial artery
a.t.r.a.	anterior tibial recurrent artery
i.a.	intercondylar artery
i.l.g.a.	inferior lateral genicular artery
i.m.g.a.	inferior medial genicular artery
j.a.t.	joins with anterior tibial artery
l.m.a.	lateral menisceal artery
l.p.a.	lateral plantar artery
m.m.a.	medial menisceal artery
m.p.a.	medial plantar artery
per.a.	peroneal artery
p.n.a.	principal nutrient artery
pop.a.	popliteal artery
p.t.a.	posterior tibial artery
sap.a.	saphenous artery
s.p.n.a.	secondary principal nutrient artery
s.s.a.	superficial sural artery
v.	opening for emissary venous sinus

It should be borne in mind that there may be two or more diaphyseal arteries supplying a bone (Fig. 2.12). For example, there are two diaphyseal arteries to the rabbit tibia (de Marneffe 1951). In the rabbit femur, the artery of the trochanteric fossa (Kistler 1935) can develop into a second afferent vessel to the diaphysis (Figs 2.26, 2.27). There may be two diaphyseal arteries present in the rat femur (Greene 1935; Brookes 1958b). Occasionally three nutrients are found in the human humerus deriving from the brachial, profunda brachii and anterior circumflex humeral arteries.

For an account of the location and variation of the principal nutrient foramina in the shafts of the lower limb bones in humans, see Sakul *et al.* (1994). The posi-

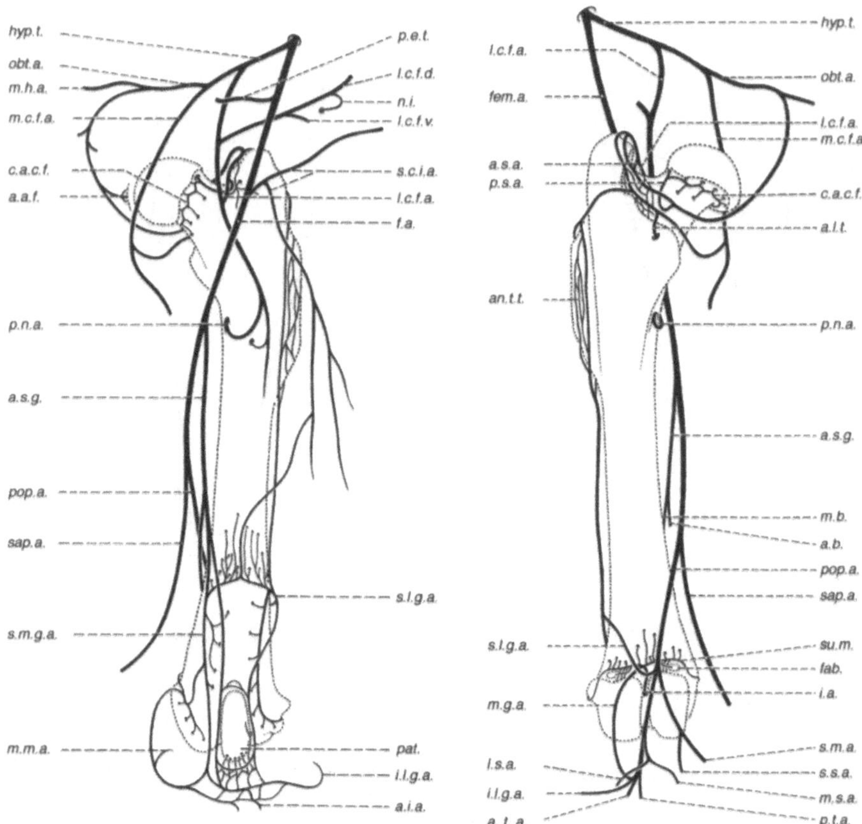

Fig. 2.5. Arterial supply of rat femur: anterior aspect.

Fig. 2.6. Arterial supply of rat femur: posterior aspect.

Key to Figures 2.5, 2.6, 2.7 & 2.8

a.a.f.	artery of acetabular fossa
a.b.	articular branch
a.c.l.	anterior crural ligament
a.i.a.	anterior intercondylar artery
a.l.t.	artery to lesser trochanter
a.s.a.	anterior subcapital artery
a.s.g.	arteria suprema genu
a.t.a.	anterior tibial artery
an.f.	anastomosis around fibula
an.t.t.	anastomosis around third trochanter
a.t.r.a.	anterior tibial recurrent artery
c.a.c.f.	circulus arteriosus capitis femoris
c.s.a.	common sural artery
fab.	fabella
f.b.p.a.	fibular branch of peroneal artery
fem.a.	femoral artery
h.f.	head of fibula
hyp.t.	hypogastric trunk
i.a.	intercondylar artery
i.l.g.a.	inferior lateral genicular artery
i.m.g.a.	inferior medial genicular artery
i.p.an.	infrapatellar anastomosis
l.c.f.	lateral circumflex femoral artery
l.c.f.a.	lateral circumflex femoral artery, articular limb
l.c.f.d.	lateral circumflex femoral artery, ascending branch, dorsal division
l.c.f.v.	lateral circumflex femoral artery, ascending branch, ventral division
l.p.a.	lateral plantar artery
l.s.a .	lateral sural artery
m.b.	muscular branch
m.c.f.a.	medial circumflex femoral artery
m.g.a.	middle genicular artery
m.h.a.	middle haemorrhoidal artery
m.m.a.	medial menisceal artery
m.p.d.	medial plantar artery, deep branch
m.p.s.	medial plantar artery, superficial branch
m.s.a.	medial sural artery
m.t.a.	medial tarsal artery
n.i.	nutrient to ilium
obt.a.	obturator artery
pat.	patella
per.a.	popliteal artery
p.e.t.	pudic epigastric trunk
p.n.a.	principal nutrient artery
pop.a.	peroneal artery
p.s.a.	posterior subcapital artery
p.t.a.	posterior tibial artery
sap.a.	saphenous artery
s.c.i.a.	superficial circumflex iliac artery
s.l.g.a.	superior lateral genicular artery
s.m.a.	superior muscular artery
s.m.g.a.	superior medical genicular artery
s.s.a.	superficial sural artery
su.l.	lateral supracondylar artery
su.m.	medial supracondylar artery
v.	opening for emissary venous sinus

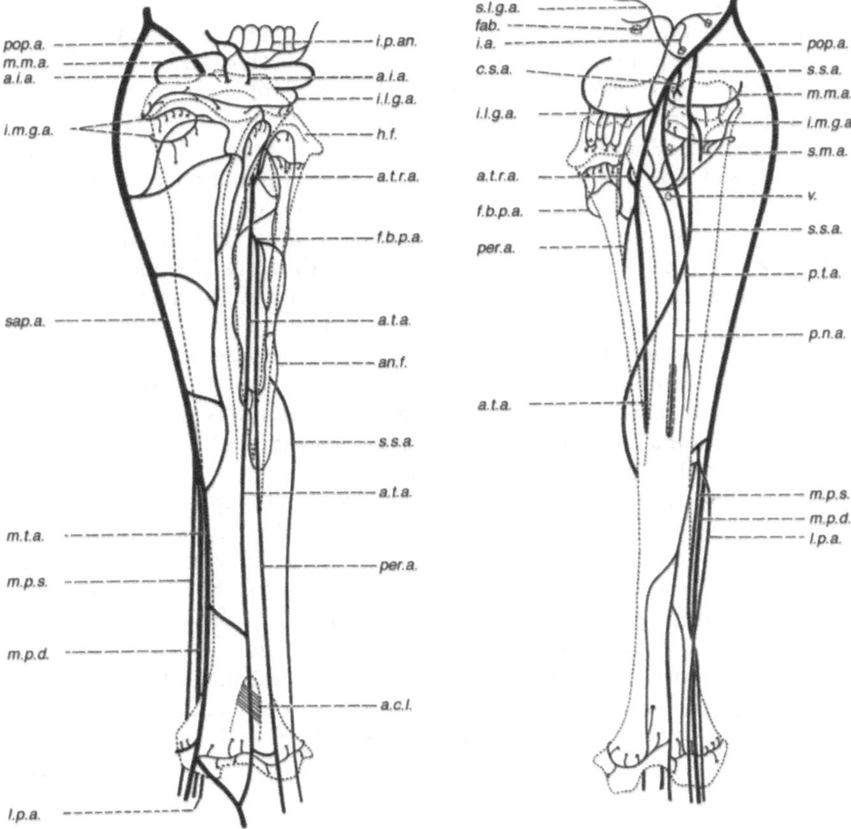

Fig. 2.7. Arterial supply of rat tibiofibula: anterior aspect. For definition of abbreviations, refer to key in Fig. 2.5.

Fig. 2.8. Arterial supply of rat tibiofibula: posterior aspect. For definition of abbreviations, refer to key in Fig. 2.5.

tion of the opening of the nutrient foramina on the bony surfaces and their distances from the proximal articular margins have been recorded by Nagel (1993). The exercise is not without clinical relevance. In the treatment of bone fractures, a precise knowledge of the position of a nutrient artery during operative exposure of a long bone for the emplacement of internal fixation devices in the human humerus, radius, ulna, femur and tibia, may help to avoid the risk of damaging a diaphyseal nutrient artery, and compromising existing bone injury.

Femoral diaphyseal nutrients

It was once held that there are usually two nutrient arteries, branches of the arteria profunda femoris, supplying the human femur. Von Haller (1763) showed this by dissection, and they were described again as an original finding by Grégoire & Carrière (1921) in their radiological examination of barium-perfused cadavers. Nowadays, it is known that the number of nutrient arteries to the human femoral diaphysis is variable, ranging from none to two. The foramina which lead into the nutrient canals are found in the linea aspera of the adult, and point obliquely upwards away from the knee. In the human fetus the two arteries are of equal size and point to the centre of the diaphysis (Fig. 2.12).

Lack of awareness of variation in the number of diaphyseal nutrient arteries can affect the interpretation placed on the results of ligation experiments and other investigations. For example, one author studied the variation in position of the nutrient foramen in several long bones of various mammals. He concluded that the adult human femur differs from the generality of mammalian femora in the frequency distribution of the foramen plotted against its measured distance along the axis of the bone. The frequency distribution was bimodal; the mammalian femora were unimodal. That the human femur might normally possess one or two diaphyseal nutrients was not mentioned.

In a recent investigation of 109 adult femora (Bridgeman & Brookes 1996), it was found that the two arteries in their canals may be equal or unequal in size (Figs 2.14–2.17). In 1.5% of cases the lesser nutrient canal was absent, possibly as a result of old trauma, arthritic change in the linea aspera, but more likely as a result of the individual's genetic endowment.

The above collection of mainly aged femora has been amplified to a new total of 194 femora (Bridgeman & Brookes 1997). Statistical analysis of these femora confirms what was unearthed in the earlier paper cited above, namely that a reciprocal statistical interaction exists between sex and side for the number of principal nutrient foramina present in the femoral diaphysis. Multivariate analysis for side shows that two-thirds of male femora have one foramen on the right side, as against one-third with two foramina (Table 2.1). Table 2.2 suggests that in female bones one or two foramina occur indifferently in both right and left sides. Similarly, in all left femora the equal presence of one or two foramina is the norm (Table 2.3). However, for right-sided femora (Table 2.4), there is a significant

Table 2.1 Effect of side in male femora

Side	1 Foramen	2 Foramina	Totals
Right	31 (64.58%)	17 (35.42%)	48
Left	20 (39.22%)	31 (60.78%)	51
Both sides	51	48	99

*Statistically significant difference: $\chi^2 = 6.31$, $P<0.01$.
Right femora are twice as likely as left to have one foramen. Left femora are twice as likely as right to have two foramina.

Table 2.2 Effect of side in female femora

Side	1 Foramen	2 Foramina	Totals
Right	16 (36.36%)	28 (63.64%)	44
Left	25 (52.08%)	23 (47.92%)	48
Both sides	41	51	92

Difference not significant: $\chi^2 = 2.27$, $P<0.13$.
There is an even chance of there being one or two foramina in mixed right and left bones in females.

Table 2.3 Effect of sex on foramen number in left femora

Sex	1 Foramen	2 Foramina	Totals
Female	25 (52.08%)	23 (47.92%)	48
Male	20 (39.22%)	31 (60.78%)	51
Both sexes	45	54	99

Difference not significant: = $\chi^2 = 1.63$, $P<0.20$.
There is an even chance of there being one or two foramina in a mixed population of male and female left femora.

Table 2.4 Effect of sex on foramen number in right femora

Sex	1 Foramen	2 Foramina	Totals
Female	16 (36.36%)	28 (63.64%)	44
Male	31 (64.58%)	17 (35.42%)	48
Both sexes	47	45	92

*Statistically significant difference: $\chi^2 = 7.24$, $P<0.01$
Chi-squared analysis shows a significant 2 : 1 chance of there being one principal nutrient foramen in males, and a 2 : 1 chance of two foramina in females; in right femora.

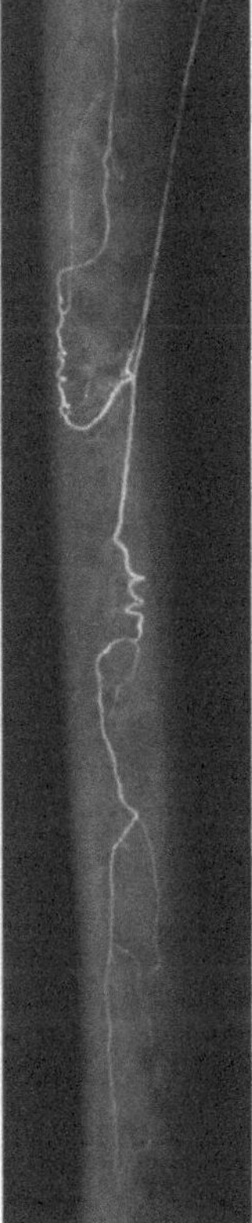

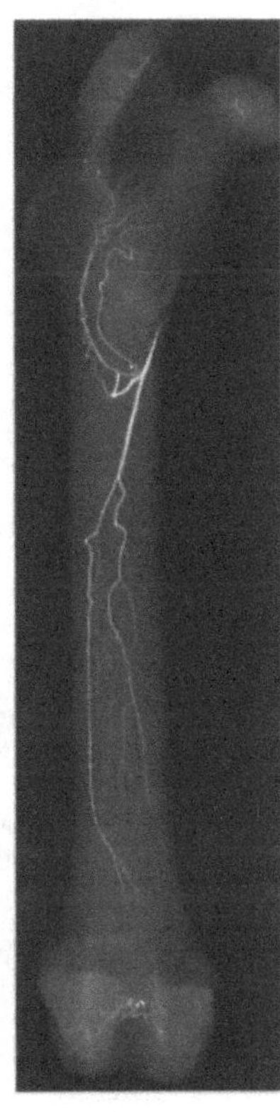

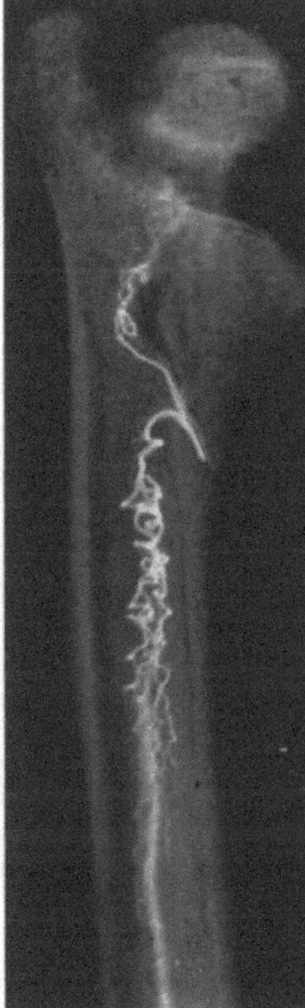

Fig. 2.9. (*left*) The principal nutrient artery and its ascending and descending branches in the medulla of a tibia amputated from a youth aged 15 years with femoral sarcoma. (Original: Natural size)

Fig. 2.10. (*middle*) Angiograph of rabbit femur after injection of undiluted Micropaque in the aorta, showing the principal nutrient artery and medullary branches. Separate supplies to greater trochanter, femoral head and inferior epiphysis are also shown. (Original magnification ×1.5)

Fig. 2.11. (*right*) Angiograph of rat femoral nutrient artery showing tortuosities in the medulla. Some venous filling is also present. (Original magnification ×6)

sexual difference, in that two-thirds of the females have two foramina while two-thirds of the males have only one, as picked up in Table 2.1 also. This analysis of 191 foraminate femora (three more had no nutrient foramina at all) shows that sex and side exert a differentiating effect on the number of principal nutrient foramina present in the human femur.

The cause of the sexual and right-sided disparities in the number of foramina present here is difficult to relate to functional differences. The dominant right femur is twice as likely to have only one foramen (and therefore principal nutrient artery), whereas the right female bones are likely to have two. Doubtless there are genetic effects, of which nothing is known, that may account for the phenotypic differences disturbing expected bilateral symmetry.

Epiphyseo-metaphyseal arteries

In his original description, William Hunter (1743) wrote:

> All around the neck of the bone there is a great number of Arteries and Veins which ramify into smaller branches and communicate with one another by frequent Anastomoses like those of the mesentery. This might be called the Circulus articuli vasculosus, the vascular border of the Joint.

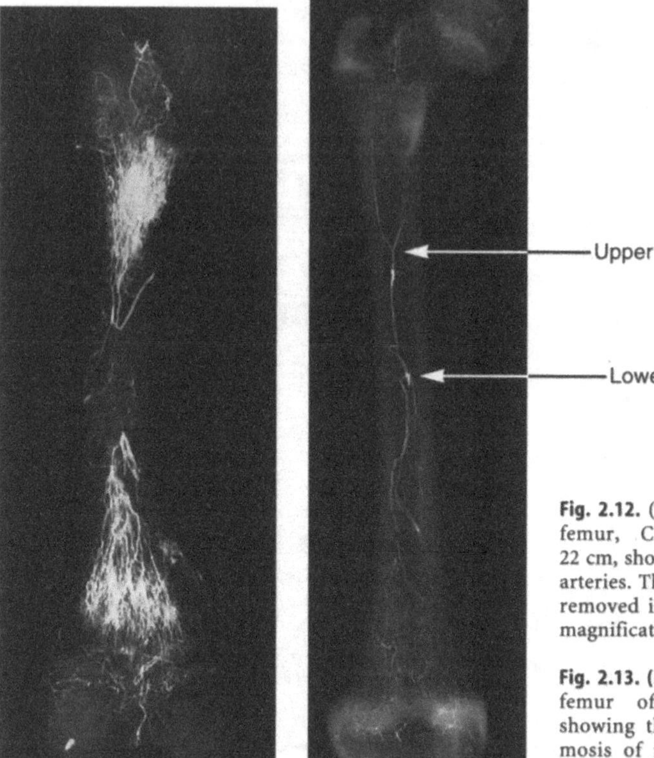

Fig. 2.12. (*left*) Angiograph of fetal femur, CR (crown-rump) length 22 cm, showing two principal nutrient arteries. The periosteum has not been removed in this specimen. (Original magnification × 3)

Fig. 2.13. (*right*) Angiograph of the femur of a 2-year-old monkey showing the intramedullary anastomosis of its two principal nutrient arteries, here seen end-on.

At the extremities of a long bone there are many nutrient foramina, some even wider than the diaphyseal nutrient foramen, as can be confirmed by examination of the surface of a degreased and dried specimen. These holes give passage to epiphyseal and metaphyseal vessels. The two groups are readily distinguished when a growth cartilage is present. The stem vessels derive from a vascular circle at the metaphyseo–diaphyseal junction.

Epiphyseo-metaphyseal arteries enter a bone extremity in localized areas. For example, it is well known that the ligamentum teres and the superior and inferior retinacula convey vessels to the femoral head and neck (obturator, medial and lateral circumflex femoral, and inferior gluteal arteries). A circumferential penetration of the cartilaginous femoral head and neck is found in the human fetus (Figs 2.18–2.20). *Metaphyseal vessels* (branches of the superior and middle genicular arteries) have been described in the lower femoral epiphysis, by Rogers & Gladstone (1950), entering anterior and posterior groups of supracondylar foramina. *Epiphyseal vessels* enter foramina on the collateral, non-articular surfaces of the condyles; the central mass of the epiphysis is supplied by middle genicular branches through foramina in the intercondylar fossa (Fig. 2.13). Some of these arteries are as large as the principal nutrient itself.

The "vascular border" on the non-articular surface of an epiphysis is actually a narrow band containing a dense, vascular anastomotic network. Its terminal capillary loops form a lace-like border at the rim of the joint cartilage (Fig. 2.21). The

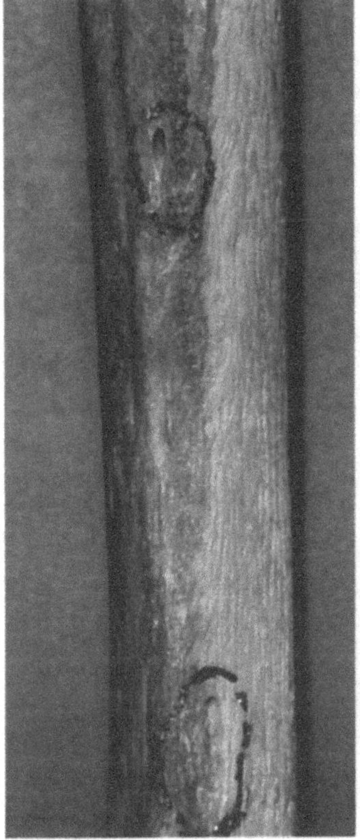

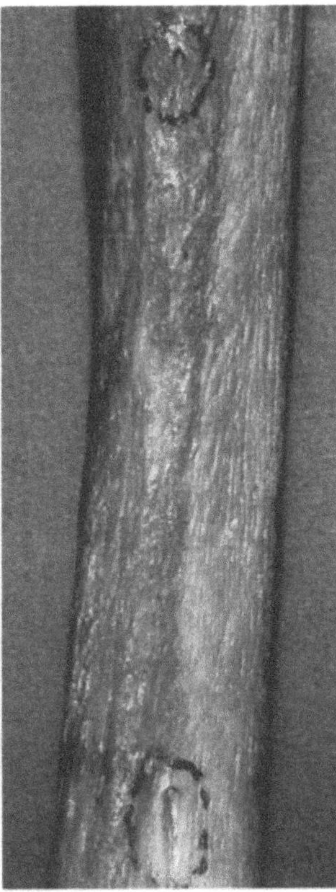

Fig. 2.14. (*left*) (*see also Colour Plate section*) Two femoral nutrient foramina of similar size on the linea aspera. (Original: Natural size)

Fig. 2.15. (*right*) (*see also Colour Plate section*) Two femoral nutrient foramina; the upper one is smaller. (Original: Natural size)

source vessels of the vascular band are Hunter's vascular circle proximal to the metaphysis, and in parallel with several other vascular rings that lie in the diaphyseal periosteum (Langer 1876). Numerous epiphyseal and metaphyseal vessels arise from Hunter's vascular circle, in addition to the complex, periarticular vessels which supply the capsule of the joint (Fig. 2.22).

Epiphyseo-metaphyseal arteries are of paramount importance in maintaining the life of long bones. Their total cross-sectional area has not been measured, but would seem to be at least equal to that of the diaphyseal nutrient artery. As pointed out above, apparently normal bones are occasionally found in cadavers in which the diaphyseal nutrient canal is absent. In these instances, the whole bone gains its blood supply in life from arteries entering solely at its extremities; from metaphyseal arteries in particular.

Diaphyseal nutrient ligation

The importance of epiphyseo-metaphyseal arteries in bone growth has been demonstrated by ligating the single nutrient artery of the femur in day-old rabbits (Brookes 1957), and obliterating the nutrient canal, thus ensuring that re-generation of the vessel did not take place. Measurements of femoral length were taken from serial radiographs of the growing animals. Final direct measurements were also taken 5

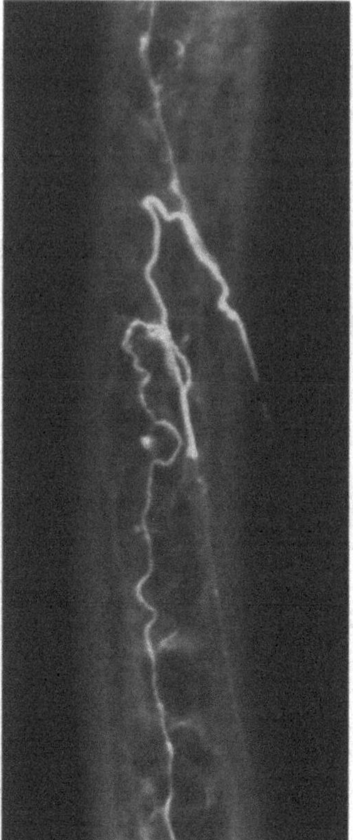

Fig. 2.16. Angiogram of a perfused femur showing two nutrient arteries linked in the bone marrow. The lower nutrient artery is much reduced in calibre. (Original: Natural size)

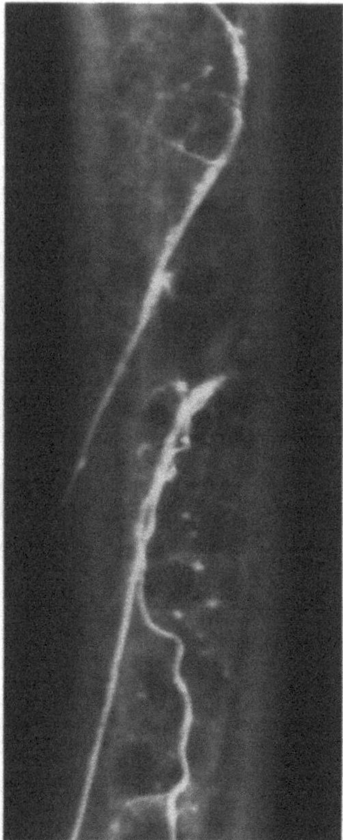

Fig. 2.17. Angiogram as in Fig. 2.16 showing absence of a medullary loop to link two nutrient arteries equal in calibre. (Original: Natural size)

months later, when the limbs were perfused intravascularly with a radiopaque medium. By means of the latter procedure the arteries of the shaft could be examined radiographically. The results showed that the defective femora still continue to grow, but nevertheless develop a 3% shortening at 5 months compared with the controls (Fig. 2.23). It was concluded that the arteries of cancellous bone are 97% adequate for growth in length of the rabbit femur from birth to maturity.

Radiography of the perfused intra-osseous vessels also showed that the metaphyseal arteries were the route by which blood reached the shaft as a whole in these experimental femora lacking a nutrient artery (Figs 2.24–2.27). In this respect, it is noteworthy that Prives and colleagues (1959) have found, by autoradiographic methods in puppies, that after ligation of the nutrient artery, red cells labelled with radioactive iron pass rapidly throughout the whole bone. Although the authors stated somewhat blandly and indifferently that their results "confirmed the existence of arterial connections in all parts of the growing long bone (diaphysis, epiphysis and metaphysis)", their findings do at least demonstrate that metaphyseal arteries can supply blood to all the shaft in the absence of the diaphyseal nutrient vessel.

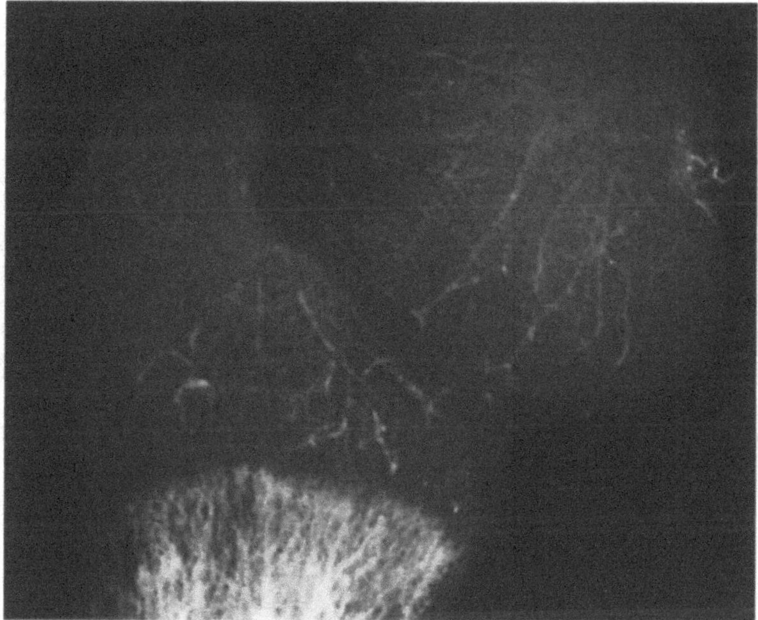

Fig. 2.18. Vascular cartilage canals in the femoral head, neck and trochanteric region of a human fetus, CR length 22 cm. (Original magnification ×5.6)

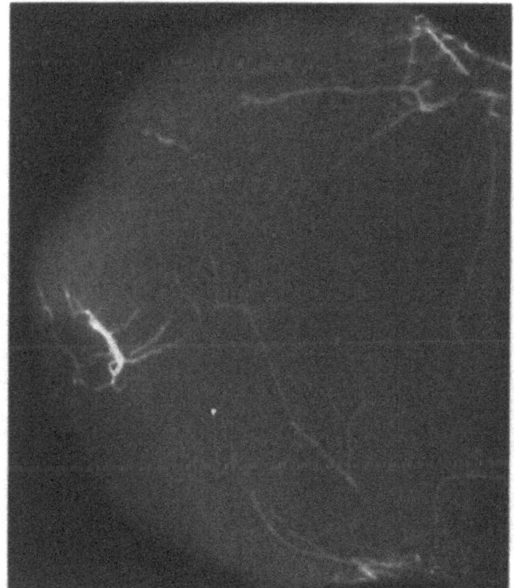

Fig. 2.19. Coronal section of head of fetal femur, CR length 28 cm, showing cartilage canals in superior, foveal and inferior groups. (Original magnification ×5.6)

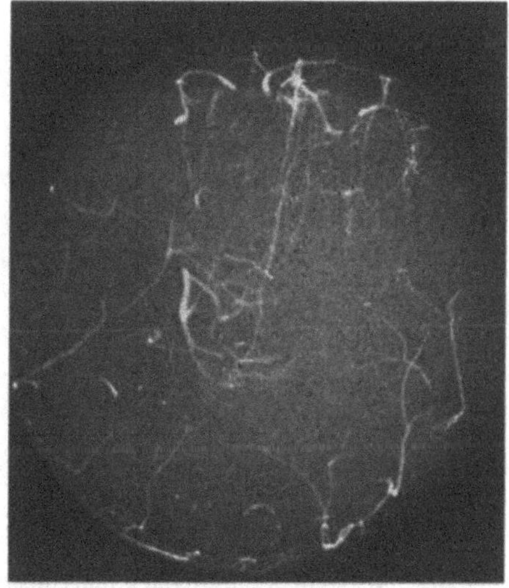

Fig. 2.20. Angiograph of isolated femoral head in a fetus, CR length 22 cm, viewed on the flat. Vascular cartilage canals penetrate from nearly all the circumference, but superior and inferior groups can be distinguished. Centrally a foveal group is present. (Original magnification ×5.6)

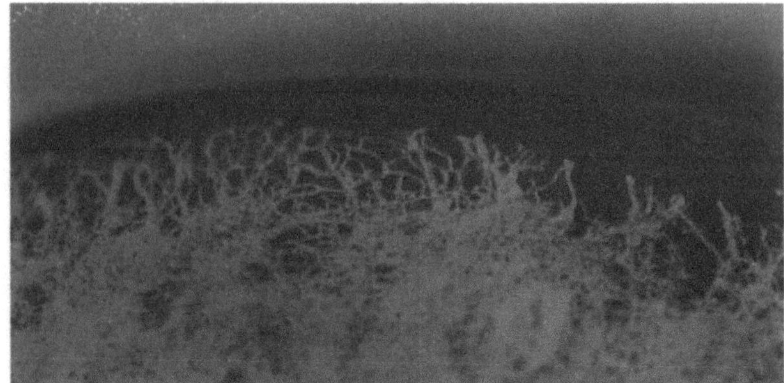

Fig. 2.21. The lace-like border of Hunter's vascular mesentery at the rim of the articular cartilage: fetal femoral condyle of human fetus, CR length 24 cm. (India ink perfusion; Original magnification ×40)

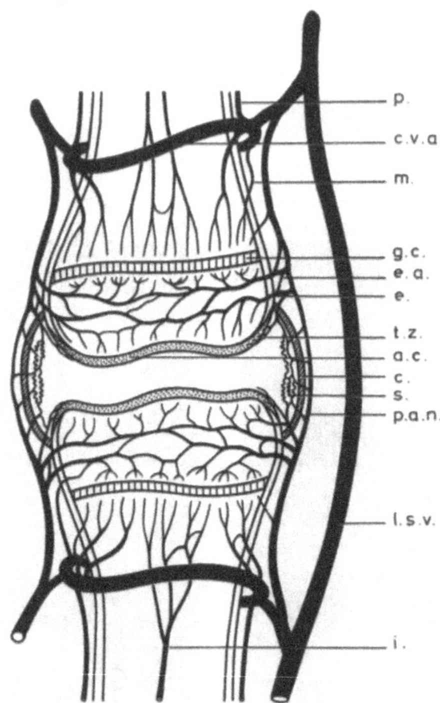

Fig. 2.22. Diagram of the arterial arrangements in a synovial joint, and the connections of Hunter's vascular circle.

Key to Figure 2.22

a.c.	articular cartilage	g.c.	growth cartilage	p.	periosteal artery
c.	fibrous capsule of joint	i.	intramedullary branches of the nutrient artery	p.a.n.	periarticular plexus
c.v.a.	circulus vasculosus articuli			s.	subsynovial plexus
e.	epiphyseal artery	l.s.v.	large systemic vessel	t.z.	transitional zone
e.a.	epiphyseal arterial arcades	m.	metaphyseal artery		

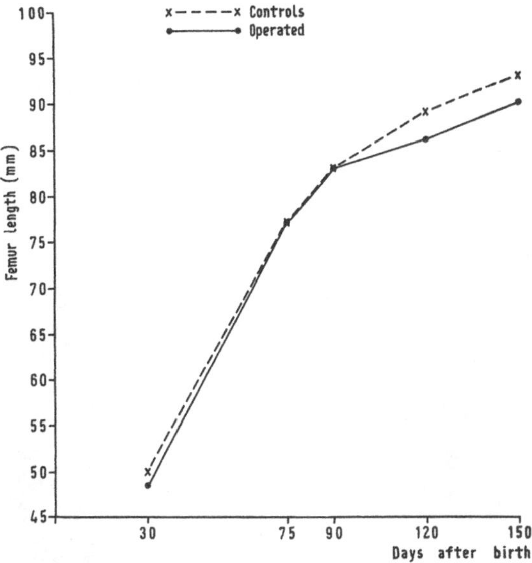

Fig. 2.23. Growth curves of rabbit femora after occlusion of the principal nutrient canal in day-old rabbits.

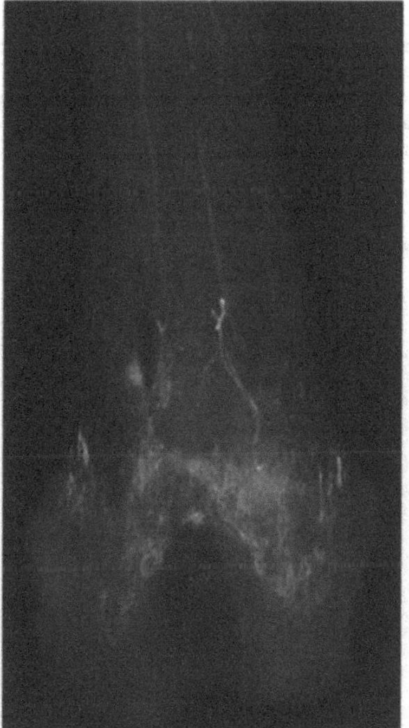

Fig. 2.24. Arteriograph of the distal part of a normal rabbit femur. (Original magnification ×2)

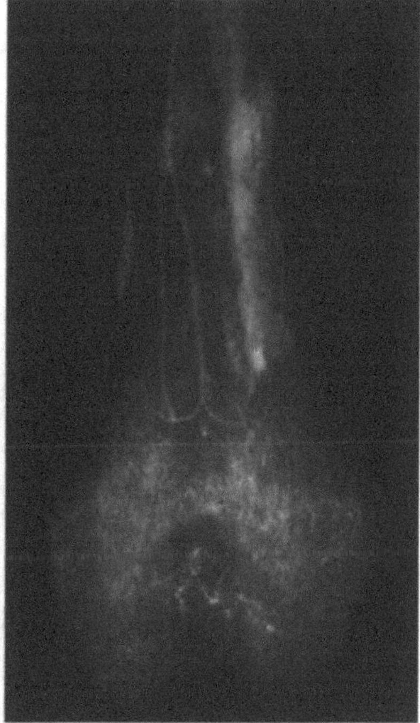

Fig. 2.25. Arteriograph of the distal part of a rabbit femur 150 days after occlusion of the principal nutrient canal, showing intra-osseous metaphyseal anastomoses. (Original magnification ×2)

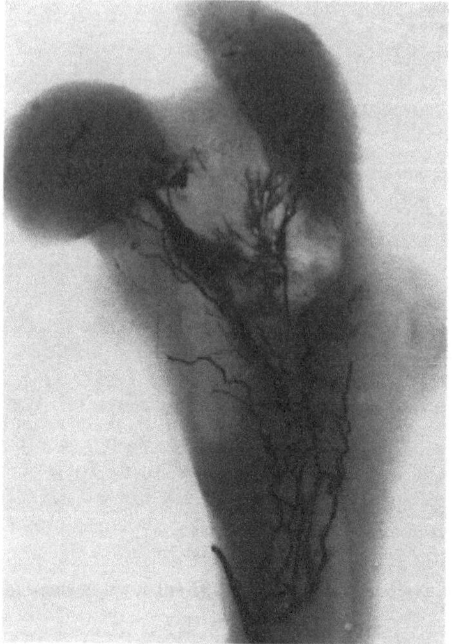

Fig. 2.26. Arteriograph of the upper part of a normal rabbit femur, showing ascending branches of the principal nutrient artery. (Original magnification ×3.2)

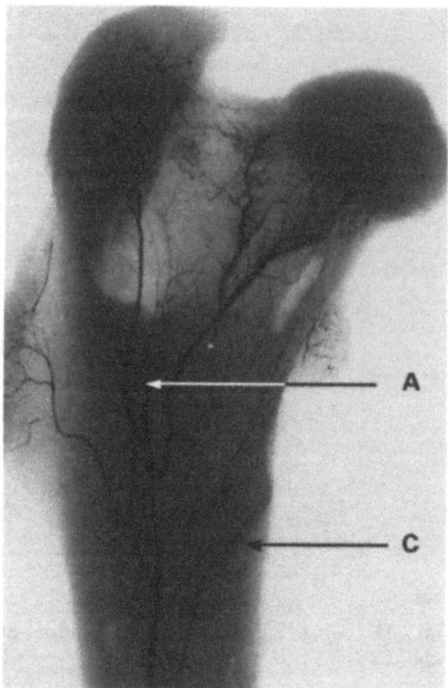

Fig. 2.27. Arteriograph of the upper part of a mature rabbit femur. The nutrient canal whose site is indicated at C, was occluded 150 days previously, a day after birth. The artery of the trochanteric fossa (A) has become a main supply channel to the medullary arterial system. (Original magnification ×3.2)

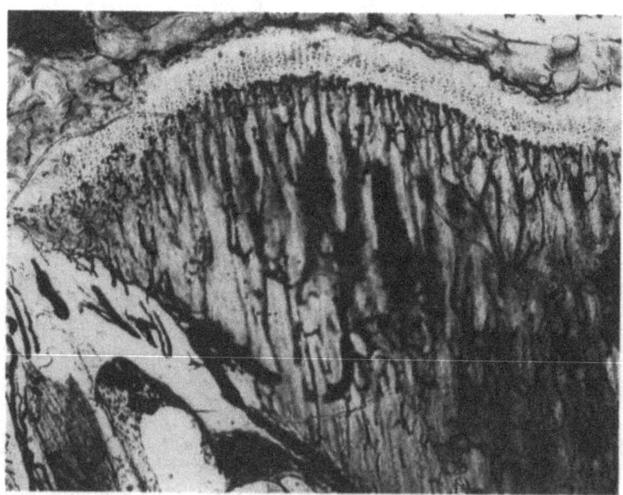

Fig. 2.28. Photomicrograph of a sagittal section through the upper part of a rat tibia, perfused with India ink, showing the growth cartilage and metaphyseal vessels orientated vertically to it. (Original magnification ×35)

Blood supply of long bone epiphyses

The cancellous extremities of a long bone are referred to as its epiphyses in gross anatomy, but consist of epiphyseal and metaphyseal parts. An important anatomical distinction between metaphyseal and epiphyseal vessels lies in the fact that the latter arise from vascular arcades "like those of the mesentery" lying on the non-articular areas of the epiphysis, and not directly from the circulus vasculosus as do metaphyseal arteries. The difference in origin between these two types of afferent vessel is in parallel with several other vascular and haemodynamic differences which distinguish epiphyseal from metaphyseal circulations. The epiphyseal arcades and anastomoses serve to lower epiphyseal blood pressure. Metaphyseal tissue pressure, as measured by electromanometers in the canine femoral metaphysis, is considerably higher than epiphyseal pressure (Stein *et al.* 1957). In the rat femur, blood flow rates were calculated in terms of pure red cell flows without the accompanying plasma content (Brookes 1971). This showed that metaphyseal red cell flow rate is higher (15 ml 100 g^{-1} min^{-1}) than in the adjacent epiphysis (9 ml 100 g^{-1} min^{-1}) confirmed by whole blood flow rate measurement using arteriolar blockade (Revell & Brookes 1993a,b). It seems that metaphyseal vessels arising directly from the circulus vasculosus deliver blood to the metaphyseal spongiosa (Fig. 2.28) at a higher blood pressure and rate of flow than the epiphyseal arteries arising from the arcades. It should also be noted that the epiphyseal arteries supply cancellous bone, whose trabeculae are orientated in rectangular array, structurally very different from the metaphyseal spongiosa with its parallel trabeculae.

Blood supply of metaphyses

In fetal life and postnatally up to maturity, the nutrient artery supplies at least the diaphysis, and epiphyseal arteries alone supply the epiphyses of a long bone. The source of the arteries in the metaphysis requires further comment.

Through preferential study of knee joint metaphyses, general opinion has it that the central region of a metaphysis, about three-fifths of its bulk, is supplied by branches of the diaphyseal nutrient artery and that metaphyseal arteries (Fig. 2.28) supply the peripheral zone (Rubascheva & Prives 1932; de Marneffe 1951; Morgan 1959; Trueta & Amato 1960; Fyfe 1964). Earlier workers, however (Lexer *et al.* 1904; Grégoire & Carrière 1921), considered that the nutrient artery contributed only to a minor extent, and that mature metaphyses were largely supplied by metaphyseal arteries alone. Possibly the perfusates they used were too viscous to reach into the finer ramifications of the principal nutrient artery.

As far as the early human fetus is concerned, the blood supply to metaphyses is derived from the nutrient artery (Figs 2.12, 9.21), and it is only later in fetal life and thereafter that metaphyseal arteries become an additional source (Lewis 1956; Brookes 1963). Perfusion results also show that the metaphysis at the "non-growing" end of a long bone is likewise supplied only by the diaphyseal nutrient artery in early fetal life.

Subsequently, metaphyseal arteries become increasingly prominent, until in the adult they ramify in and supply the whole of the "non-growing" metaphysis, as in the head and neck of the femur or the lower end of the tibia. Indeed, the superior metaphysis of the femur, which includes more than half the bulk of the head as well as the neck, is unexceptional in its blood supply, notwithstanding the voluminous literature on the subject. It is normally supplied by metaphyseal arteries, branches of the medial and lateral circumflex femoral vessels, with variable reinforcement from the cruciate anastomosis.

In summary, in fetal life up to 6 months, all metaphyses are supplied by the diaphyseal nutrient artery alone. With the advent of remodelling of the bone extremities, metaphyseal vessels are acquired peripherally (third trimester). Later, in postnatal long bones, it is necessary to distinguish between the "growing" and "non-growing" ends of the bone. The metaphyses at the "growing" end have a dual arterial blood supply from diaphyseal and metaphyseal vessels; "non-growing" metaphyses are supplied by metaphyseal arteries alone.

Chapter 3

Modes of bone growth: disposition of the nutrient artery

Inequality of longitudinal bone growth

In birds and mammals, the principal nutrient foramen is commonly nearer one extremity of a long bone than the other; and the nutrient canal usually lies obliquely in the bone cortex. It is also well known that in the human embryo a vascular irruption takes place (8th week) into the cartilaginous precursor of a long bone, at the centre of the shaft and at right angles to the bone's long axis. These facts raise some important problems concerning bone morphogenesis. The displaced location of the nutrient foramen and the obliquity of the nutrient canal and its vessels are usually explained in that:

1. longitudinal growth occurs only at bone extremities, and
2. growth at one end exceeds that at the other.

These fundamentals of bone growth were known to the Rev. Stephen Hales (1727), who wrote of them in a brilliant digression in his treatise on plant physiology, *Vegetable Staticks*, as follows:

> And as in vegetables, so doubtless in animals, the tender ductile bones of young animals are gradually increased in every part that is not hardened and ossified; but since it was inconsistent with the motion of the joynts to have the ends of the bones soft and ductile as in vegetables; therefore nature makes a wonderful provision for this at the glutinous serrated joyning of the heads to the shanks of the bones; which joyning while it continues ductile the animal grows, but when it ossifies then the animal can no longer grow. As I was assured by the following Experiment, viz. I took a half-grown Chick, whose leg-bone was then two inches long, and with a sharp pointed Iron at half an inch distance I pierced two small holes through the middle of the scaly covering of the leg, and shin-bone;two months after I killed the Chick, and upon laying the bones bare, I found on it obscure remains of the two marks I had made at the same distance of half an inch: So that that part of the bone had not at all distended lengthwise since the time that I marked it: Notwithstanding the bone was in that time grown an inch more in length, which growth was mostly at the upper end of the bone, where a wonderful provision is made for its growth at the joining of its head to the shank, called by Anatomists Symphysis.

Bérard (1835) was the first to point out that the nutrient canals were obliquely disposed in *human* long bones, and pointed towards the elbow in the upper limb

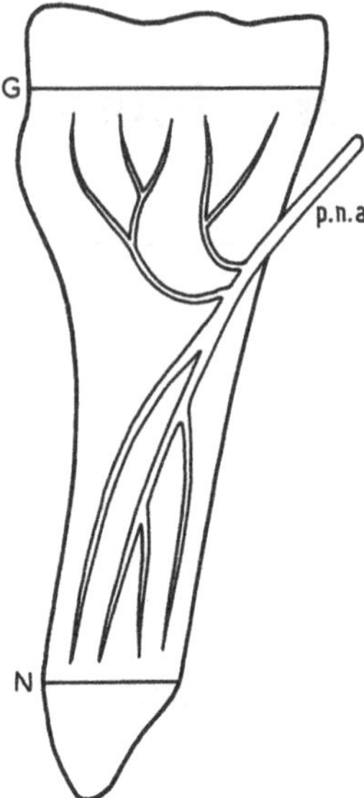

Fig. 3.1. According to Bérard, the principal nutrient artery (p.n.a.) points to the non-growing end (N). Larger branches pass to N, causing earlier epiphyseal fusion than at the growing end (G). Inequality of elongation is a result of a nutrient arterial imbalance within the marrow cavity.

and away from the knee in the lower limb. As the familiar dissecting room jingle has it, in the original French:

Au coude je m'appuis,
du genou je m'en fuis.

He also noted an unequal division of the nutrient artery into an ascending and a descending branch in the medulla. In his view, a *larger* branch passed to that extremity where growth normally ceased first, thereby causing an unequal contribution to bone elongation (Figs 2.9, 3.1). He suggested that the basis of the earlier demise of the growth cartilage was its increased blood supply.

Nowadays, only Bérard's rule of canal direction would be accepted, and it must be emphasized that while it applies to humans and many mammals, there are numerous exceptions (Ollier 1867). Even in human bones, a small percentage of cases can be detected where the nutrient canal does not obey Bérard's rule (Lütken 1950; Shulman 1959). Furthermore, it is generally held that the basis of inequality of elongation in long bones, resides, in the first instance, in different rates of growth at the growth cartilages and not, as Bérard supposed, in a continuation of growth at one end after growth has ceased at the other.

Differential growth at the epiphyses

There is considerable evidence for this in postnatal bones (Keith 1919; Payton 1934; Aries 1941), and Digby (1916) devised a method to demonstrate the fact. He pointed out that the site of primary ossification of the shaft could be gauged in a given long bone by observing where its long axis was intersected by a line drawn through the principal nutrient canal. Measurements made from this point to the growth cartilages, then give an estimate of the length of the shaft contributed by each. In growing bones, the ratio of these two measurements for a specific bone is roughly constant, and quantifies the differential rates of growth at the two extremities.

Fetal bone elongation

As yet there is only sparse information concerning the rate of bone elongation during the fetal period in mammals. Bisgard & Bisgard (1935), utilizing a radiographic method in goats, and Felts (1954), applying Digby's method to the human femur, noted the absence of any marked disparity in growth rates at the two extremities of fetal long bones. Brookes (1963), studying cortical capillary networks in the long bones of the fetal lower limb, concluded that growth rates are equal at proximal and distal growth cartilages. Yet, although the indications are that fetal bones elongate equally at their extremities, attention is drawn to the human fetal tibia whose nutrient foramen is normally displaced and whose vessels run an oblique course during fetal life. The nutrient vessels do, however, pass to a central marrow point (Fig. 3.2, *overleaf*).

The conclusion must therefore be drawn that inequality of longitudinal bone growth alone is insufficient to explain the normally oblique course of the nutrient artery in postnatal bones. In particular, the lie of the vessel can be displaced from its original embryonic position even in fetal bone, in which there is no "growing end", that is, the rate of growth at one end does not predominate over the other.

Interstitial growth of the periosteum

Another morphogenetic mechanism that was early invoked (Humphry 1861) to explain nutrient artery obliquity, was that while a long bone grows by apposition both in length at the growth cartilages (Hales 1727) and in breadth at the periosteum (Duhamel 1743), the latter membrane itself grows interstitially. Humphry made use of the technique of feeding pigs with madder root. The vegetable was formerly boiled by dyers to extract its red dye for use in the wool trade. John Belchier (1736), surgeon at Guy's Hospital, London, observed that the skeletons of pigs were red when they had been fed on the refuse of the dyers' vats. Duhamel (1739) then made use of intermittent madder feeding in order to show that the periosteum was osteogenic. In this way he was able to distinguish layers of newly deposited *red* periosteal bone, from the *white* bone formed when madder was withheld. The root acts by virtue of its contained alizarin which is incorporated into bone mineral. By means of madder feeding, Humphry was also able to demonstrate unequal growth at the ends of a long bone, and proposed that the cause of nutrient artery obliquity was the unequal drag exerted on the periosteum at each epiphysis (Fig. 3.3, *overleaf*). Many authorities have supported and amplified Humphry's position, which emphasizes bony appositional and periosteal interstitial growth (Kölliker 1873; Schwalbe 1876; Piollet 1905). The manner in which these affect the disposition of the diaphyseal nutrient vessels in postnatal bones has been expounded by Lacroix (1951) as follows (Fig. 3.3, *overleaf*).

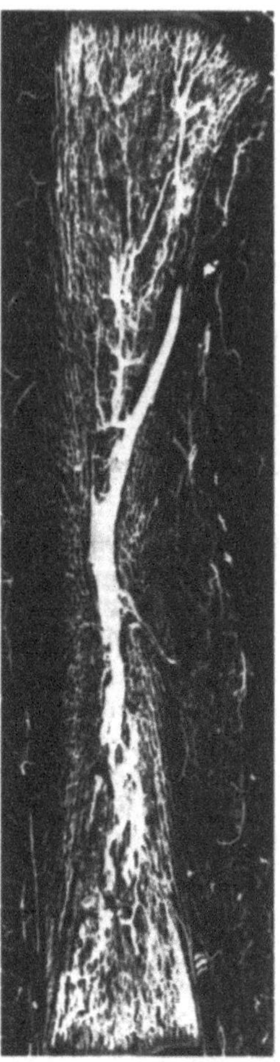

Fig. 3.2. Microangiograph of a longitudinal section, 300 μm thick, of a human fetal tibia, CR length 22 cm. Two diaphyseal nutrient arteries are shown; also the radiating pattern of capillaries in the bone cortex. (Original magnification ×3.7)

The periosteum is attached at each end to the growth cartilages. As these become wider apart during growth in length of the shaft, the periosteum elongates like an elastic sleeve from each side of a fixed point: this is central in position if bone growth at each end is equal, and is displaced away from the "growing end" if one is present. It is emphasized that periosteal growth is only analogous to the elongation of a stretched elastic membrane. It is in fact a fibrocellular structure, all parts of which grow, that is, it grows interstitially. Nor can it be said to slide over the surface of the shaft during growth, because it is attached down to the bone by numerous microscopic fibres, the perforating fibres of Sharpey (1848). Nevertheless, the fixed point (Fig. 3.3) is a region of minimal tension in the growing membrane, away from which the periosteum elongates, and whose position is determined by the rates of bone apposition at the two growth cartilages.

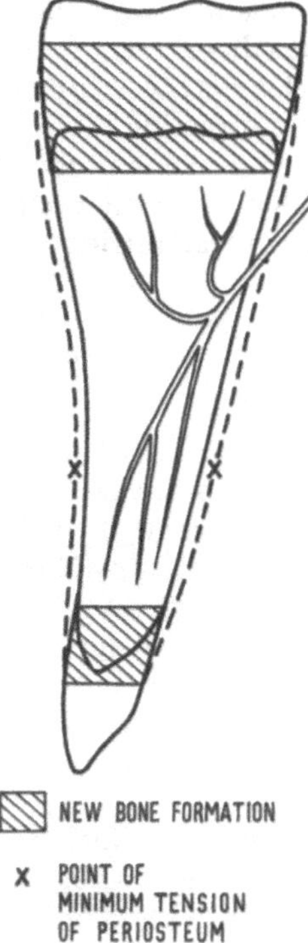

Fig. 3.3. Nutrient artery obliquity according to Humphry and Lacroix. Rate of bone apposition at the growing end exceeds that at the non-growing end. The periosteum, however, grows interstitially and drags the artery towards the growing end, causing the vessel to point away from it.

In postnatal bones, at any rate where there is a growing end, nutrient vessels affixed to the growing periosteum will tend to be dragged away from the fixed region of minimal tension and pulled towards the "growing end". Hence, they come to lie obliquely in relation to the surface of the shaft. Periosteal deposition of bone, which increases the breadth of the shaft, will then take place around the obliquely lying vessels. This process, continuing until growth ceases, will result in an oblique nutrient canal pointing away from the growing end, as is the usual case.

Muscle traction on the periosteum

If the above were the whole explanation, then there should be no exceptions to Bérard's rule. Lacroix (1948), who was a strong supporter of the view that canal direction is an expression of differences in modes of growth of bone and periosteum, investigated the direction of the nutrient artery in the rabbit femur; this passes anomalously towards the knee, the growing end (Figs 2.10, 2.11). The femoral nutrient foramen lies just below the lesser trochanter, to which the muscle psoas major is attached. Lacroix sectioned the muscle in young rabbits and found that the nutrient canal in the adult animals then pointed away from the knee. He postulated that peculiarities in the pull of the psoas muscle on the periosteum below the lesser trochanter, were the reason why, in this animal, the nutrient canal had an anomalous direction.

The action of attached muscles may well influence local periosteal growth, in certain instances. Yet the normal direction of the canal in animals such as the rat (Fig. 2.11), whose femoral nutrient canal is situated in a similar location to that of the rabbit, makes it probable that other factors also participate in determining the site and direction of the diaphyseal nutrient vessels.

Bone remodelling

Payton (1934) studied growing long bones in pigs fed with madder root. His observations led him to introduce two new factors into the discussion. He showed that in the pig's ulna an actual movement of the canal occurred towards the growing end, which was not accounted for by Humphry's explanation. He considered that the site of the canal and its direction were independent of each other, and that the movement of the canal was due to partial internal remodelling of the shaft, whereby bone was removed from one wall of the canal and new bone was deposited on the other. The direction of the canal was also, according to Payton, an expression of the manner in which bone is deposited at the surface of the shaft in order to preserve its shape.

During growth in length, new periosteal bone in Payton's material was deposited in such a way that the nutrient artery was caught up between two distinct bone deposits: on the one hand, a bevel of newly deposited bone lying on the side of the vessel away from the nearest growth cartilage; and on the other hand, the old bone forming the shaft surface on its other side (Fig. 3.4). This mechanism might explain those anomalous cases where the nutrient artery points towards the growing end and the canal is sited nearer to the other, as in the pig's humerus and femur (Fig. 3.5), both of which disobey Bérard's rule. In the pig's

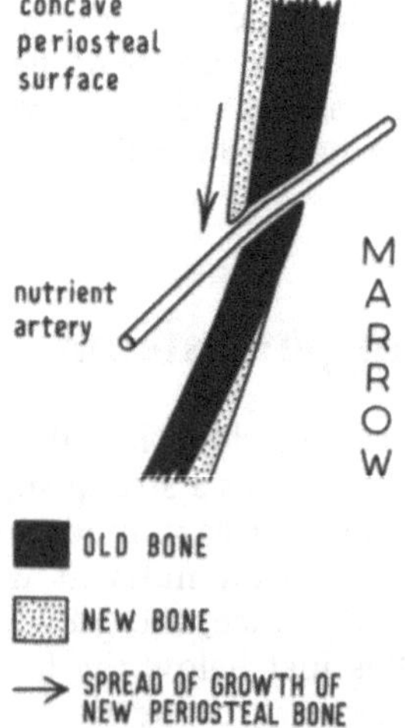

Fig. 3.4. Nutrient artery obliquity according to Payton. The spreading edge of new surface bone pushes the artery increasingly into obliquity during development.

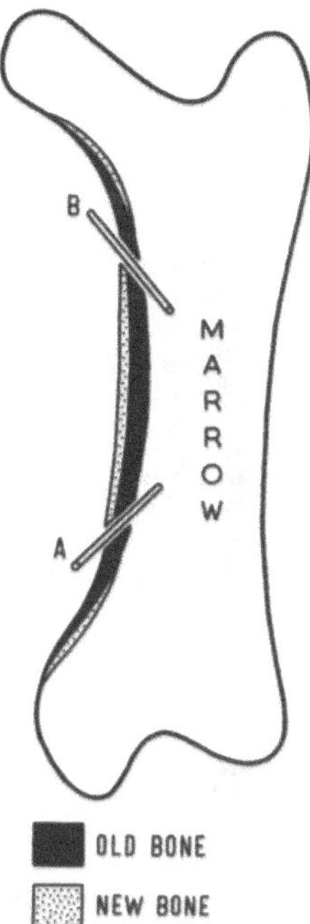

Fig. 3.5. According to Payton, the final direction of the nutrient artery depends on whether it is near the "growing end" (A) or "non-growing end" (B). The latter is normal in the rabbit's or pig's femur.

ulna, however, the canal is nearer to the non-growing end and points towards it. Payton pointed out by way of explanation that the anterior convex surface is situated in this bone canal and that, during growth, endosteal deposition occurs. The nutrient artery is trapped between this and the old bone of the shaft, and made to point towards the elbow (Fig. 3.6, *overleaf*).

Hence, in Payton's view it would seem that mechanisms controlling the remodelling of bone and preserving its surface contour are important factors determining the site and obliquity of the nutrient artery.

Interstitial growth of systemic vessels

Hughes (1952) introduced another factor into the discussion which just missed being represented in the idiosyncratic schema (Fig. 3.7, *overleaf*) of Wood-Jones (1949), namely the growth of the parent artery giving origin to the nutrient vessel (Fig. 3.8, *overleaf*). Hughes examined the long bones of a wide variety of avian and mammalian species and was able to confirm that, in general, nutrient canals obeyed Bérard's law. Anomalies of direction, when they occurred, affected particularly the canals of the femur (in several avian species as well as the horse, sheep, elephant and others), and also the radius (dog, camel, llama and others).

Hughes argued that if the parent vessel of the nutrient artery grew interstitially, then obliquity of the extra-osseous nutrient vessel would automatically result,

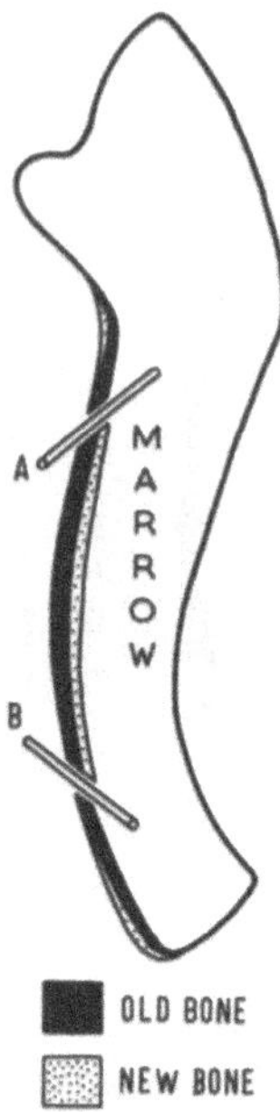

Fig. 3.6. In Payton's theory, when the nutrient artery enters a convex surface, anomalies may arise because endosteal new bone pushes the vessel into obliquity. The usual nutrient artery direction (**A**) occurs when the vessel is near the non-growing end (ulna of man); an unusual direction occurs when the vessel (**B**) is near to the growing end (ulna of a pig).

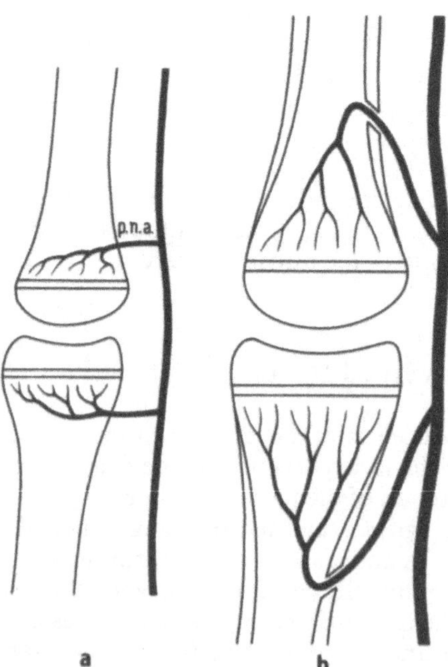

Fig. 3.7. Wood-Jones' theory of nutrient artery obliquity applies to the knee but not the elbow joint. It assumes an initial position of the vessel (p.n.a.) in the metaphysis **a**, and that growth of the bones by apposition imposes obliquity on the nutrient vessel **b**.

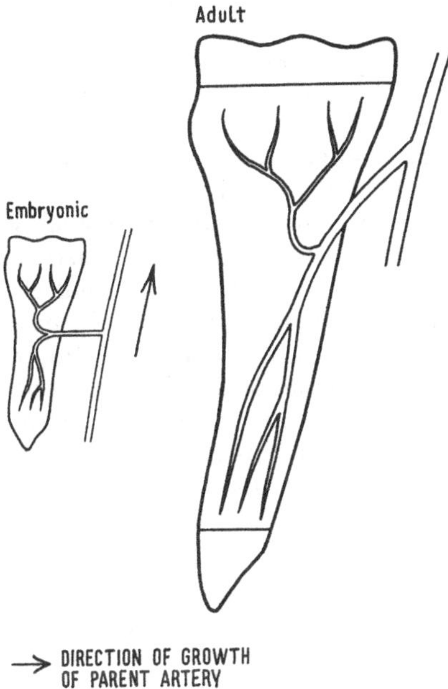

Fig. 3.8. Hughes' theory. Interstitial growth of the parent vessel causes an increasing obliquity of its branch, the nutrient artery, during appositional bone growth.

because its site of entry was fixed in the bony shaft lengthening by appositional growth alone. New periosteal bone would be deposited around the oblique vessel during growth in thickness of the shaft, resulting in an oblique nutrient canal (Fig. 3.8). He discounted the notion of nutrient arterial obliquity being produced by the tug of the growing periosteum because, as he rightly pointed out, it may well be that normally the tissue of this membrane simply grows around the artery traversing it, exercising no drag at all.

Hughes' suggested mechanism helps to explain obliquity of the canal in the fetal tibia, where inequality of longitudinal bone growth is absent. In this case, the fixed point according to the theory of periosteal slip is central, and hence no tendency to periosteal drag on the nutrient vessels exists. Interstitial growth of a systemic artery can still in these circumstances impose obliquity on its nutrient branch, fixed at its distal end in bone tissue.

Variant systemic arterial pattern

Some other specific anomalies may be due to a changed arterial pattern of the limb, especially where the parent vessel does not so much run parallel with the bone, as across it. Hughes refers to the lateral circumflex femoral artery, which in many animals is the source of the femoral nutrient. Growth of the parent artery here would exercise little influence on canal direction, but would account for the maximal incidence of canal anomalies occurring in the femur.

Nevertheless, it would be difficult to apply Hughes' theories to account for several specific anomalies of canal direction which he describes in the radius, where the parent vessel *does* run parallel with the bone. Furthermore, if two nutrient arteries are present in the human fetal femur, then they point to the centre of the bone, that is, they have contrary directions (Fig. 2.12). However, the upper one postnatally has a changed direction towards the head of the bone, so that both nutrient arteries in the adult "flee the knee". Such a change in canal direction is more easily explained by invoking periosteal slip in conjunction with the known change from fetal equality to postnatal inequality of growth rates, at the ends of the femur. On the other hand, a postnatal change in the pattern of interstitial growth of the a.profunda femoris, which is the source of both nutrient arteries in the human femur, cannot be excluded. Again, in some cases the nutrient artery pursues a winding or sinuous extra-osseous course, for example (Fig. 3.9) upwards before passing downwards into a straight nutrient canal (in the canine femur (Parouti 1962)). In this instance it seems doubtful whether the extra-osseous lie of the nutrient artery has any influence at all in determining the direction of its canal.

Temporal variability of growth patterns

Finally, Piollet's solution (1905) of the problem of the nutrient canal which changes direction during growth and development may be alluded to. In the human femur, radius and ulna (Figs 2.12, 3.10a), it is apparent that the nutrient canal may have different directions in embryonic, fetal and adult life. Piollet reminded us of the possibility that at different times in the life span, different growth patterns, especially of the extra-osseous soft parts, may be dominant.

A further example may be added on here of directional change in a neurovascular foramen. Warwick (1950) pointed out that the mental foramen in the human fetus opens on to the surface inclined upwards and forwards (Fig. 3.10b). In the adult jaw, the foramen and the issuing vessels and nerve point upwards and backwards. This major change in the direction of the mental

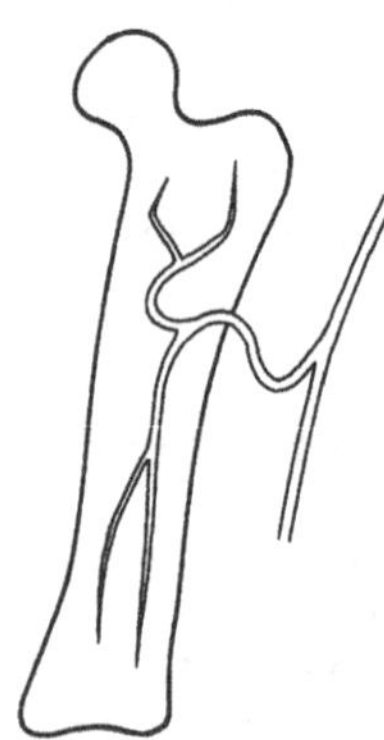

Fig. 3.9. Hughes' theory is difficult to apply when the nutrient artery has a sinuous extra-osseous course.

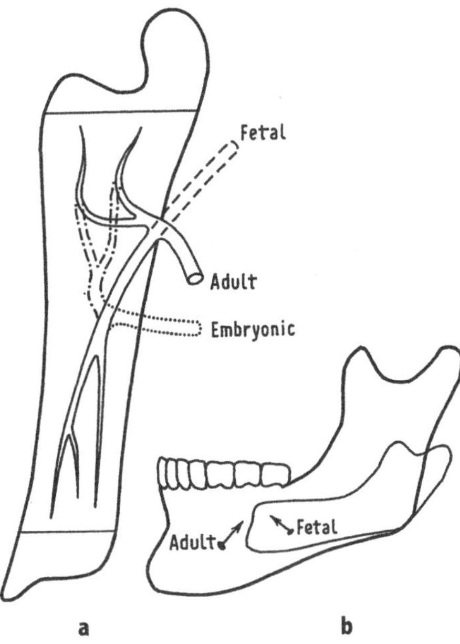

Fig. 3.10. Piollet is of the opinion that variable growth patterns of the extra-osseous soft parts may change the direction of the nutrient artery during development and growth. Examples are shown in the human radius or ulna **a** and mandible **b**.

foramen actually takes place in early postnatal life and is presumably related to the development of the chin.

The mechanism whereby the change occurs is uncertain. It is recalled that Tomes (1882) took this foramen as a fixed point when assessing directions and surfaces of bone accretion during mandibular growth. Nowadays its fixed character would no longer be conceded. It is thought that in the first place, the change of direction of the mental foramen is brought about by an eccentric deposition of periosteal bone in relation to the opening of the foramen on the surface of the mandible. This recalls Payton's observations on the movement by remodelling of nutrient canals during growth of long bones. From Brash's experiments (1924) with madder feeding of growing pigs, it is also known that the mandible grows, as it were, backwards: that is, by accretion at the posterior border of the ramus and removal at its anterior border. Presumably there is periosteal drag towards the ramus of the mandible. If this is so, then possibly the theory of periosteal slip is adequate to account for the eccentric bone deposition during growth, demarcating the mental foramen and causing it to point backwards.

Periosteal slip could also be invoked to account for the upward component in the direction of the mental foramen, since Brash has shown that alveolar bone is incorporated into the body of the mandible and little or no accretion takes place at the inferior border. In this way the direction of the foramen in postnatal life is explicable. But how can its direction in the fetal jaw be accounted for? Presumably another mechanism is at work in the fetal period causing the forward direction of the foramen, for which growth of the mandible at the symphysis menti may possibly be conjectured.

Conclusion

A variety of mechanisms have been put forward to account for the site and obliquity of the diaphyseal nutrient vessels of tubular bones. These include the different modes and rates of growth of bone and periosteum; interstitial growth of systemic vessels giving off nutrient branches; and remodelling processes. Selected growth mechanisms may be active only at specific periods during growth and development. A combination of factors may be involved in a given case. It must be borne in mind that the various factors affecting the disposition of the nutrient artery in the cortex of long bones are likely to influence the disposition of all the fine vessels present in compact bone, i.e. the vascular scaffold of the cortical microcirculation.

Chapter 4

Early development of nutrient vessels

Diaphyseal vessels

In the 5th week after conception, the human skeleton is blastemal in structure, consisting of mesenchyme cells in a tissue fluid matrix. In the 7th week, the skeleton of the human embryo is cartilaginous, the long bones consisting of a shaft, enlarged at both ends into the epiphyses of the embryonic bone. Surrounding the shaft of the cartilage model is a *vascular perichondrium* made up of inner osteogenic and outer fibrous zones (Fig. 4.1). At the beginning of the 8th week

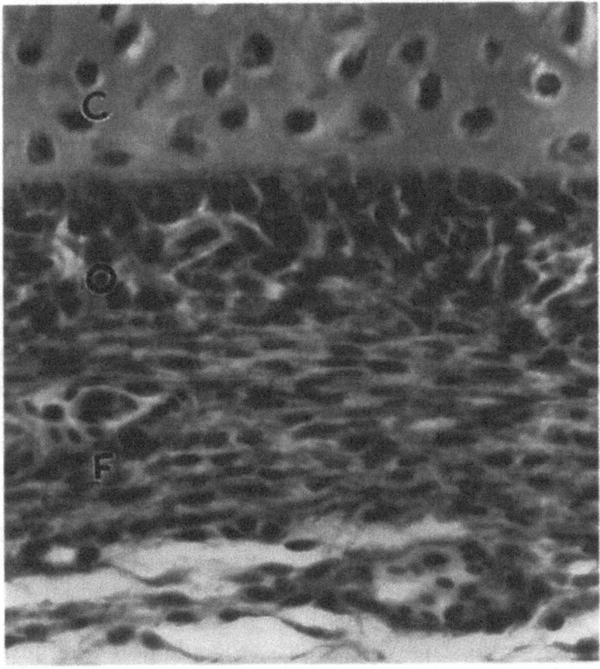

Fig. 4.1. Longitudinal section through the femoral primordium of a chick embryo, showing the cartilaginous shaft (C), and osteogenic layer (O) and fibrous layer (F) of the perichondrium. (Original magnification ×240)

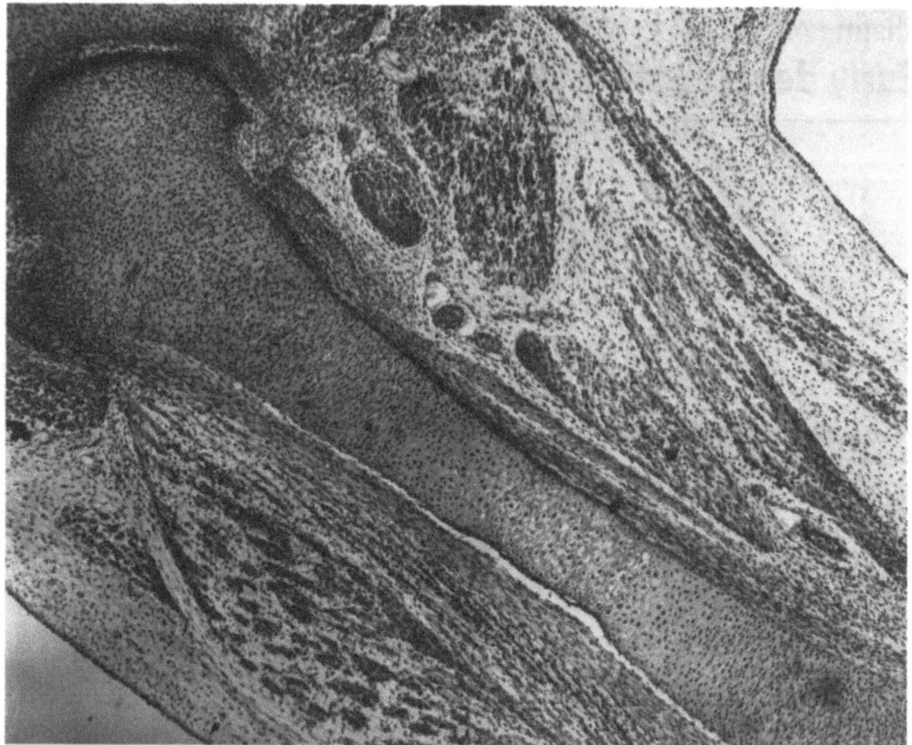

Fig. 4.2. The cartilaginous primordium of the human femur 7 weeks after conception, showing hypertrophic cells in the centre of the shaft prior to vascular irruption. This ossific centre is coated with the primary bone lamella of Lovén. (Original magnification ×37)

(3.5 cm CR length) the centre of the shaft shows chondrocyte hypertrophy, immediately followed by the laying down of a cylindrical *primary lamella of bone* (Lovén 1863) (Figs 4.2, 4.3). The lamella of Lovén is the first deposit of bone tissue to appear in tubular bones. It is on the primary lamella that a *perichondrial collar* of bone trabeculae (Ranvier 1875) is then laid down (Figs 4.4, 4.5, *overleaf*).

The diaphyseal nutrient vessels are first indicated in the 8th week by a leash of vessels, growing in the trabecular spaces of Ranvier's perichondrial collar. A localized *primary vascular irruption* then takes place into the middle of the cartilaginous primordium, and at right angles to it. Subsequently a single arterial channel differentiates from the irrupting leash. Other vessels differentiate into a nutrient vein or leash of veins closely accompanying the artery in the newly formed nutrient canal.

The fine vessels of the irrupting leash, i.e. the sinusoids linking the artery and veins, are intimately associated with mesenchyme cells, with a potentiality to differentiate into cells forming bone, cartilage, fibrous tissue and haemopoietic cells. Together, the vessels and cells constitute a typical example of an *osteogenic blastema*, i.e. vascular mesenchyme with osteogenic potentialities. The blastema also has chondrolytic powers, removing cartilage as it invades the cartilaginous shaft. Bone trabeculae are then deposited in the shaft *in* the space now made available (Figs 4.6–4.8, *overleaf*).

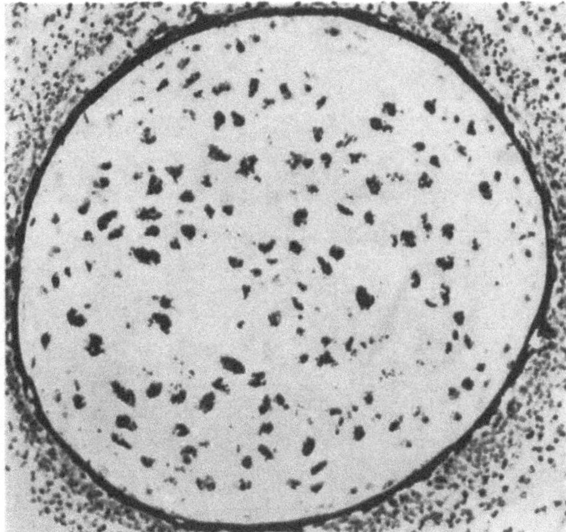

Fig. 4.3. Cross-section through a chick embryonic femur (10th day of incubation) showing the primary bone lamella. (Silver impregnation; Original magnification ×50)

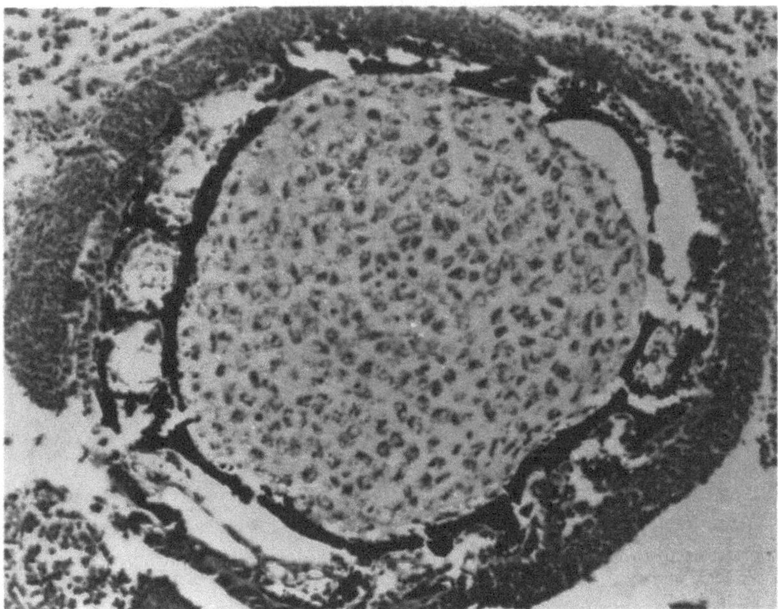

Fig. 4.4. A stage later than Fig. 4.3, showing the bone trabeculae of Ranvier's perichondrial collar. (Silver impregnation; Original magnification ×60)

The concept of removal of the cartilage model preceding bone formation within it, was established more than two centuries ago by Von Haller (1763). It was so well attested that Bell (1823) averred that the cartilage primordium was neither a bone nor its precursor, but was entirely removed by the "absorbent

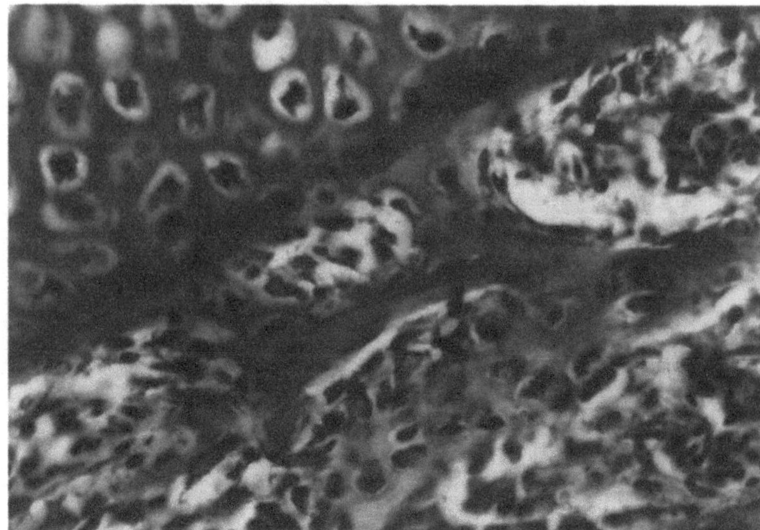

Fig. 4.5. Chick embryo: perichondrial collar of bone showing highly vascular and cellular intertrabecular spaces. (Original magnification ×248)

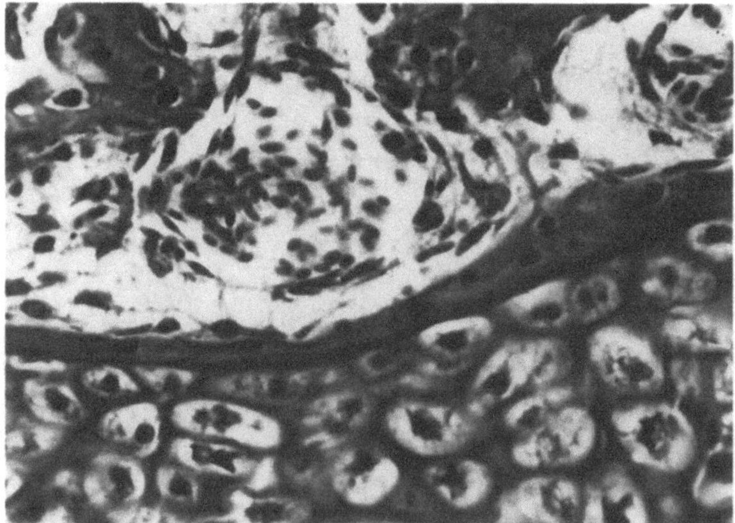

Fig. 4.6. Chick embryo: vascular irruption into the cartilaginous shaft is imminent. (Original magnification ×155)

vessels", that is, the sinusoids. It is repeatedly necessary to emphasize, like Wolff (1868) and many others, that bone is not derived from cartilage but is a connective tissue *sui generis*.

The osteogenic blastema irrupts into an *ossific centre* [where bone will be formed] in the middle of the cartilaginous shaft, where the cells exhibit hypertrophy and calcification (Fig. 4.1). This central core of calcified cartilage precedes

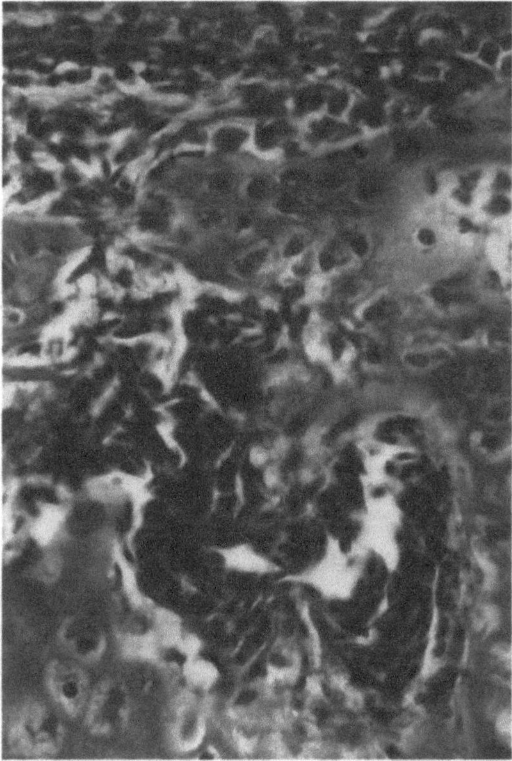

Fig. 4.7. Primary vascular irruption into the cartilage primordium of the chick femur. (Original magnification ×155)

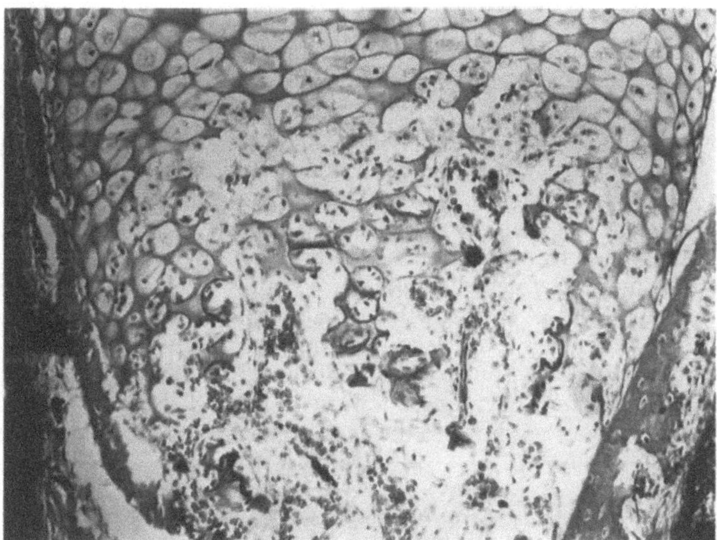

Fig. 4.8. Longitudinal section through the head of a fetal metatarsal II (13 cm CR length), showing primary spongiosa embraced by the ossification ring. The hypertrophic cells of the growth zone are arcuate. (Original magnification ×175)

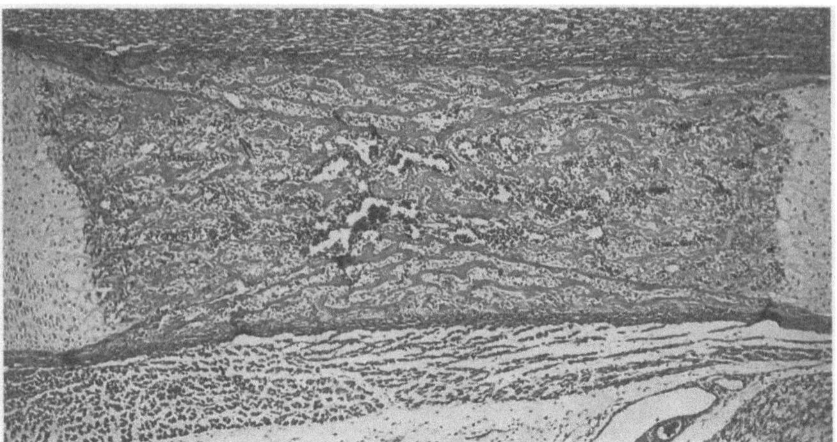

Fig. 4.9. Fetal mouse femur showing periosteal bone trabeculae forming a cortex, and endochondral bone trabeculae forming two conical regions of primary non-haemopoietic marrow. Note cartilage growth zone at each end of the long axis. (Original magnification ×29)

and seemingly evocates (in an embryological sense) the deposition of Lovén's primary bone lamella, Ranvier's perichondrial collar of bone, and then the primary vascular irruption. The chondrolysis which the latter entails results in the separation of proximal and distal *cartilaginous growth zones*, the immediate descendants of the original single ossific centre of cartilage.

Formation of bone marrow

At first the growth zones are separated by an area occupied by the osteogenic blastema and a few spicules of bone which have already been formed on cartilage matrix debris. This is the *primary centre of ossification* [where bone is formed]. Its proximodistal expansion is brought about by continual chondrolysis of the growth zones (Fig. 4.9). Each zone is simultaneously renewed by its basal proliferating layer of germinal cells immediately adjacent to the cartilaginous epiphysis.

In this way, a *primary non-haemopoietic marrow* replaces at an early stage (9th week) the embryonic cartilaginous shaft. After completion of the primary vascular irruption, bone formation and its concomitant bone removal, both a function of specialized mesenchyme cells, take place mainly on the outer and inner surfaces of the shaft and at the growth cartilages. By the end of the 3rd month, a *haemopoietic marrow* is established in the fetal medullary cavity, persisting throughout childhood. At puberty most of the appendicular skeletal marrow is transformed into a non-haemopoietic *fatty marrow*. Blood formation is thereafter, in health, largely confined to the axial skeleton.

Bone growth in girth and length

A cortex of periosteal bone trabeculae continues to be laid down after the centre of ossification has formed. *Lateral expansion* of the marrow cavity is brought

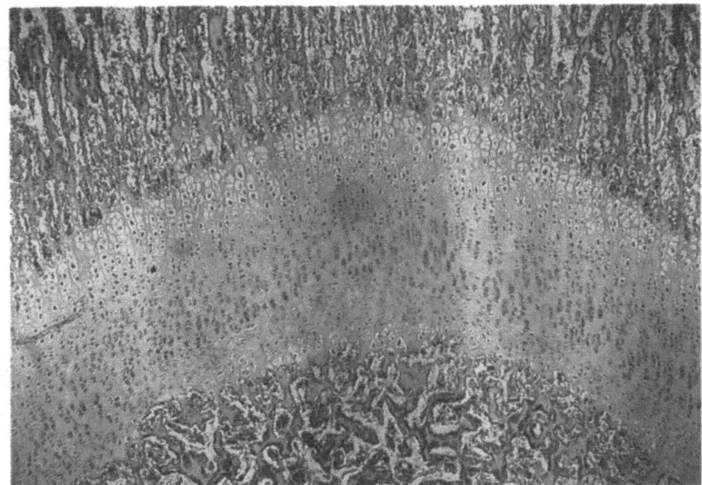

Fig. 4.10. Secondary centre of ossification in the lower femoral epiphysis of a yearling monkey. A growth cartilage separates epiphysis from metaphysis. The cartilage cells are vertically orientated on each side of the cartilage, and also the metaphyseal bone trabeculae. The epiphyseal trabeculae are irregular. The trabecular pattern is a result of vascular pattern, not chondrocyte pattern. (Original magnification ×40)

about by erosion from within by osteoclasts, and bone deposition externally from the periosteal osteoblasts. *Growth in length* of the young bone is assured by erosion of the cartilaginous growth zones by marrow chondroclasts and their replacement with endochondral bone trabeculae by marrow osteoblasts (Fig. 4.9). The cartilaginous epiphyseal extremities persist and enlarge for a considerable period extending into childhood, before a *secondary centre of ossification* appears within them (Fig. 4.10).

In the formation of a diaphyseal primary marrow (Fig. 4.11) the vessels of the osteogenic blastema differentiate into medullary vessels, i.e. arteries and

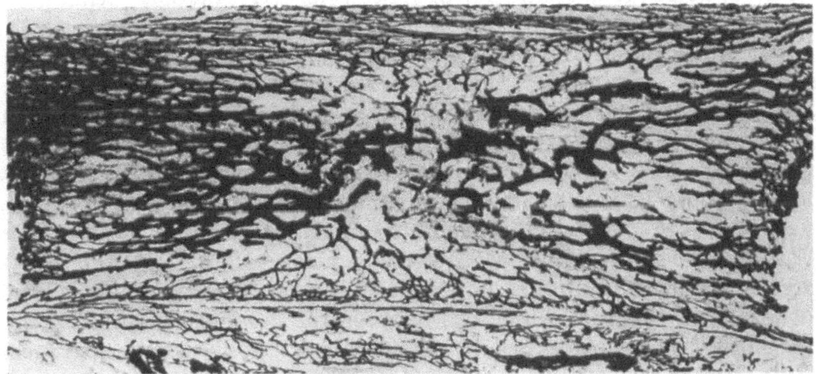

Fig. 4.11. Fetal mouse femur showing highly vascular marrow and cortex. A marrow cavity has not yet formed. The medullary vessels have a metaphyseal pattern and are in two conical groups, joined by their apices at the waist of the bone. A diaphyseal marrow is absent. Cf. Fig. 4.9. (India ink, Original magnification ×29)

sinusoids, drained by venous sinuses and nutrient veins. With expansion of the medullary cavity, the *medullary vessels* become confluent with *cortical vessels*, around which bone trabeculae are deposited during growth in girth of the shaft (periosteal bone deposition) (Ham 1953; Brookes 1964). The medullary and cortical circulations remain separate, until the primary bone lamella of Lovén (Figs 4.3, 4.6) is removed by internal erosion.

Epiphyseal vessels

These make their first appearance at the beginning of fetal existence, at the 4.5 cm CR length stage of human development (9th week). Fine perichondrial vessels are incorporated into the enlarging cartilaginous epiphyses, resulting in the formation of vascular *cartilage canals*. The vessels in the canals are the forerunners of the vessels of the bony epiphysis, which replaces the cartilaginous precursor. Their developmental history is discussed separately in Chapter 9.

Formation of the metaphysis

There is no large body of information available on the genesis and further development of metaphyseal vessels, as there is on their diaphyseal and epiphyseal counterparts. It is known (Lewis 1956; Brookes 1958a) that they are present in the proximal and distal regions of human fetal long bones in the third trimester. Before that, the diaphyseal nutrient artery perforates the fetal cortex, and it is the ramifications of this vessel alone which are in the marrow of the shaft of young fetal long bones (first and second trimesters).

Hunterian remodelling

Lovén's perichondrial bone lamella rapidly extends proximally and distally to surround the rims of the nascent growth zones (Fig. 4.12), thereby forming at each site Ranvier's ossification ring. For a short time, the *ossification ring* and perichondrial lamella are in continuity. Hence the diaphyseal nutrient vessels growing into the growth cartilage are separate from those in the periosteum. During *growth in girth* of the shaft in the second trimester, the cortex overlying the newly formed spongiosa next to the growth zone is continually removed by *bone remodelling* (Hunter 1772), in order to conserve the overall shape of the bone (Fig. 4.13). Remodelling also leaves the ossification ring isolated on the rim of the growth cartilage (Fig. 4.14, *overleaf*): between the ring and shaft cortex a circumferential *ossification groove* is now present, covered over by perichondrium (Fig. 4.14).

External Hunterian remodelling then exposes a metaphyseal bone surface (of endochondral formation) which lies between the ossification ring and the diaphyseal cortex (of periosteal origin). The periosteal capillaries are then incorporated into the metaphyseal spongiosa and undergo vascular differentiation, giving rise to the definitive metaphyseal arteries and veins.

Kölliker (1873) described in the humerus of an 8-day-old rabbit how resorption cavities appeared in the cortex of what he named the *metaphysis*: the part of

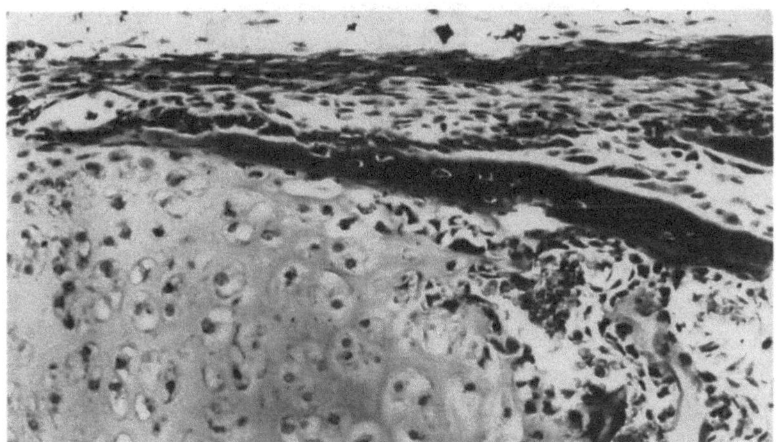

Fig. 4.12. Ranvier's ossification ring overlies the hypertrophic zone of the growth cartilage and metaphyseal spongiosa. (12-week human fetal phalanx; Original magnification ×300)

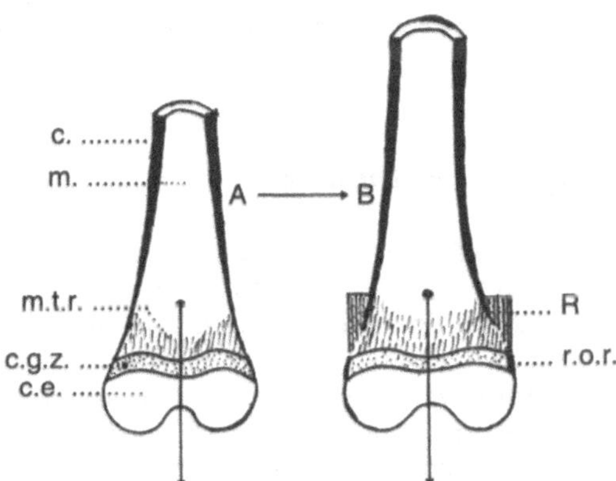

Fig. 4.13. The shape of a bone increasing in size from **A** to **B** is conserved, by external Hunterian remodelling. **c.**, Cortex; **m.**, medulla; **m.t.r.**, metaphyseal trabeculae; **c.g.z.**, cartilage growth zone; **c.e.**, cartilage epiphysis; **r.o.r.**, ossification ring; **R**, the mass of new metaphysis which would accrue during growth in length, if not removed by remodelling.

the shaft composed of endochondral bone trabeculae (*spongiosa*) adjacent to the growth zone. The cavities initiated on the periosteal surface uncovered the spongiosa within. Bone resorption was brought about by multinucleate giant cells, which he named *osteoclasts*. These formed, however, only a fraction of the mononuclear cells and vascular tissue which filled the resorption cavities. According to Kölliker, the periosteal blood vessels anastomosed with those in the young metaphyseal spongiosa. Hence it would appear that the disposition of the metaphyseal vessels lies in those remodelling phenomena which conserve bone shape, particularly at the metaphysis.

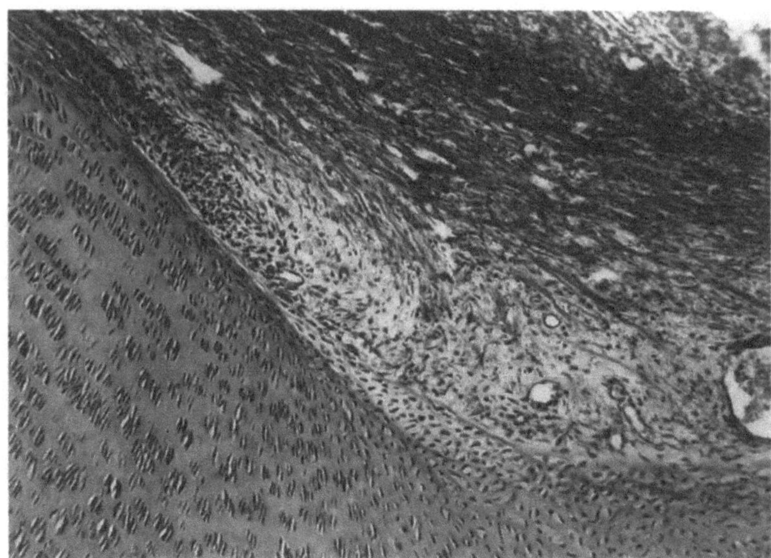

Fig. 4.14. The ossification ring is visible in the top left-hand corner, overlying the growth zone. Remodelling has removed the cortex between ring and diaphysis, forming an ossification groove spanned by perichondrium. (Fetal humerus, 22 cm; Original magnification ×80)

Constancy of pattern of metaphyseal vessels

The manner in which metaphyseal vessels maintain their position in the metaphysis and their relationship to the rest of the bone during bone elongation, must now be discussed. The possibility of continual formation of new metaphyseal nutrients during bone growth can be excluded, on the grounds that the pattern of metaphyseal vascular foramina is much the same in a fetal as in an adult bone. Without the intervention of some mechanism maintaining the constancy of pattern of metaphyseal vascular penetration of the bone, there would result in the adult condition a bony *diaphysis* covered with large foramina, giving passage to nutrient arteries and veins. But the surface of the diaphysis is comparatively smooth, without numerous large foramina of metaphyseal type. Only one or two diaphyseal nutrient foramina are normally present.

Consider the fate of a group of metaphyseal arteries near the knee joint in a fetal femur. Arising from pre-existing periosteal capillaries incorporated into the metaphysis during early growth and external remodelling, they subsequently differentiate into peripheral metaphyseal vessels. Once given off from the circulus vasculosus, this group passes directly into the metaphysis (Fig. 4.15a). However during appositional growth in length of the bone, the metaphysis is incorporated into the diaphysis (Pratt 1957). The circulus vasculosus might maintain its relationship to the epiphyseal plate by interstitial growth of the systemic vessels (Hughes 1952) which give rise to it. However, this would in no way affect the tendency for the point of entry of the vertical nutrient vessels to come to lie more and more distant from the growth zone/cartilage; if their entry into the bone is fixed (Fig. 4.15b, m, m).

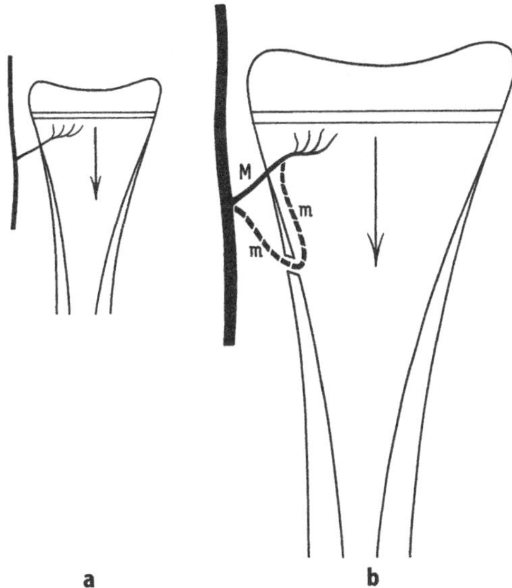

Fig. 4.15. Diagrams to illustrate internal remodelling to maintain a constant relationship between metaphyseal arteries and the metaphysis: **a** young epiphysis; **b** Postnatal epiphysis. M, Normal metaphyseal artery; mm, displaced artery in the absence of remodelling.

It follows therefore that the constancy of pattern of metaphyseal vessels during growth, results from *internal remodelling* of the metaphysis. Contrasting bone deposition and removal occurs on opposite, i.e. proximal and distal, faces of the metaphyseal foramina. This allows the fully differentiated metaphyseal arteries and veins lodged in them to slip down towards the growth cartilage, from which they would otherwise be increasingly removed (Fig. 4.15b). Payton's (1934) demonstration in growing pigs that the diaphyseal nutrient foramen actually moves along the shaft because of internal remodelling, lends support to this.

Constancy of pattern of fibromuscular attachments

Internal remodelling of the metaphysis may also provide the mechanism whereby constancy of pattern of *muscle and tendon attachments* to a bone is preserved. For reasons analogous to those detailed above in respect of the arteries, growing muscles and tendons affixed to the metaphyseal cortex, itself being incorporated into the diaphysis, would tend to drift away from the growth cartilage unless the fibrous attachments were relocated. *Collagen fibre renewal* at an ultrastructural level using ^{14}C-labelled proline has been demonstrated to occur in the periodontal ligament (Thomas 1967). In this case, collagen removal and relocation is essential in order to maintain the oblique disposition of the ligament between the lamina dura of the tooth socket and the cementum of an erupting tooth. It might also account for the process of tooth eruption itself.

Chapter 5

Blood supply of irregular bones – 1: Vertebral column

The vertebral column (Nomina Anatomica 1989) is familiar to all as the spine, run through by the spinal cord, and operated upon by spinal surgeons. It has seven cervical, 12 thoracic and five lumbar vertebrae, and a sacrum formed by the fusion of five sacral segments, and ending in a diminutive coccyx (fusion of four segments). At birth, the column is concave ventrally; from childhood onwards, the cervical and lumbar regions are convex.

The body of an adult vertebra can be likened to an abbreviated *long bone*, but it lacks a diaphysis and consists of two conical parts joined together at their apices. The vertebral body is composed of spongy bone trabeculae of endochondral origin, with haemopoietic marrow filling the intertrabecular cancelli. As in long bone metaphyses, the blood vessels of the vertebral body branch profusely and diverge towards the bony epiphyses. The entire vertebral body is encased in a thin shell of corticalis. Posteriorly, the neural arch of the vertebra is classified anatomically as a *flat bone*. It has a thick cortex enclosing a marrow cavity and is joined to the body by right and left pedicles. Various bilateral processes are also present in the neural arch; transverse, spinous, articular and mammillary.

Vertebral development

Blastemal phase

Precursor vertebrae first appear in the human embryo in the 5th week, straddling the ventral and lateral aspects of the neural tube (Fig. 5.1). Each is subdivided into a *centrum* incorporating the related part of the *notochord*; a *costal process* grows ventrally in the body wall; and two *neural processes* grow dorsally which only later fuse (second trimester) to form the neural arch.

For more than a century, it has been held that a vertebra derives from the fusion of four sclerotomic masses, i.e. from *two pairs* of adjacent somites (Remak 1855; von Ebner 1888; von Bochmann 1937; Töndury 1958). The vertebral primordia were said to be divided transversely by intervertebral fissures, allowing the caudal two-thirds of a blastemal vertebra to fuse with the cranial third of the next. This makes each bony vertebra *intersegmental* in value, and related to cervical spinal, thoracic intercostal and lumbar and sacral arteries.

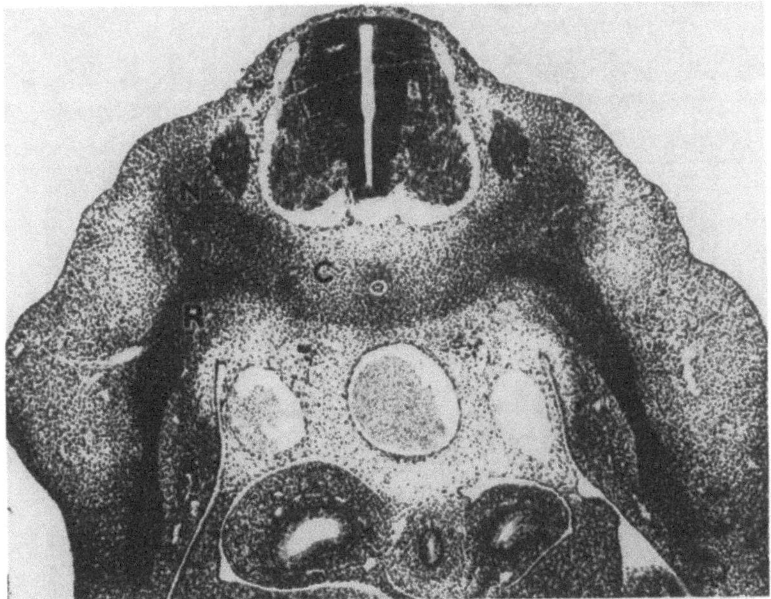

Fig. 5.1. Blastemal vertebra in a mole embryo, showing the centrum (C) and neural (N) and costal (R) processes. The neural tube, notochord, dorsal aorta, trachea and lung buds are also well displayed. (Original magnification ×56)

This is denied by Verbout (1974, 1985) in sheep, mouse, rat, rabbit and man, and also by Christ (1975) in birds. They insist that in general the whole vertebra originates from a *single pair* of sclerotomes and therefore is *segmental* in value; the vertebrae lie caudal to a pair of segmental spinal nerves, which correspond numerically with them; "Neugliederung" (rarely translated correctly, if at all, in the literature: it means "reorganization") of the blastemal vertebrae does not happen; and the vertebral bodies and their processes as well as the intervertebral discs, from the start arise in their *definitive* sites in relation to the myotomes, without relocation. The caudal part of a blastemal vertebra develops into the whole bony vertebra: the cranial blastema develops into the *dura mater* of the spinal cord, and the *annulus fibrosus* of the *intervertebral disc* (but not its nucleus pulposus which is a notochordal remnant).

Cartilage phase

Chondrification of blastemal vertebrae begins in the 7th week, transforming them into cartilaginous vertebrae (7 weeks) (Fig. 5.2, *overleaf*). The cartilaginous costal processes are distinct and separate from the rest of the vertebrae in the thoracic series and give rise to ribs. Costal processes which do not develop into ribs persist as costotransverse bars in cervical vertebrae, or as phenotypic transverse processes of lumbar vertebrae, or as the anterior transverse masses of the sacrum. The cartilaginous vertebral column persists into the second trimester of fetal life.

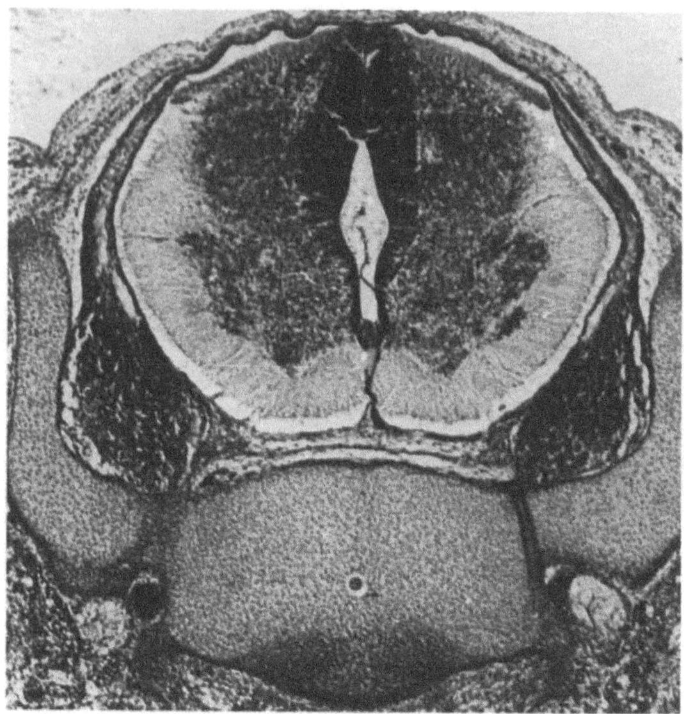

Fig. 5.2. Cartilaginous vertebra, showing the centrum (with the notochord right in its middle) and two neural processes growing dorsally to embrace the fetal spinal cord and dorsal root ganglia. (Human, 7 weeks; Original magnification ×35)

Osseous phase

From the 4th month of fetal life, a wave of ossification starting at C2 and T1 (neural processes) and at T10 and L1 (centra) spreads up and down in the vertebral column (Figs 5.3, 5.4). For a time the three fundamental parts of a growing bony vertebra are separated by three growth cartilages; one uniting the *laminae* at the apex of the arch, and one each at the feet of the *pedicles* forming cartilaginous neurocentral joints or *synchondroses*. The laminae fuse dorsally (at 3 years), an apical growth cartilage allowing for elongation of the vertebral spine. Fusion of the pedicles with the centra is complete in the 6th year.

Vessels of the vertebral column and spinal cord

The source of the nutrient arteries of the vertebral column includes the spinal branches of the intracranial vertebral arteries, and the spinal branches of the vertebral and deep cervical arteries in the neck, and below this, of the spinal branches of the intercostal, lumbar, ilio-lumbar and lateral sacral arteries. The spinal arteries enter into the spinal canal through the intervertebral foramina to supply both spinal cord and vertebral column. Venous drainage is by means of extrinsic and intrinsic longitudinal venous plexuses and segmental veins. The

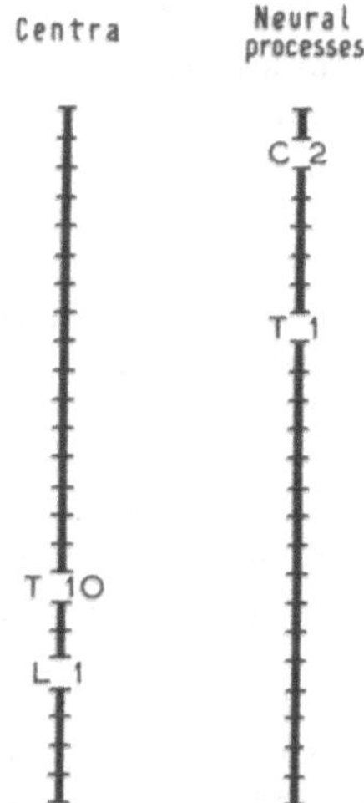

Fig. 5.3. Ossification centres first appear in fetal cartilaginous vertebrae in the numbered sites, and spread up and down the column until at birth three centres are present in each vertebra. (After Noback and Robertson 1951.)

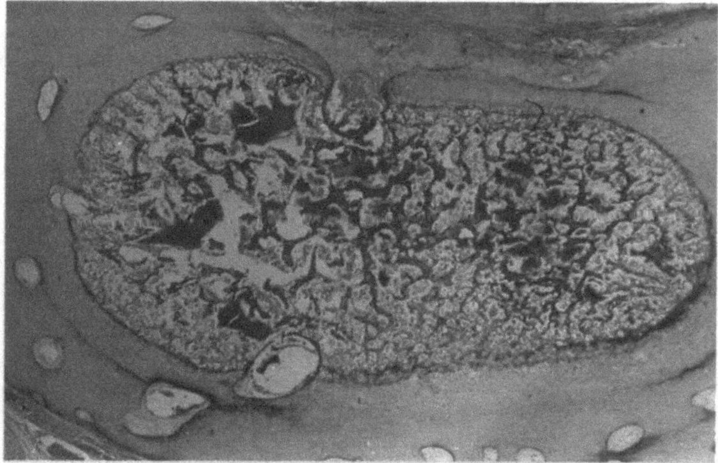

Fig. 5.4. Ossification in the centrum of a human fetal lumbar vertebra (26 cm CR length). Note the presence of anterolateral cartilage canals in the non-ossified primordium and the dorsally situated basi-vertebral foramen. (Original magnification ×18)

anterior and posterior longitudinal venous chains unite the intracranial with the veins of the vertebral column.

Blood supply of the neural process

Each *spinal artery* in an intervertebral foramen has a small *prelaminar branch* which supplies the periosteum of the corresponding neural process, and is also the source of its *nutrient artery.* The nutrient vessel pierces the inferior border of the arch where lamina, pedicle and transverse process meet. Intra-osseous twigs then ramify in the subdivisions of the neural process, the cortex being irrigated by capillaries from the marrow which connect with those of the periosteum.

As long as the three basic parts of the young vertebra, centrum and two neural processes, are separated by cartilage, typical metaphyseal vascular patterns are formed in association with the growth cartilages at the feet and apex of the neural arch. Bony fusion of the neural processes dorsally unites the two laminar circulations. But the dorsal growth cartilage persists, and is found at the tip of the developing *spinal process* projecting from the neural arch (Fig. 5.5). This cartilage, and others found at the tips of growing *transverse, articular* and *mammillary processes,* are functionally equivalent to the growth and epiphyseal cartilages of long bones.

Metaphyseal-type vascular territories form from the branches of the neural nutrients, and provide a mechanism for increase in length of the bony processes of the neural arch. Judging from the numerous vascular foramina found in the adult vertebral arch, it seems certain that fine arteries pierce the cortex of the laminae and are auxiliary to the single nutrient artery, whose branches ramify in the neural marrow cavity. By the 6th year, vascular union and *neuro-central synostosis* unite the centrum and pedicles.

In adolescence, secondary centres of epiphyseal ossification appear (16–18 years) in the cartilages at the tips of the bony spines and neural processes. For a short while distinct cartilaginous growth plates are present in these situations, but are soon lost by *epiphyseo-metaphyseal synostosis* (18–21 years).

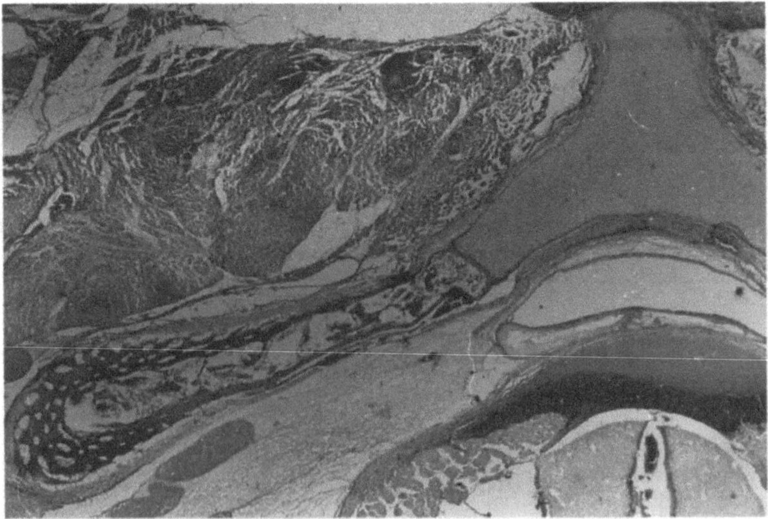

Fig. 5.5. Section through an ossifying lamina of the vertebra shown in Fig. 5.4. Note cartilaginous growth zone at dorsal extremity of the ossicle. (Original magnification ×18)

Arteries of the vertebral body

Spinal arteries are the source of *basivertebral arteries*, two of which commonly enter the dorsum of a vertebral body through a large foramen, in whose depths they then divide into four basivertebral arteries correlated with its genesis from a single pair of sclerotomes (Verbout 1974), or from adjacent segmental and bilateral sclerotomes (Willis 1949). The basivertebral arteries diverge and branch profusely, forming an extraordinarily rich sinusoid network in the cancelli of the spongiosa. More *metaphyseal arteries* enter the anterior and lateral aspects of the vertebral body, as well as dorsal groups additional to the basivertebral arteries. All these arteries, as in a typical long bone, help to form looped juxta-epiphyseal sinusoid plexuses in contact with the upper and lower growth cartilages, which separate a growing vertebral body from the adjacent intervertebral discs (Fig. 5.6).

There are two *ventral longitudinal anastomoses* between the spinal arteries of the column. *Transverse anastomoses* behind the vertebral bodies also occur between pairs of spinal arteries. They form median V-shaped junctions whose apices point inferiorly, and can give rise to a *median longitudinal arterial chain* (Quain 1894). The longitudinal and transverse anastomoses are found postcentrally, i.e. in front of the spinal theca, in the spinal canal. The transverse anastomoses, or median longitudinal chain, are the source of the basivertebral arteries which can be observed in cleared sections of perfused preparations (Figs 5.4, 5.6).

In late childhood, the vertebral body acquires bony epiphyseal plates. The epiphyseal nutrients which appear at this time are probably offsets of the ventral longitudinal anastomotic chains behind the vertebral bodies and also of the intersegmental arteries lying anterolaterally. Amato & Bombelli (1959) denied the existence of anterolaterally located epiphyseal or metaphyseal vessels in the vertebral body, in rabbit vertebrae, and described only a single dorsal nutrient for the discoid epiphyses in this animal. Indeed, these writers were of the opinion that nutrient vessels to the vertebra as a whole emanate solely from within the spinal canal. On the other hand, direct photography of careful dissections of young rabbit and monkey material (Stilwell 1959) showed that both anterolateral (metaphyseal)

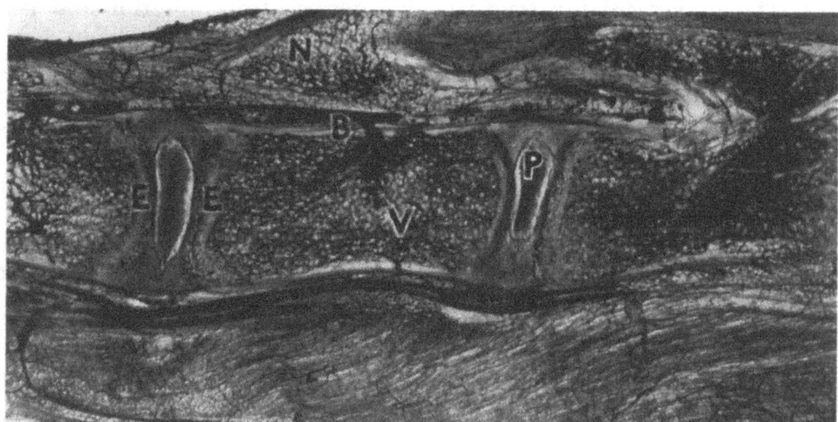

Fig. 5.6. India ink preparation of mouse sacral vertebrae in longitudinal section, showing basivertebral veins (B), vascular plexuses in epiphyseal bone plates (E) and neural processes (N). Vertebral body (V) and nucleus pulposus (P) are also indicated. (Original magnification ×12.0)

vessels as well as dorsal groups supply the vertebral bodies. His material, however, was not old enough to have developed epiphyses. In man at any rate, the bony epiphysis is usually annular (Schmorl 1929; Bick & Copel 1950), and deficient posteriorly (Bick 1951) as in the dog (Haas 1939). This suggests that the vessels of the thin flat annular epiphyseal bone plates enter circumferentially, at the rim, but dorsal inputs into the exiguous bone plates from the transverse anastomoses in the vertebral canal are not excluded (Kushkhabiev 1993). At maturity the vertebral body synostoses with its epiphyses, thereby uniting the individual vertebral circulations. Oki *et al.* (1994) using scanning electron microscopy (SEM) have examined the microcirculation abutting against the vertebral epiphyseal bone plate, in rabbits. They describe how capillaries from an individual arteriole form loops returning into the veins. The authors suggest that these capillaries, or vascular buds, are important in the nutrition of intervertebral discs.

Intervertebral joints

Symphyses

The intervertebral discs separating vertebral bodies, are made up of a central myxomatous *nucleus pulposus* encased in the *inner fibrocartilaginous zone* of the *annulus fibrosus.* The *outer zone* of the annulus is composed mainly of collagen and elastin fibres (Hickey & Hukins 1981; Johnson *et al.* 1985). The elastin fibres possibly hold in the disc at the rim, as if it were like a corset resisting horizontal pressures derived from axial compression forces in the upright posture. Superiorly and inferiorly a hyaline cartilage microplate affixes the annulus to the epiphysis of the vertical body.

The intervertebral discs are not normally vascularized, although of course they must have a supply of nutriment. Presumably ionic diffusion from the periarticular vascular plexus lying on the surface of the rim of the annulus is one source. Menck & Lierse (1990) in newborns find lateral branches of the spinal arteries penetrate the rim of the disc and would name these vessels rami disci intervertebrales. The periarticular vascular plexus derives from anterior and lateral branches of the spinal arteries on the outer surface of the vertebral body. A spinal arterial branch in 92% of cases examined descends downwards to ramify on the inferior disc and join in with the anterior and lateral arteries supplying the lower vertebra (Kushkhabiev 1993). In addition, nutrient diffusion from the sinusoid plexuses in the attached vertebral bodies (Brodin 1955), passing through the hyaline cartilage plates and inner fibrocartilaginous zones, are presumably important. The cartilage plates bounding human lumbar discs, and their rim tissue, have a glucose diffusion coefficient of 2.5 $cm^2\ s^{-1}$ as in articular and other hyaline cartilages (Maroudas *et al.* 1975), suggesting that the disc has a metabolism comparable to that of hyaline cartilage.

Diarthroses

The synovial joints between the *articular processes* of adjacent vertebrae have not been intensively studied from the vascular viewpoint. It is known that twigs from dorsal intersegmental and spinal vessels are important in the formation of the periosteal network of the neural arch (Quain 1894; Stilwell 1959), and are intimately conjoined to the vessels of the numerous muscles attached to the vertebral column. Offsets from these vessels, together with ventral branches of the *vertebral, intercostal* and *lumbar vessels*, form the vascular net of the capsular tissues of these small synovial joints. Vascular foramina found on the articular processes of the neural arch suggest that they are pierced by a few fine arteries which join intra-osseous branches of the neural nutrient vessel, to form an epiphyseal circulation, terminating in a subarticular network.

The vertebral column as a whole

As described above, the blood supply to the vertebral column is dependent on numerous small twigs from a variety of systemic arteries. Nevertheless, the nutrient pattern to vertebrae does not depart radically from that found in typical tubular bones. One may point to the discrete localized areas which give access to blood vessels, such as single centrally placed vessels (neural nutrients), metaphyseal type vessels (basivertebral, anterolateral and dorsal groupings) and numerous epiphyseal arteries supplying vertebral epiphyses. The internal arterial anastomotic chains which are a noticeable feature of the arteries to the vertebral column are paralleled by external anastomoses across synovial joints between the circuli vasculosi of long bones (Fig. 2.22). The vessels to vertebral bodies show similarities to the vascular arrangements in long bones, which can be recognized even at the level of the specialized subchondral circulations.Yet vertebral bodies lack a diaphyseal-type bone marrow, and their medullary vessels have a bi-metaphyseal pattern.Their terminations abutting the intervertebral discs are presumably end-arteries as in metaphyseal vessels in tubular bones. Positron emission tomography (PET) scanning has shown that the blood flow rate in the marrow of young lumbar vertebrae is brisk at 17.6 ml min^{-1} 100 g^{-1} (Kahn *et al.* 1994)

Parke *et al.* (1994) examining spinal arteries arising below the bifurcation of the aorta pointed out that the arteries to the intervertebral foramina L4–L5 and L5–S1, are not related to the dorsolateral zones of the discs where lateral surgical approaches are best accomplished and are to that extent safe. They also point out that the posterior division of the internal iliac artery is often the source of the spinal arteries for L4, L5 and all the sacral foramina. Interruption of blood flow in the internal iliac during pelvic surgery might explain the occurrence of spinal chord ischaemia in these circumstances.

Blood vessels of the spinal cord

Because of the surgical intimacy of the vertebral column and the spinal cord, a brief account of the vascularization of the spinal cord is necessary. *Anterior and posterior spinal arteries* branch off from the vertebral arteries in the cranium, and pass down through the foramen magnum into the spinal canal. The anterior spinals fuse and form a median longitudinal vessel, the anterior spinal artery, passing down the length of the cord in the anterior median sulcus. The anterior spinal artery (the artery and its branches) was noted in 78% of thoracolumbar myelograms, and it was possible to identify the anterior spinal system visible over several segments (Sartor 1978).

The two posterior spinal branches of the vertebral arteries do not fuse, but form similar longitudinal vessels related to the dorsal roots of the spinal nerves. The same *segmental spinal arteries* which supply the vertebral column, and derived from the cervical vertebral, deep cervical, intercostal and lumbar arteries, reinforce the longitudinal arterial columns, and also supply the cord directly. Segmentally, a radicular artery enters the spinal nerve in the intervertebral foramen and divides into posterior and anterior radicular branches in the nerve roots. The posterior branch also supplies the dorsal root ganglion and on each side helps to form twin posterior spinal arteries running above and below the origin of the dorsal nerve roots (Fig. 5.7).

The anterior spinal artery supplies the ventral grey column and also the base of the dorsal grey column and adjacent white matter. Its central branches supply about two-thirds of the cross-sectional area of the cord. The rest of the dorsal grey and white columns, and peripheral parts of the lateral and ventral white columns, are supplied from the posterior spinal arteries and the arterial plexus built up in the pial membrane (Fig. 5.7).

Venous drainage of the cord is by means of six longitudinal veins. One is in front of the anterior spinal artery in its anterior median sulcus; another is posterior to the posterior median septum; and a venous channel accompanies the anterior and posterior nerve roots. The six longitudinal venous plexuses communicate with the longitudinal intrinsic venous plexuses of the vertebral column, which drain through segmental veins corresponding to the spinal arteries (Figs 5.7, 5.8).

Vertebral venous plexuses

Several extraordinarily capacious venous anastomotic chains are found in association with the vertebral column. The *extrinsic veins* lie *anterolateral* to the vertebral bodies and postlaminar with respect to the neural arches. This group receives numerous veins from the external surfaces of the vertebral body and from the processes of the vertebral arch. Two *intrinsic chains* lie extradurally behind the bodies. They drain in particular the large basivertebral veins which issue, on each side of the posterior longitudinal ligament, from the corresponding foramina.

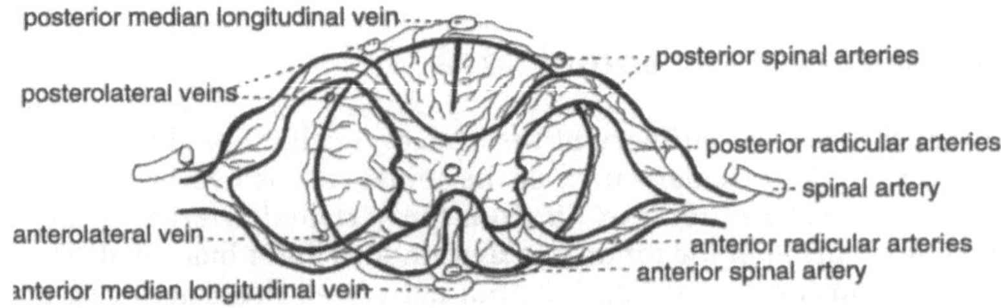

Fig. 5.7. (*see also Colour Plate section*) Plan of the spinal cord and its intrinsic blood vessels, united by longitudinal arterial and venous columns. (Based on Gray 1989.)

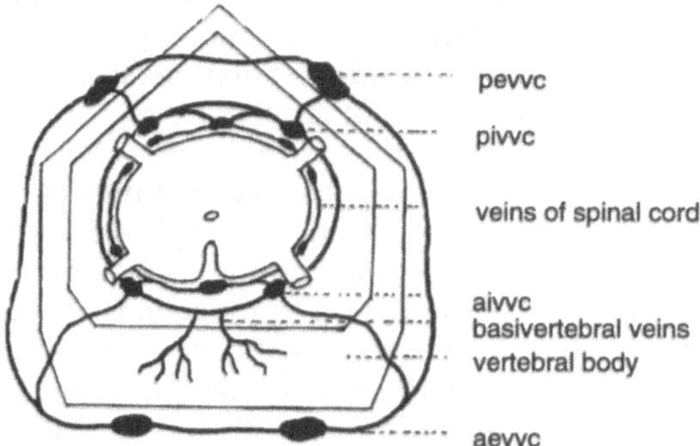

Fig. 5.8. (*see also Colour Plate section*) Plan of the three great venous circles around each vertebra and the spinal cord, showing **pevvc** and **pivvc**, posterior external and internal vertebral venous columns; **aevvc** and **aivvc**, corresponding anterior columns;and the innermost venous circles of the spinal cord and their longitudinal anastomoses. The caval, azygos, abdominal and pelvic venous systems communicate with the vertebral veins.

These *ventral longitudinal venous anastomoses* are freely connected with other intrinsic *dorsal longitudinal venous plexuses* posterior to the spinal theca, providing an additional drainage route for the laminae and spines (Fig. 5.8).

The intra-osseous venous vascular pattern of vertebral bodies does not differ fundamentally from the arrangement of metaphyseal veins in cancellous tissue elsewhere. The richness of the venous net converging on to the basivertebral veins is matched by a similar profusion of dilated sinuses in the extremities of long bones. On the other hand, the profusion of veins in and around the vertebral column is distinctive, and their connection with intracranial venous sinuses and the posterior body wall has been remarked on by several authors (Batson 1940; Anderson 1951; Bowsher 1954).

Batson, using radiographic methods, emphasized the free communication between the *prostatic venous plexus* and the vertebral venous plexuses, and suggested that here lay the route for *spinal* and *intracranial metastasis* of prostatic carcinoma. Such a blood route is retrograde with respect to the veins of the bone in which the metastasis lodges. Breschet (1829) held that there were no valves in the internal vertebral venous plexuses, nor in the *azygos system* of veins with which they communicate (Vesalius 1555), except for an incompetent valve in the arch of the vena azygos major.

The direction of blood flow in these veins, according to Breschet, is not constant. It is probable that there are normal fluctuations in vertebral venous flow varying with posture and with variations in the circulation elsewhere. Konerding & Blank (1987), investigating the blood supply of the vertebral column in rats, have identified blood flow regulating sphincters which can be identified in all parts of the arterial and venous systems of the column. If applicable to man this fact seems to be of great importance with respect to degenerative and possibly regenerative processes in intervertebral discs and synovial articular joints.

Suzuki *et al.* (1991, 1992) have examined the connections between prostatic vessels and the vertebral venous system in dogs. They find that prostatic veins drain in part into the posterior vena cava of the dog, but also into the vertebral venous system. The latter has direct connections with the posterior vena cava, and freely anastomoses with the common iliac, internal iliac and internal pudendal veins. Gowin (1983) points out the anatomy of the venous connections of the kidney, lung, mammary gland, genitals and thyroid with the vertebral veins, which would account for the spread of spinal metastases from these sites. Aubin *et al.* (1976) have also pointed out other major connections with the vertebral venous system, especially in what they term the prespinal system, i.e. vertebral, right superior intercostal, hemi-azygos, azygos (and its arch), ascending lumbar and lumbar veins, all of which can be explored by catheterization. Multiple impediments in the afferent connections can change intraspinal flow direction, or result in venous stasis in the vertebral venous plexuses. Major *et al.* (1980) point out that vertebral heterotopic ossification complicating paraplegia and other neurological disorders, is remarkably similar to the pattern of metastases in the vertebral venous system of Batson. Stasis consequent to immobilization, combined with skeletal demineralization, are postulated as main factors which promote the precipitation of calcium salts in the musculo-tendinous tissues around the vertebral column.

The fluctuating nature of venous flow may not be peculiar to vertebrae alone among the bones of the skeleton, because there are experimental grounds for believing that retrograde venous flow is a possibility in the veins of cancellous tissue in the limb bones (Vanderhoeft *et al.* 1963; Brookes 1966). These observations, taken with the profuse arterial supply to vertebrae and their capacious venous drainage, suggest that the oxygen tension of the blood in vertebrae is relatively high, which presumably is linked to the *haemopoietic function* of the vertebral marrow and the trabecular character of the bone in the vertebral bodies.

Barnett *et al.* (1958) in particular have emphasized the diversion in diving animals of inferior vena caval blood into the vertebral venous networks during submersion. According to these workers, the great blood-holding capacity of the *vertebral venous plexuses* is normally exploited for maximum oxygen utilization in Pinnipedia and Cetacea, permitting them to remain under water for unusually long periods (30 minutes). Burger & Estavillo (1977) in chickens have emphasized venous connections in the lungs with the vertebral venous system, and intercostal, inferior mesenteric and splenic veins. Hence, pulmonary and vertebral blood volumes are in communication regulated by pressure gradients and sphincters.

It is particularly striking that adjacent bones of the vertebral column are united by large extra-osseous veins in the spinal canal which are in continuity with the spinal veins. Because the veins unite one vertebra with its neighbours, extensive regions of the column can be regarded from the vascular standpoint as a unit. It is also probable that venous drainage of the vertebral column is promoted by the pumping action of the muscles which have such extensive attachments, particularly to the neural arch and its processes. It is noteworthy that *rheumatoid* and *ankylosing spondylitis* affect not isolated parts but considerable lengths of the vertebral column. It seems likely that venous impediment is a factor in the progress of these disorders, because the beneficial effects of physical medicine in their treatment can be attributed in no small measure to the promotion of venous drainage from the vertebral column.

Wardle (1964) and Helal (1965) demonstrated radiographically in cases of *osteoarthritis* of the knee that venous congestion of the cancellous bone is present. They suggested that the beneficial effects of *osteotomy* in the surgical treatment of osteoarthritis, particularly the relief of pain when severe deformity has developed in the joint, seems to be due to surgical decompression of the veins of cancellous bone. As is well known, osteoarthritis of the spine affects not one but many joints, possibly because of the diffuse venous drainage of the vertebral column which takes in many joints in one vascular territory. It is this anatomical, venous factor which gives osteoarthritis of the spine its generalized distribution, as distinct from that of the appendicular skeleton, where it is common for large joints to be singly attacked by the disease process.

Chapter 6

Blood supply of irregular bones – 2: Carpal and tarsal bones

The nutrient vessels of the carpus and tarsus may be likened to the epiphyseal nutrients of tubular bones. These small masses of cancellous bone are covered with articular cartilages and limited areas of thin compact bone largely taken up by ligamentous attachments. Like long bone epiphyses, they are supplied by a number of small vessels rather than by a single major nutrient, the nutrient veins outnumbering the arterial vessels. For the talus and calcaneum, the sinus tarsi is an important site for the entry and exit of nutrient vessels (Haliburton *et al.* 1958; Montis & Ridola 1959a,b; Crock 1967). In their intra-osseous course, the arteries and venous sinuses radiate towards the articular surface where typical *articular vascular plexuses* are formed. When a growth cartilage is present in the calcaneum, typical subchondral circulations are found on each side of it, indistin-

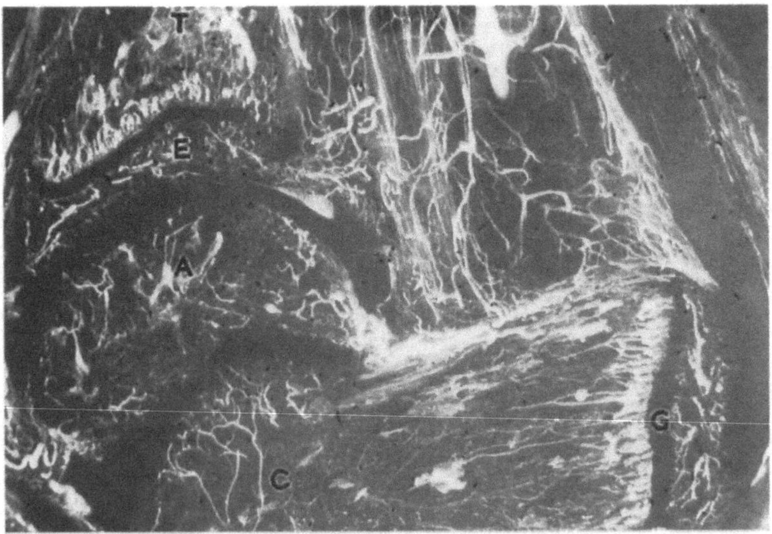

Fig. 6.1. Arteriograph of rat ankle joint and heel, showing lower tibia (T) and its epiphysis (E), the body of the talus (A), and the calcaneum (C). Note the contrasting metaphyseal and epiphyseal patterns associated with the growth cartilage (G) of the calcaneum. Vascular patterns in tarsals and carpals are usually epiphyseal in type. (Original magnification ×14)

guishable from those associated with the growth cartilages of long bones (Fig. 6.1). The predominantly venous character of the vessels in human tarsal bones has been noted by Vsevolodov (1959) and by Haliburton *et al.* (1958) in studies of preparations perfused with India ink, allowing the venous side of the circulation to be appreciated. In particular, these workers have shown innumerable capillaries and venules traversing the junctional region comprising the periosteum, cortex and cancellous bone in non-articular areas of the calcaneum and other tarsal bones.

Carpals and tarsals, like the vertebrae, are subject to juvenile osteochondrosis, as in:

- apophysitis of the calcaneum (epiphyseal ischaemic necrosis)
- the lunate bone (Kienböck's disease, 1910)
- the navicular bone (Köhler's tarsal scaphoiditis, 1908).

All of these and Scheuermann's disease of vertebral epiphyses, are forms of avascular necrosis, but with specific aetiologies. A knowledge of the blood supply of these irregular bones is important both for diagnosis and particularly in the treatment of their fractures and other disorders. A detailed account of the carpus and individual carpal bones is presented here.

Vessels of the carpus

There is considerable diversity of opinion as to the pattern of vascularization of the bones of the wrist, possibly because of genetic, racial and extrinsic factors which cannot be detected in analyses of small groups of individuals. In addition, arteriography and digital angiography, the conventional methods of examining the carpus, are unable to eliminate the effects of superimposition of views in this highly mobile region; dissections are difficult and are likely to produce significant artefact. Three-dimensional reconstructions of the carpus have only lately become possible (Oberlin *et al.* 1992). Compare the following accounts given by Mestdagh *et al.* (1979), Gelberman *et al.* 1983) and Panagis *et al.* (1983).

In examination of more than 50 specimens injected intra-arterially with coloured dyes followed by dissection, Mestdagh *et al.* (1979) described two different patterns of arterialization of the carpal bones. The outer scaphoid, trapezium, trapezoid, capitate and lunate were supplied from the radial and dorsal and palmar interosseous arteries. The inner bones triquetral, hamate and pisiform are primarily supplied by palmar branches derived almost exclusively from the ulnar artery. The posterior carpal arch was derived from the dorsal carpal branch of the radial artery, which crosses the carpus transversely and is joined in 50% of cases by the posterior interosseous artery. A contribution to the posterior carpal arch from the ulnar artery was restricted to 25% of cases. The dorsal arch lay on the distal row of carpals and gave off short branches running proximally to enter the posterior aspects of the proximal row of carpal bones. The carpals of the distal row received several short twigs penetrating their dorsal surfaces. In particular, the dorsal carpal arteries were smaller but more numerous than the palmar vessels.

In contrast, Gelberman *et al.* (1983) have a triple approach to carpal vascularization. They found the carpal bones were supplied from an anastomotic network of three dorsal and three palmar arches, connected at their medial and lateral borders by the radial and ulnar arteries, and also by dorsal and palmar branches of the anterior interosseous artery. Two recurrent arteries, radial and ulnar, consistently arose from the concavity of the deep palmar arch, and frequently anastomosed with the terminal branches of the anterior division of the anterior interosseous artery, which in the authors' view provided the major collateral circulation about the wrist. The same authors (Panagis *et al.* 1983) went on to divide the carpal bones in the above material into three groups based on size and location of nutrient vessels, and dependence of large bony masses on single intraosseous vessels. Group I comprised scaphoid, capitate and 20% of the lunates; each had large areas of bone dependent on a single vessel and was considered at risk to develop avascular necrosis following fracture. Group II included the trapezoid and hamate, both of which have two areas of vascular entry but lack intraosseous anastomoses. Group III comprised the trapezium, triquetrum, pisiform and 80% of the lunates; these had more than one non-articular surface, consistent intra-osseous anastomoses and a lack of large areas dependent on a single vessel. Groups II and III were not at risk of avascular necrosis.

Gelberman & Gross (1986) in their extra- and intra-osseous studies of carpal vascularity (75 specimens) have modified the findings of Panagis *et al.* (1983) in that they found only 8% of the lunates in Group I were dependent on a single vessel, and 92% of the lunates were better placed in Group III. The latter as well as Group I were at risk of avascular necrosis, but unlike Group I (and including the talus in the foot) required severe vascular injury to succumb to avascular necrosis.

Vessels of individual carpal bones

Hamate

Avascular necrosis of the hamate is a rarity. The distal part of the bone, its base, is well supplied by palmar and dorsal nutrients. Its proximal part is wedge shaped and largely enclosed by the cavity of the mid-carpal joint and on account of that is totally dependent on the basal vasculature, i.e. the wedge is dependent on an intra-osseous nutrition (van Demark & Parke 1992). Fracture separating the base from the wedge can therefore bring about avascular necrosis of the wedge of this unciform bone. The hook of the hamate however is often broken. Its blood supply is from two sites: the radial base of the hook has large foramina for nutrient vessels; the tip of the hook has small foramina which may be absent in 30% of specimens. Hence, fracture at the base of the hamate process can compromise its blood supply and hinder the healing process (Failla 1993).

Capitate

Isolated capitate fractures resulting in avascular necrosis of its proximal pole are uncommon. Palmar vessels and some dorsal nutrients enter the distal part of the capitate and cross its waist to supply the proximal pole, in much the same way as the blood supply of the scaphoid. Fracture through the waist may result in polar necrosis of the capitate (Vander Grend *et al.* 1994).

Pisiform

Vascular foramina are situated on its lateral border in the proximal half of the ridge occupied by the ulnar artery. Others are found on the medial border and the distal tip of the bone. In 34 injected specimens the pisiform nutrients were traced from the ulnar artery and its dorsal carpal and deep palmar branches. The pisiform nutrients anastomose and form an intra-osseous arterial circle in the bone (Mestagh *et al.* 1984). This is reminiscent of a similar arterial circle found in the much larger sesamoid bone, *the patella*. From the intra-osseous patellar ring arise radial branches which support the cancellous tissue and articular cartilage (Bridgeman & Brookes 1990). The dorsal carpal artery is the main vascular pedicle of the pisiform and can be used for pisiform replacement of the lunate.

Triquetrum

This pyramidal bone is supplied in its medial and dorsal aspects by twigs derived from the dorsal branch of the ulnar artery. They are intimately associated with the main vascular pedicle of the pisiform, and much vascular variation is common in this site (Kuhlmann *et al.* 1982).

Lunate

Gelberman *et al.* (1980) have studied the vascularization of the lunate, using specimens injected with latex and cleared by the Spalteholz method. Extra-osseous vascularity derived from dorsal and palmar vessels, three or four of each, which fed into dorsal and palmar plexuses. One or two nutrient vessels entered both dorsal and palmar poles of the bone, anastomosed and supplied the cancellous trabeculae and articular cartilages. Trabecular bone fracture from repeated compression was held to be a cause of Kienbock's disease. On the other hand, Koken (1975) believed that when the wrist is extended the dorsal vessels to the lunate are caught as in a vice between the radius and the capitate bones. Vascular compression up to complete occlusion may be brought about. For Koken, vascular compression rather than bone compression is the cause of Kienbock's avascular necrosis.

Carpal scaphoid

The carpal scaphoid has often been investigated with respect to its blood supply, because of the frequent occurrence of fracture, its susceptibility to malunion and, unusually, to avascular necrosis during treatment. Obletz and Halbstein (1938), utilizing a radiographic and vascular perfusion technique, pointed out that there is considerable variation in the site of the nutrient foramina in the dorsal non-articular area which corresponds to the waist of this bone. Their results have been confirmed by direct examination of the nutrient foramina in macerated and dried specimens by Watson-Jones (1952). Usually the foramina are distributed fairly evenly on the waist proximodistally, but in about one-third of cases they tend to be aggregated on and near the tubercle of the scaphoid. The proximal pole of the scaphoid is then dependent for its nutrition on vessels traversing the waist. Hence, fractures through the waist can interfere with the blood supply of the proximal fragment. On the other hand, the rapid union of fractures through the tubercle can be correlated with the constant retention by this fragment of a nutrient blood supply of its own.

The above account of the blood supply of the scaphoid has been repeatedly confirmed, e.g. by Oehmke (1987). He describes carpal vascular plexuses, dorsal and palmar, which supply numerous stems passing through the dorsal and palmar radiocarpal ligaments. In two out of three cases in his experience the scaphoid is uniformly vascularized so that after fracture both fragments retain their blood supply. But in a third of all cases only one end of the scaphoid has an arterial input, and it is the poorly vascularized fragment that frequently becomes necrotic. The same account applies to the progressively ossifying scaphoid of the child. Diagnosis of scaphoid fracture may be difficult when it occurs through the osteochondral interface. Non-union and ischaemic necrosis of the proximal pole may occur in children as in adults (Larson *et al.* 1987). Fracture of the tuberosity of the scaphoid is common and usually without incident, because of its rich blood supply (Mody *et al.* 1993). Occasionally, non-union occurs in this situation if sufficient violence has been exercised and crushed the nutrient vessels.

Gelberman & Menon (1980) find that the major blood supply to the scaphoid is from the radial artery. Branches from the radial artery enter the bone through foramina in the dorsal ridge, and supply up to 80% of the intra-osseous vessels and the entire proximal pole. The rest of the bone in the region of the distal tuberosity receives blood from branches of the radial artery in the palm. The anterior interosseous artery provides an efficient collateral circulation to the scaphoid through its dorsal and palmar branches (see Oehmke 1987). Two extracapsular vascular pedicles are constant (Kuhlmann & Guérin-Surville 1981); a lateral pedicle in the anatomical snuff-box, and an anterior pedicle arising in the area of the radial pulse which passes behind the flexor carpi radialis.

Handley & Pooley (1991) have used injected coloured latex to add an extra detail to scaphoid vascular anatomy. They find that the venous drainage of the scaphoid is through the dorsal ridge of the bone emptying into the venae comitantes of the radial artery.

Radio-ulnar articular disc

This triangular articular cartilage arises from the inferior radial notch and is inserted into the styloid process of the ulna. Peripherally, the cartilage contains longitudinal collagen bundles where it is subject to tensile stresses. The central part of the disc is made up of a basket work of oblique collagen fibres where multidirectional stresses occur. The radial origin of the disc is reinforced by horizontal collagen bundles penetrating the cartilage for 2 mm (Chidgey 1991).

Bednar *et al.* (1991) in their account of the blood supply of the articular disc in 10 cadaver specimens, describe small vessels penetrating the fibrocartilage in a radial fashion from the palmar, ulnar and dorsal attachments of the joint capsule. The vessels supply from 10 to 40% of the cartilage periphery. The central area right up to the radial attachment is avascular. Tears at the radial attachment or centrally, for want of a blood supply, are unlikely to heal without surgical assistance. Similar findings have been reported by Mikic (1992) in 24 dogs. Vascular penetration of the disc is extensive in puppies, but in adults it ranges from 15 to 25% of the discal width. The source of the blood supply is given by Mikic as from the palmar and dorsal branches of the anterior interosseous artery.

Chapter 7
Blood supply of flat bones

Bones of the skull

These may consist of only a thin lamella of hard tissue, as in the case of the *nasal conchae* covered with a mucous membrane. India ink perfusion shows that the bony plates in these instances get their blood supply from the overlying periosteal vessels. The two periosteal vascular plexuses, sandwiching a bony conchal lamina, are only infrequently joined together by solitary perforating capillaries. Usually, flat bony laminae, however thin, consist of two bony plates with an interposed medullary layer, as for example, the perpendicular plate of the ethmoid and the vomer in the *nasal septum* (Fig. 7.1). Their vascularization is analogous to that of the much thicker flat bones of the cranial vault.

Membrane bones

Development of the calvaria

In the human embryo,the calvaria is represented by a bladder-like *brain capsule* suffused with a rich capillary plexus. At the end of the embryonic period (8th week), several islands of ossification appear in the vascular membrane encapsulating the growing brain. A cartilage precursor is not present; the bones of the calvaria are examples of *intramembranous ossification*. The membrane bones (Nesbitt 1736) of the cranial vault are at first without cortical tables or diploë, but are made up of a few trabecular plates stacked together in an imbricated way. One or two *nutrient arteries* derived from the dural vessels then penetrate the bones in their inner aspect at the sites where ossification first appeared. Branches of these nutrient arteries have been observed in radiographic preparations to radiate peripherally in the fetal period from the ossification centres towards the sutural boundaries of the frontal, parietal and occipital bones (Fig. 7.2). Examination of the skull vault also shows a fine guttering of both inner and outer surfaces which is incised in the bones of the vault in a radial pattern. The guttering and the slit-like openings of vascular canals in the floor of the furrows indicate that the trabeculae of a fetal cranial bone and the intervening vessels are obliquely arranged with respect to the tangential plane.

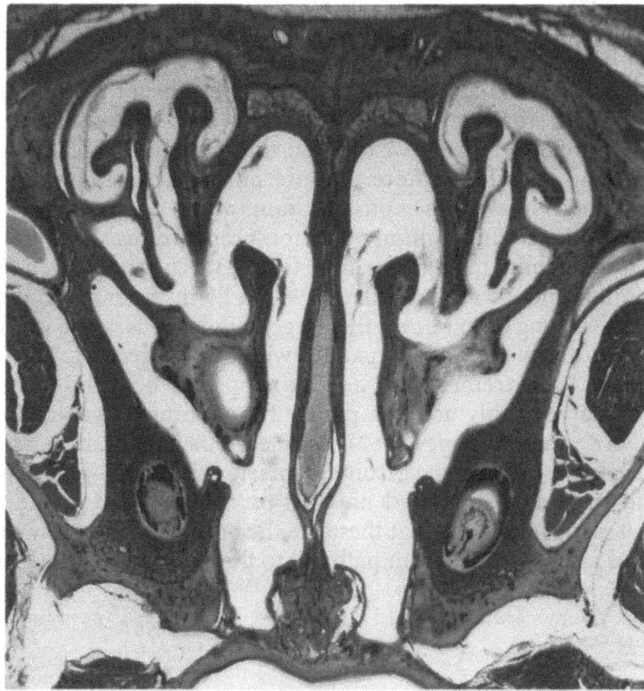

Fig. 7.1. Frontal section through the head of a mouse, to show two bony plates in the nasal septum and thin laminae in the nasal conchae. (Original magnification ×15)

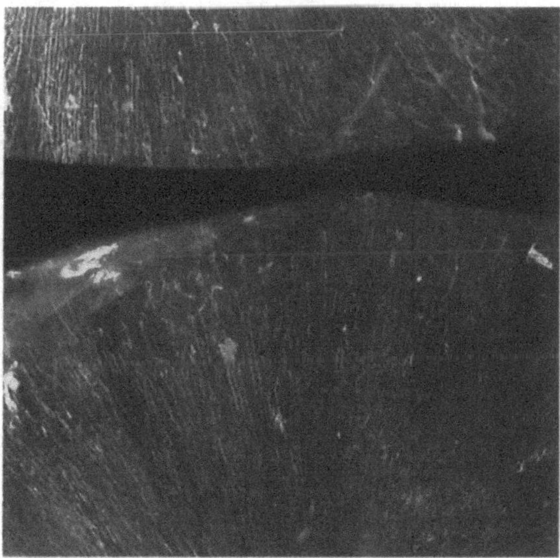

Fig. 7.2. The two parietals of a fetal skull, perfused with Thorotrast, have been cut apart through the sagittal sutural membrane and laid flat on an X-ray plate. The vascular radiations between the imbricated trabeculae making up the bones are shown. (Original magnification ×5)

Veins of the calvaria

Breschet (1829) thought that all the vessels in the fetal calvaria were veins, but Langer (1877), in a meticulous study of the blood vessels of the skull vault and the dura mater, demonstrated that an arterial as well as a venous network was present in the cranial bones. He also noted that characteristically, fine arteries joined large venous radicles without the interposition of capillaries; that is, the fetal calvaria was rich in *arteriovenous anastomoses.*

In the diploë of the adult cranium, perfusion preparations show that the diploic venous sinuses are highly irregular in calibre (Fig. 7.3). They are united to the vessels of the pericranium and dura by capillaries which lie in the inner and outer tables (Figs 7.3, 7.4). It has long been known that large diploic sinuses, the *veins of Breschet* (Breschet 1829), lie fairly close to and parallel with the sutures (Fig. 7.5). The walls of the diploic sinuses are extremely thin, and are supported here and there by fine trabeculae which may possibly act as a poorly functioning valvular mechanism to promote venous drainage (Sappey 1867). They leave the outer table of the skull vault in a few named diploic foramina (frontal, anterior temporal, posterior temporal, occipital); and in several unnamed nutrient foramina found in the inner table. Nevertheless, it is most unlikely that these are the only efferent pathways or that the nutrient arteries are the sole afferent pathway to the flat bones of the cranium.

Sutural vessels

Near the sutural borders, where both dura and pericranium are firmly attached, there are innumerable fine foramina containing arteries and veins. These *juxta-*

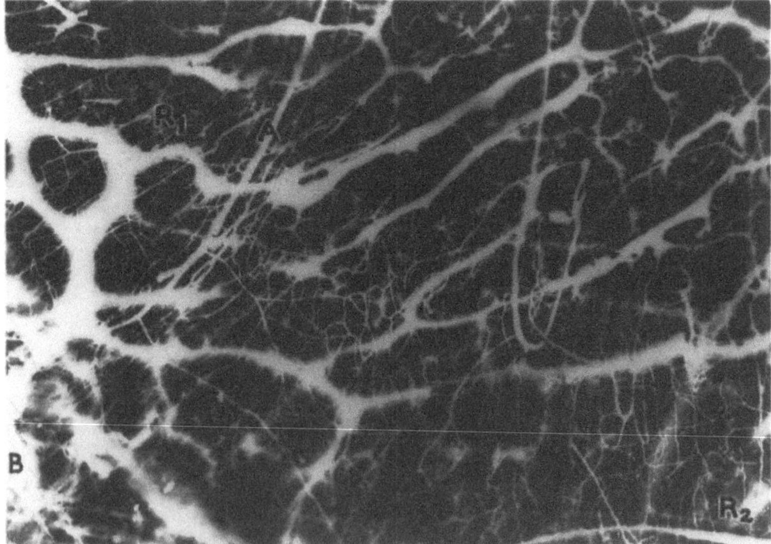

Fig. 7.3. India ink preparation of a cleaned parietal bone of a young monkey, showing the Breschet veins (B) draining diploic venous sinuses. Diploic arteries (A) are visible, as well as a fine vascular radiation in the inner and outer tables. Note the change in orientation of these tabular vessels between R1 and R2. (Original magnification ×9)

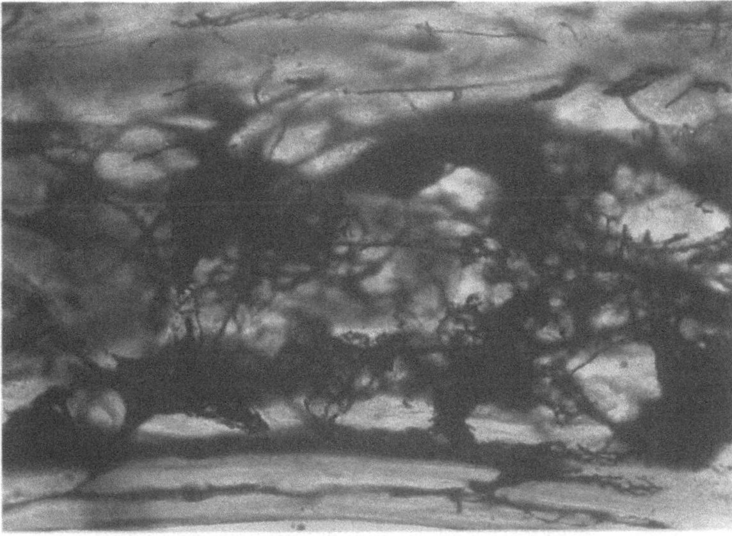

Fig. 7.4. India ink preparation of an incised monkey parietal bone, showing diploic vessels sandwiched between the inner and outer tables. (Original magnification ×28)

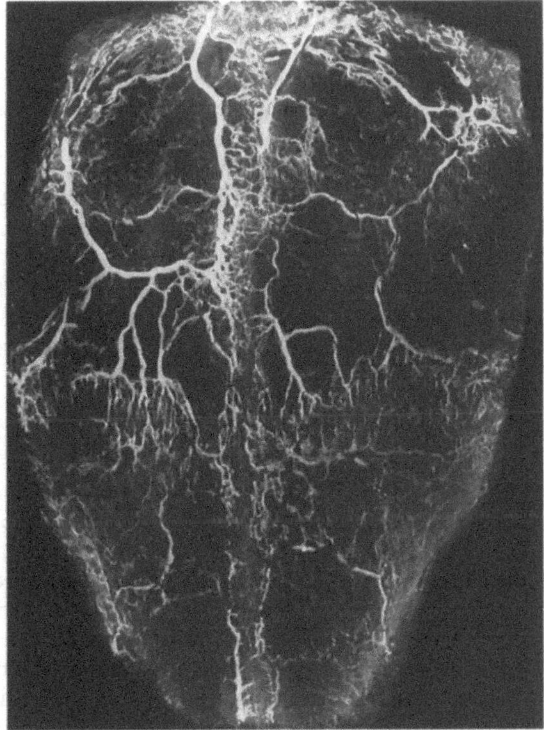

Fig. 7.5. Venogram of the vault of a rat's skull, showing the Breschet veins and their trans-sutural connections. (Original magnification ×4)

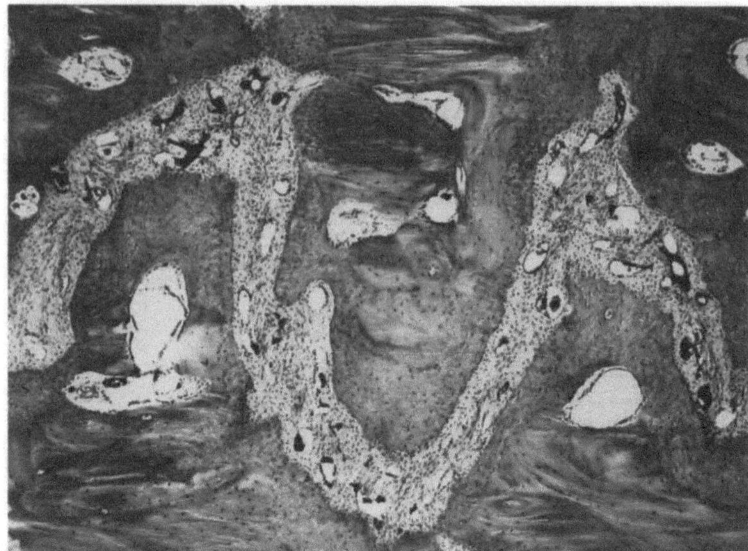

Fig. 7.6. Tangential histological section through the parietofrontal suture of a rat injected with India ink. The fibrous tissue in the suture is highly vascular. (Original magnification ×81)

sutural vessels, like long bone metaphyseal vessels, are important for the growth in surface area of individual flat bones. Moreover, the sutural fibrous tissue is unusually well provided with sutural veins (Fig. 7.6). In the serrated edges of the bones there are numerous holes for the passage of veins which unite the Breschet veins of one bone with those of its neighbours, trans-suturally. The sutures also unite the vessels of the dura with those of the pericranium.

After closure of the sutures (from within outwards) in middle-aged individuals, it is to be noted that although the skull vault may appear to be smooth, it is nevertheless covered with tiny foramina observable with a hand lens. The capillaries lodged in these foramina (Fig. 7.4) unite diploic with pericranial capillaries. Similarly, fine vessels pass through the inner table and join diploic to dural vessels.

Dural blood vessels

The dura is often said to consist of two layers, but it is most doubtful whether their existence can be demonstrated even by histological methods. Langer (1877), however, described two distinct vascular networks in the dural membrane. The *inner vascular plexus*, consisting of arteries, veins and an intervening capillary network, he held to be the primary dural plexus. Its arteries are derivatives of the intracranial *meningeal vessels*, and the veins freely communicate with venous plexuses in the *outer vascular plexus* of the dura, where the meningeal arteries ramify. Perfusion of the middle meningeal artery results in filling all the dural vessels and even the ophthalmic and carotid arteries. The meningeal veins in the outer dural layer join the large intracranial venous sinuses. Langer placed heavy emphasis on the fact that the finest arteries in the outer layer normally enter venous radicles directly; in effect, the dural outer vascular plexus consists of a fine arterial network, freely anastomosing veins, and abundant arteriovenous anastomoses.

Meningeal arteries

The cranial meningeal arteries indeed supply the dura and leptomeninges and are abundant in the anterior, middle and posterior cranial fossae where they freely anastomose. They include the ophthalmic, internal and external cerebral, middle meningeal and vertebral arteries to name only the more familiar. But the name is largely a misnomer in the skull, because here the meningeal vessels mainly supply the bony cranium, and not the meninges of the brain. In the vertebral column, the meningeal vessels largely supply the spinal cord and its meninges as well as giving nutrients to the vertebral column.

Michel (1872), on the basis of perfusion studies carried out on dogs, held that the outer dural plexus was entirely venous in accord with Breschet's view of the vascularization of the fetal skull. This concept seems to have influenced neurosurgical opinion until quite recently. Rowbotham and Little (1962), working on the brain–scalp circulation, failed to mention an artery at all either in their description or their diagram of this region. The same authors (1965), however, later revived and confirmed Langer's account of the vascularization of the dura mater, complete with emphasis placed on the arteriovenous anastomoses in the outer dural layer. Nevertheless, the author (M.B.) has been unable to detect two vascular layers in the perfused dural membrane of the adult monkey. A single plexus is present consisting of arteries and their venae comitantes, united by numerous arteriovenous anastomoses and somewhat incompletely developed capillary beds (Fig. 7.7, *overleaf*).

The pericranial vascular plexus, on the other hand, is somewhat exiguous. Perfusion preparations in monkeys and other animals do show that it is comparable to the vascular plexus in the periosteum of a long bone. It is connected by means of arteries and veins passing through the juxtasutural foramina with the internal vasculature of the cranial bones. In addition, as pointed out above, the capillaries in the outer table also intervene between the diploic veins and those of the pericranial membrane.

Blood supply of cranial flat bones

In review of the available evidence it would seem that nutrient arteries piercing the inner table, and others entering the outer table close to its sutural borders, comprise the afferent pathway to the diploic sinusoids of a cranial flat bone. Venous drainage takes place through nutrient and diploic veins; veins leaving the juxtasutural foramina; and capillaries leaving the inner and outer surfaces of the bone generally. There is free and extensive communication between dural meningeal veins, the veins of the skull vault and those of the pericranium.

The question arises as to which aspect, dural or pericranial, is normally the more important for the blood supply to the cranium. No firm answer can be given as yet. Humphry (1858) thought that the arterial supply came largely from the dural meningeal vessels, while Langer (1877) gave in his account equal

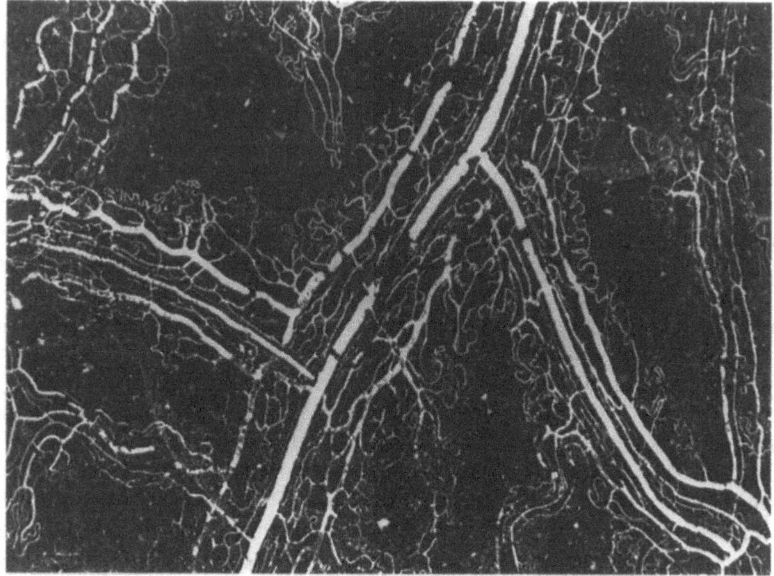

Fig. 7.7. The dural membrane of a monkey, perfused with India ink. Numerous arteriovenous anastomoses are present. Avascular areas are bordered by capillary loops. (Original magnification ×8.5)

prominence to dural and pericranial afferent routes. Nevertheless, the fact that bone survives in an osteoplastic flap, when it is nourished solely through existing vascular connections between the outer table and pericranium, indicates that the pericranial arteries are a sufficient afferent pathway for bone survival, and that the capillaries of the outer table generally, and the juxtasutural veins in particular, constitute an adequate pathway for venous drainage.

Flat bones developing in cartilage

Pectoral girdle

This ancient supporting mechanism of the forelimb was once represented by three bony elements: a flat dorsal element and two ventral elements represented by coracoid and precoracoid bars of bone. The three elements met centrally to form a joint cavity articulating with the humerus. In humans, only the dorsal and one ventral element are represented by the scapula.

Development

According to Frazer (1940) the scapula is present in mesenchyme in the 5th week, undergoing chondrification in the 7th week, and ossifying in the lateral border of the blade of the bone (8th week). At birth, this primary centre of ossification representing the dorsal moiety has spread to form most of the bony scapula, but not the peripheral acromion, coracoid process, vertebral border, lower angle and glenoid fossa which are all still cartilaginous. A second primary centre of ossification (an ancestral ventral element of the pectoral girdle) appears in the 1st year, and accounts for the ossification of the upper one-fifth of the glenoid fossa and the adjoining base of the descriptive coracoid process. Additional peripheral centres appear from 10 to 14 years (including the rest of the glenoid fossa) which all coalesce from 18 to 21 years.

Vessels of the scapula

The blood supply of the scapula is by means of a primary nutrient branch of the *subscapular artery*. It pierces the lateral pillar of bone in the subscapular fossa (or the "infrascapular" fossa (Crock 1996) or the infraspinous fossa (Lexer *et al.* 1904)). From Crock's cleared specimens of the scapula in a child aged 8 weeks and a boy aged 11 years, the artery divides into upper and lower branches repeatedly forming extended biconical vascular areas irrigating much of the bone. Another primary nutrient artery is present, a branch of the *suprascapular artery* in the supraspinous fossa. Here, it pierces the base of the scapular spine at its medial third and then divides into medial and lateral vascular cones supplying the scapular spine. Peripherally, the borders and angles of the bone are supplied by periosteal arteries. The scapular coracoid, spine and acromion are also well marked with foramina, some of which are presumably vascular. Sections of India ink preparations of these bones also show that the two tables of compact bone are irrigated by capillaries, uniting the intra-osseous sinusoids with periosteal capillaries.

Pelvic girdle

The three primary elements articulating with the hind limb are fully represented in the pelvic girdle; a dorsal element or ilium; and two ventral elements,the ischium and pubis. The three elements comprise the hip bone, and meet centrally to form the acetabulum, which with the head of the femur are encapsulated in a synovial joint, the hip joint.

Development

The hip bone begins as a mesenchymal mass at the base of the hind limb bud (5th week), relates to the blastemal lumbosacral vertebrae (6th week) and chondrifies (7th week) from three primary centres corresponding to its fundamental parts. By central fusion of the three elemental bars a shallow acetabulum is already in place at the end of the 7th week and two plates of condensed mesenchyme unite the cartilaginous hip bones ventrally. Three primary centres of ossification are initiated near to the acetabulum; the first for the ilium (8th week), another in the ischium (late 3rd month) and a third primary centre in the pubis (4th month). At birth, each bone is represented in the otherwise cartilaginous acetabulum, as are also the iliac crest, greater sciatic notch, iliopectineal eminence, ischiopubic ramus and the symphyseal region.

Ossification spreads slowly in the peripheral cartilage, the ischium ossifying with the pubis in the lower ramus in the 8th year, followed by centres in the triradiate cartilage in the acetabular floor. The acetabulum is consolidated by puberty, but peripherally areas of cartilage persist. Secondary centres of ossification then appear from 15 years in at least seven listed sites during adolescence, with the iliac crest and ischial tuberosity being the last to show separate epiphyses. Fusion is not complete until after 25 years.

Vessels of the hip bone

The *iliolumbar artery* gives off a principal nutrient artery which enters the iliac fossa postero-inferiorly. A principal nutrient artery also enters the ischium from the *medial circumflex femoral*, and another for the pubis, possibly from the *obturator artery*. In the three elements of the hip bone in a 10-day-old boy the nutrient artery divides and ramifies into an extensive "double fan-like distribution of fine arteries which terminate in capillary networks of metaphyseal type around the edges" (Crock 1996). The pattern of distribution of these fan-like vessels in the flat ilium, biconical vessels in the ischium and pubis, is unmistakeably identical to the pattern of vascularization in the shaft of long bones. With increasing age the outer areas of the hip bone are clearly supplied from the periosteal vascular network, reinforced by branches of the *superior and inferior gluteal arteries*, and *superficial and deep circumflex femoral vessels*. The perfused hip bone of a 17-year-old girl (Crock 1996) clearly shows the major dependence of the bone on the *periosteal vessels* which perforate the cortical surfaces everywhere, and ramify in the bone marrow. Numerous foramina close to the acetabulum, iliac crest, and the spines and processes of the hip bone suggest the presence of an additional supply of small perforating arteries through these areas as well as an important venous drainage route.

Acetabulum

Fischer *et al.* (1977) emphasized the presence of many anastomoses above the acetabular area. Katthagen *et al.* (1995) examined 30 human hips, 16 with barium sulphate perfusion, and 11 with a solution of resin and lead powder; three more were excluded on account of extravasation (a rare confession). They found the central parts of the acetabulum were vascularized by the *obturator artery*, the craniolateral part by the *superior gluteal*, and the ischial part by the *inferior gluteal artery*. In 53 fetal acetabula studied by Damsin *et al.* (1992), it was found that the acetabular branch of the obturator artery is distributed to the cartilage-free acetabular fossa and the triradiate cartilage, and ends in the three primary bone components. The superior and inferior gluteal arteries, internal pudendal and obturator arteries all form a peri-acetabular vascular circle. It is clear that acetabular vascularity is abundant, and massive necrosis is unlikely in the child if there is a need for triple osteotomy of the pelvis. Kirkpatrick *et al.* (1990) using CT scans pointed out that the *iliac vessels* are at risk, if surgical penetration of the inner cortex of the pelvis occurs in the anterosuperior region of the acetabulum; and the obturator vessels are at risk if the antero-inferior quadrant is penetrated.

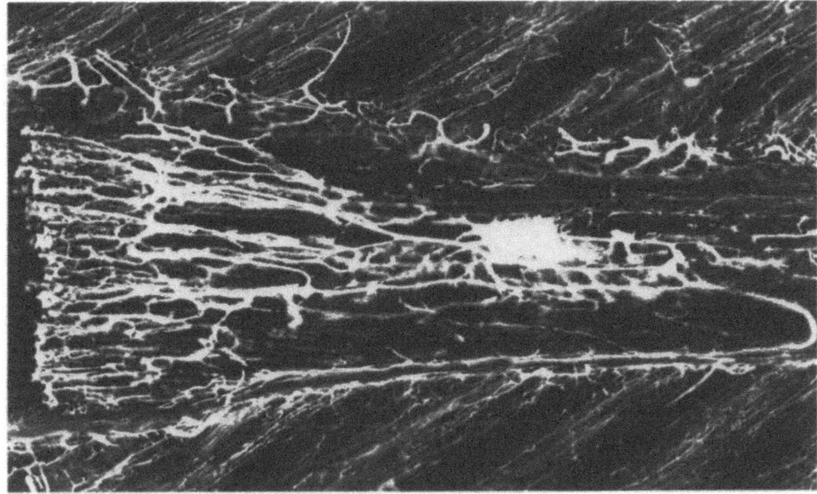

Fig. 7.8. Section through the rib of a rat, perfused with India ink. Capillaries and venules in the attached intercostal muscles are in free connection with periosteal vessels. (Original magnification ×4)

Vessels of the ribs

A nutrient artery enters just beyond the tubercle and sends branches proximally to the head and distally along the elongated body. However, numerous foramina on the head, neck and tubercle as well as close to the costochondral junction suggest the presence of arteries and veins equivalent to the metaphyseal nutrient group of typical long bones (Fig. 7.8). Ostrup *et al.* (1976) pointed out that the neck and tubercle of ribs are supplied by branches of the principal nutrient artery. The rib head, however, received an additional supply from two groups of epiphyseal arteries deriving from the posterior intercostal artery.

The extent to which the general costal cortex is supplied by the medullary system or the periosteal vessels has been assessed by Hendel *et al.* (1982). Canine bone grafts were made in the absence of the nutrient artery or the overlying periosteum. In both situations the grafts were fully viable, there being no demonstrable difference in the blood supply to the rib cortex. Their findings suggested to them that the rib cortex was supplied equally by the medullary and periosteal circulations.

It will be seen in the vascularization of flat bones in the above examples, whether cartilaginous or membranous in development, the vascular pattern includes:

- A central principal nutrient artery;
- Many small metaphyseal type nutrients at the periphery;
- A significant, if not dominant, periosteal arterial supply, adjuvant to nutrient input;
- Profuse sinusoids in the contained marrow, associated with persistent haemopoiesis.

The total vascular pattern of a flat bone departs significantly from the vascular organization of a young long bone (Figs 9.29–9.31), in that there is a considerable *periosteal* blood supply to flat bones which is lacking in young long bones. With the ageing of long bones, there is an increasing dependence on a periosteal blood supply.

Chapter 8

Blood vessels in bone marrow

Several important features of the vascular organization of bone marrow were early established by means of light microscopy of thin unstained sections, particularly of material perfused with Prussian blue and vermilion suspensions (Langer 1876; Ranvier 1875). In modern times light microscopy is still an indispensable technique, but electron microscopy, especially at low powers of magnification (2000–20 000), is increasingly being applied to the study of the vascular endothelium in bones.

Methods of investigation

Notable advances have been made in the study of bone vascularization, particularly in the borderland between macro- and microanatomy, where both naked-eye and microscopic observations formerly proved inadequate. This has been largely brought about by modifying the eighteenth century technique of intravascular perfusion.

Intravascular perfusion

The problem with this technique was to prevent extravasation, and confine the coloured injectate to the small vessels under examination. To this end *injection vehicles* were devised in the nineteenth century, especially warm gelatin suspensions or cold glycerine solutions, which are still used today in the dissection halls of medical schools (Lee 1924). These carry coloured *injection masses* which make the vessels visible. Ferric ferrocyanide is the chief ingredient of the Prussian blue injection mass (Langer 1876), sometimes used in conjunction with copper sulphate rather than ferric chloride. Vermilion, i.e. mercuric sulphide suspensions (Ranvier 1875) and other coloured masses based on salts, such as silver nitrate (Hoyer 1882) and lead chromate (Thiersch 1865) were all available in the late nineteenth century for the investigation of small vessels in bone.

Microradiography

Intravascular perfusion was fundamentally changed with the discovery of X-rays by von Roentgen (1895). As early as 1904, Soulié was able to utilize bone angiography in dogs, and pointed out the absence of an anastomosis between medullary arteries in bone cortex and the arteries of the periosteum. Grégoire & Carrière (1921) perfused human femora with a barium sulphate suspension in water and by the use of X-rays emphasized the metaphyseal blood supply to the bone shaft and its associated growth cartilage. Improved X-ray definition of small vessels in bone had to await the development of suitable microfocal X-ray apparatus capable of delivering soft X-rays continually (Daniels 1952).

Nowadays a limb or other body part for vascular investigation is typically perfused at 34.5 kPa (5 p.s.i.) with a 40–50% suspension of barium sulphate powder in water (Brookes & Harrison 1957; Brookes 1971; Bridgeman & Brookes 1996) in order to reach and fill the arterioles of the osseous circulation and lend contrast to the blood vessels in bone. After fixation in a 10% phosphate buffered formalin solution (3 days for a rat; 3 weeks for a cadaveric limb), the bone is decalcified in a 5% nitric acid in 5% formalin solution in tap water. Decalcification depends on the ambient temperature and the absolute amount of fluid used in relation to the volume of the bone or bones being investigated. The end point of decalcification is usually reached after 1 week (rat limb) or up to 6 weeks (human). After decalcification and whole bone radiography, 400-μm-thick sections are then cut by hand on a microtome and microradiographed, utilizing a microfocal X-ray unit. For the numerous microradiographs exhibited in this book the contact mode of radiography has been used (Fig. 8.1) at low voltages and prolonged exposure times (12 kV, 20 minutes). This is followed by subsequent photography of the X-ray film to show the separate arterial, venous and capillary fields, depending on the viscosity of the perfusate and the mode of perfusion, arterial or retrograde venous in direction.

Macroradiography

This is dependent on the *projection mode* of radiography. Here the object is far removed from the X-ray film but is fairly close (*c.* 5 cm) to the X-ray source (Fig. 8.1). Macroradiography requires a specialized microfocal X-ray apparatus and adept manual focusing of the X-ray beam. Although not commonly used, it yields a ×5–10 magnification on film with ease, allowing bone blood vessels to be directly examined, without the intervention of photography (Buckland-Wright *et al.* 1990).

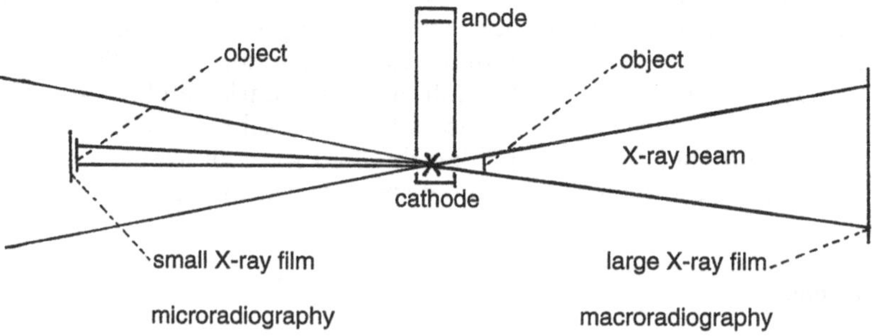

Fig. 8.1. Diagram to show the basic difference between contact and projection modes of magnification radiography.

3D-CT scans

Recently, three dimensional computed tomography (3D-CT) has become available to display and compute vascular fields. Resin and lead salt powder mixtures have been used to enhance vascular contrast (Bachmann *et al.* 1993; Katthagen *et al.* 1995), but they have not displaced the much more convenient barium sulphate suspension in water. Anatomically, 3D-CT scans of cadaveric bone blood vessels using resin-lead powder injection masses (Bachmann *et al.* 1993) offer an alternative mode of defining arterial arborizations in bone. They have the advantage of permitting the isolation of corrosion casts of blood vessels after maceration. There is still a need for a precise description of 3D vascular patterns in bone and a mathematical elucidation of their organization.

Alkaline corrosion casts

Limbs have occasionally been perfused intravascularly with Neoprene latex (de Marneffe 1951) and other plastic, and coloured injection masses, then macerated in potash, and examined under the light microscope. Recently, this method has been revived by perfusion of methyl methacrylate in the human fetus. After complete polymerization of the resin, the bones are isolated, decalcified in trichloroacetic acid, macerated in potassium hydroxide and thoroughly washed in running hot water. The casts are finally coated with gold and examined in the SEM. Such material reveals the density of capillaries and sinusoids in bones (Irino *et al.* 1975; Miodonski *et al.* 1981; Ohtani *et al.* 1982; Skawina *et al.* 1994a,b).

Light microscopy

In modern times, light microscopy (LM) with its panoply of fixation, embedding, sectioning and tissue staining techniques in the service of powerful microscopes with camera attachments and connections to image intensifiers, is indispensable for biological study. It has not been displaced by electron microscopy.

Electron microscopy

At low powers of magnification (2000–20 000) the electron microscope (EM) comes into its own, and should facilitate vascular studies enormously, with respect to the vascular endothelium of bone marrow, the origins of bone cells and the content of Haversian canals.

Spalteholz process

The bones are first perfused with India ink suspension. Fixation and decalcification are followed by clearing and celloidin embedding. Whole bones or sections are then examined under the microscope. The Spalteholz process (1911) is still very useful for investigating capillary and sinusoid layouts at a fraction of the cost of some modern microscopic technologies.

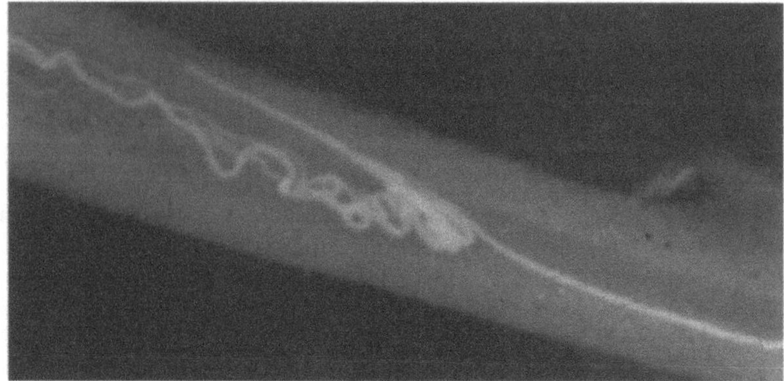

Fig. 8.2. Principal nutrient artery and its main branches. The ascending group is on the left. (Rat tibia; Original magnification ×7)

General features of the osseous circulation

Arterial supply

In the diaphyseal marrow of tubular bones, the nutrient artery divides into medullary branches, both ascending and descending (Fig. 8.2). Together with branches of the metaphyseal and epiphyseal arteries (Figs 8.3, 8.4) ramifying in the cancelli of spongy bone, these vessels form the *afferent limb* of the osseous circulation and are responsible for the supply of blood to fatty and haemopoietic marrow, compact and cancellous bone tissue, and articular and epiphyseal cartilages.

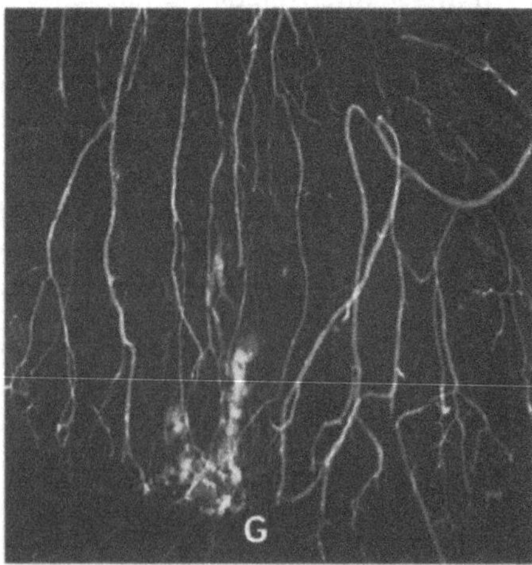

Fig. 8.3. Metaphyseal arteries approaching the growth cartilage (G) in the lower femur of a rat. (Original magnification ×20)

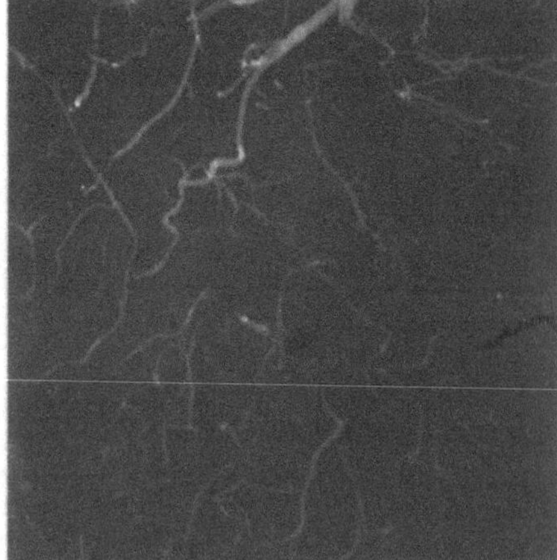

Fig. 8.4. Epiphyseal arteries in a rat femoral condyle. (Original magnification ×20)

Sinusoids and capillaries

The medullary arteries feed into dense networks of sinusoids (Figs 8.5–8.7), the functional vascular lattice of bone marrow. In normal bones the arteries also supply the functional vascular lattice of the cortex, represented in this case by capillary networks (Figs 8.8, 8.9, *overleaf*). Cortical capillaries and medullary sinusoids are in continuity at the cortex–marrow interface.

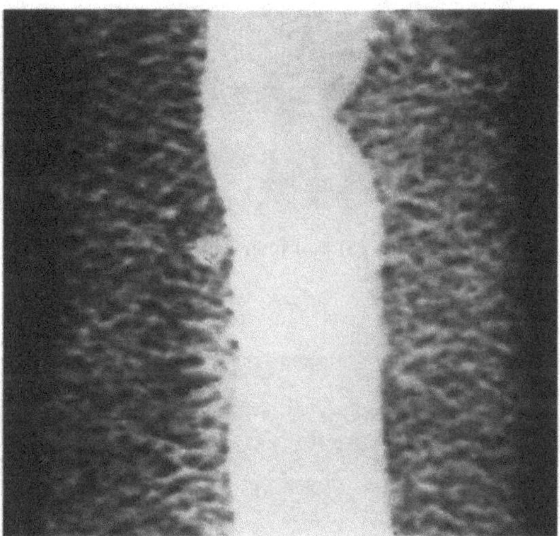

Fig. 8.5. The central venous sinus draining tiered sinusoids in the diaphyseal marrow of the rat femur. (Original magnification ×30)

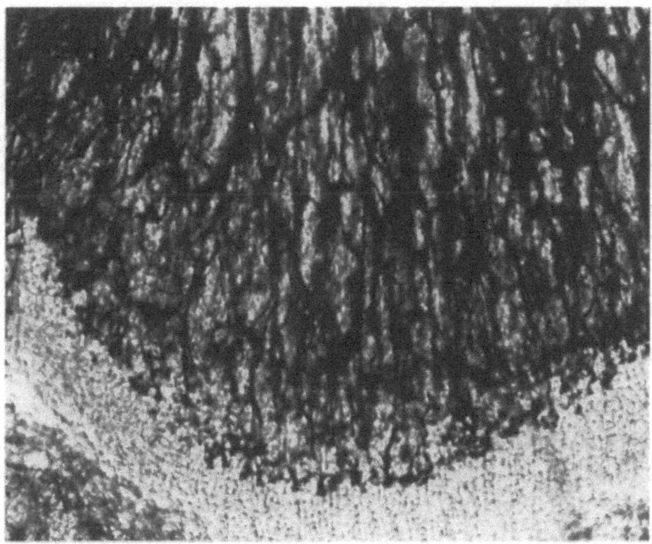

Fig. 8.6. Dense metaphyseal sinusoids vertical to the growth cartilage. (Original magnification ×53)

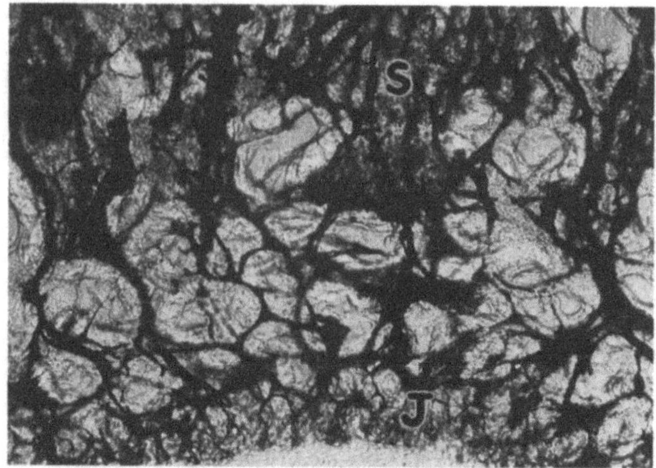

Fig. 8.7. Irregular epiphyseal sinusoids (S) and finer articular sinusoids (J). (Rat femur, India ink preparation; Original magnification ×78)

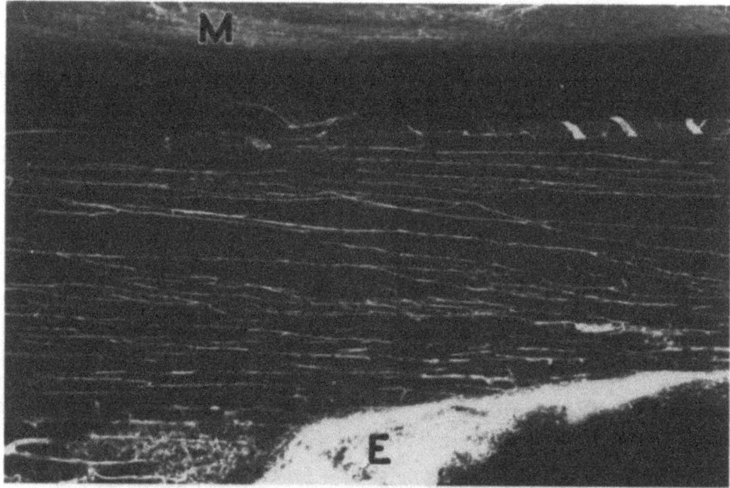

Fig. 8.8. Longitudinal section through the cortex and adjacent muscle (M) and marrow (E) of a monkey femur, showing typical long and wide cortical capillaries. (Original magnification ×22)

Venous drainage

By confluence the sinusoids of bone marrow form numerous collecting sinuses (Fig. 8.10), tributaries of the central venous sinus of the diaphyseal marrow (Figs 8.11–8.13). The venous sinuses communicate directly with extra-osseous, i.e. nutrient and metaphyseal, veins. The cortical capillaries, on the other hand, are in continuity with the capillaries in the osteogenic layer of the overlying periosteum and with periosteal and intramuscular veins (Figs 8.9, 8.14, 8.15).

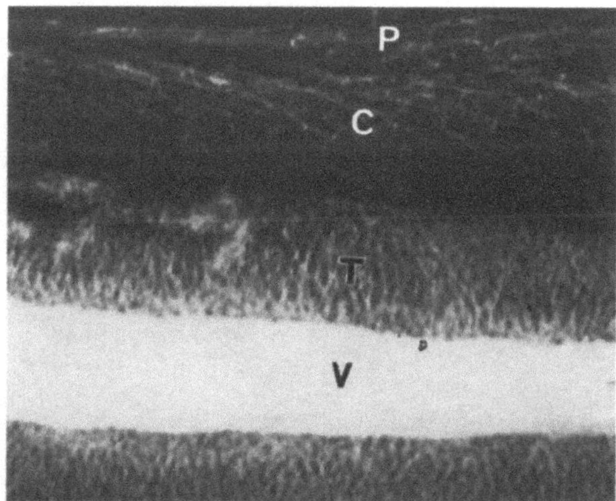

Fig. 8.9. Microradiograph of a rat perfused with Thorotrast through the veins, showing continuity between the periosteum (P), cortex (C), marrow sinusoids (T) and central sinus (V). (Original magnification ×30)

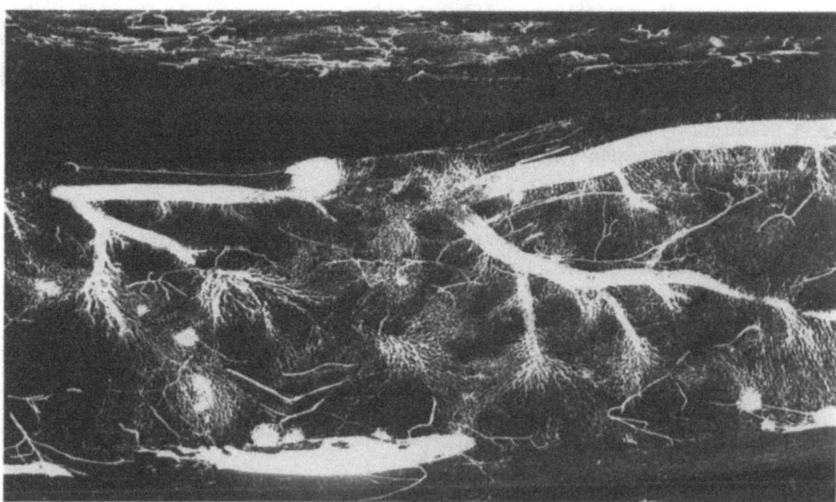

Fig. 8.10. Angiography of a longitudinal section through a rabbit humerus; the opposite bone had been fractured. The animal was perfused with Micropaque through the heart. This section shows lobular groups of sinusoids draining into large collecting sinuses in the marrow. Scattered fine arterial channels are also visible. (Original magnification ×6.2)

Arteries and arterioles

There are two types of *afferent vessels* in bone marrow. The first type, represented by the nutrient artery and its main branches, consists of typical *small arteries* as found elsewhere in the systemic circulation (Fig. 8.16). In the cardiovascular system generally, the peripheral resistance to the circulation of the blood is exercised in the main at *arterioles* (Starling's hypothesis). Neurohumeral

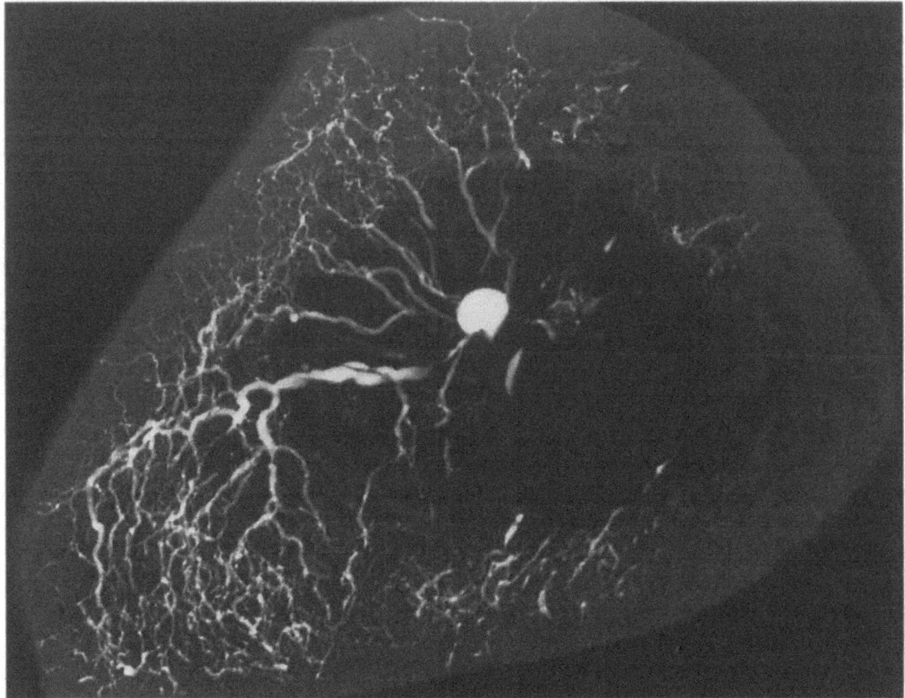

Fig. 8.11. Central venous sinus and collecting vessels in a cross-section of a human tibia. (Micropaque, retrograde venous perfusion; Original magnification ×3.2)

mechanisms, by varying the calibre of the arterioles, can alter the peripheral resistance. The lumen of these fine vessels is variable in diameter, but is usually of the order of 30–70 μm. The vessel wall has a smooth muscle coat, so that normally in the passage of arterial blood through arterioles, its pressure drops from about 80 mmHg in small arteries to 30 mmHg on entering the capillaries.

Bone marrow arterioles

Branching abruptly off the small arteries in bone marrow are peculiar *straight arterioles*, whose mural structure is two layered, consisting of an endothelial tube covered by a single layer of cubical or spindle cells, possibly smooth muscle elements (Figs 8.17, 8.18). The change from small artery to straight arteriole is without a gradual transition from one type to the other (Hashimoto 1936; Yoffey 1962). In small mammals such as the rat, even the larger branches of the nutrient artery are of this fine variety, with an internal diameter of only 30 μm or so. Although a muscular tunica media is not conspicuous, the straight vessels are directly innervated by non-myelinated sympathetic nerve fibres (Thurston 1982). The individual fibres are some 2 μm in diameter, and can be traced in close contact with the vessel wall (Fig. 8.22). They probably represent the arterioles of bone marrow, feeding into the medullary sinusoids and cortical capillaries: in both cases the double-walled arteriole gives way to a single-walled endothelial tube (Fig. 8.19).

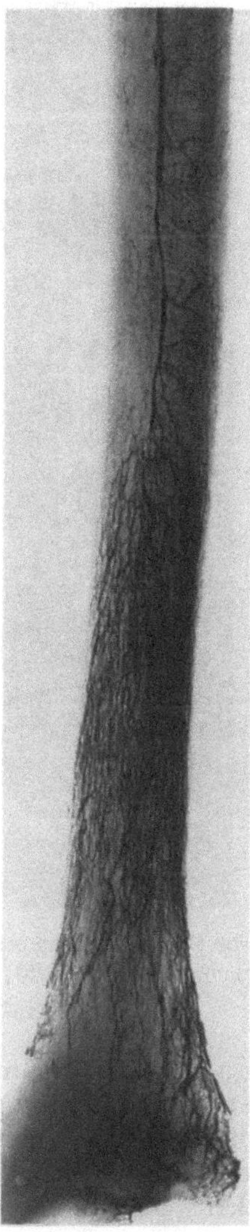

Fig. 8.12. Central venous sinus in the marrow of a human tibia, breaking up into a spray of vessels in the cortex of the lower third of the bone. (Original: Two-thirds natural size)

Arteriovenous junctions

The junction between the terminal arterial vessels and the sinusoids in bone marrow is very difficult to demonstrate. von Rustizky (1872) measured the narrowest medullary arterioles (5 μm) and venules (15 μm), as he called them, that he could see, and assumed that a funnel-shaped junction existed between the two. Reichel (1947) gives a drawing of such a connection. This shows an abrupt funnel-shaped junction between arteriole and sinusoid. In laboratory animals, however, India ink preparations of bone marrow indicate that the transition from arteriole to sinusoid is not as abrupt as von Rustizky surmised and as others (Testut &

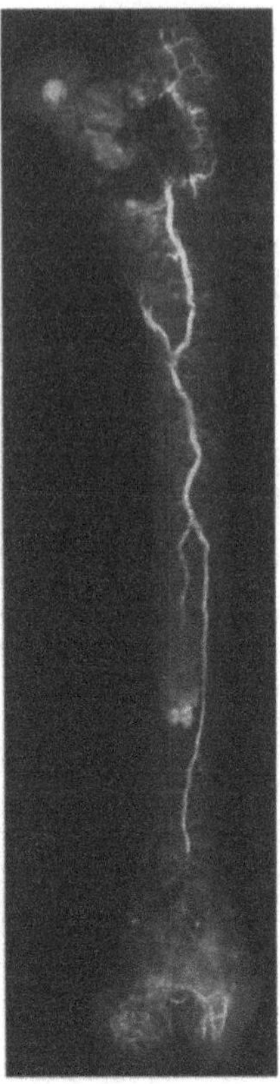

Fig. 8.13. Central venous sinus in a rabbit femur, making connection with the nutrient vein and the vein of the trochanteric fossa. (Original magnification ×1.25)

Latarjet 1948) state, but rather a gradual widening from one to the other occurs which may take place over two or three microscopic fields.

The venous sinuses of bone marrow have a very tenuous wall (Fig. 8.16). In the largest of them it is only three or four cells thick and muscular elements appear to be absent. The adventitia thickens considerably when a sinus passes through a foramen in the cortex and becomes an extra-osseous vein.

Nerve supply of bone marrow

In larger laboratory animals (rabbit, cat, dog) substantial bundles of nerve fibres accompany the nutrient vessels and have been followed into the marrow cavity. In the nutrient canal, the nerve bundles associate with the artery, running a straight course on its adventitia. Once in the marrow cavity the nerve bundles divide (Fig. 8.20), following the arterial branching pattern and generating plexuses spiralling around the small arteries of bone marrow (Fig. 8.21) (Ottolenghi 1902; Kuntz and Richins 1945; Calvo 1968; Duncan & Shim 1977; Thurston 1982).The two-layered straight arterioles, however, are associated with only one or two reduced nerve bundles, containing up to four nerve fibres per bundle in close contact with the

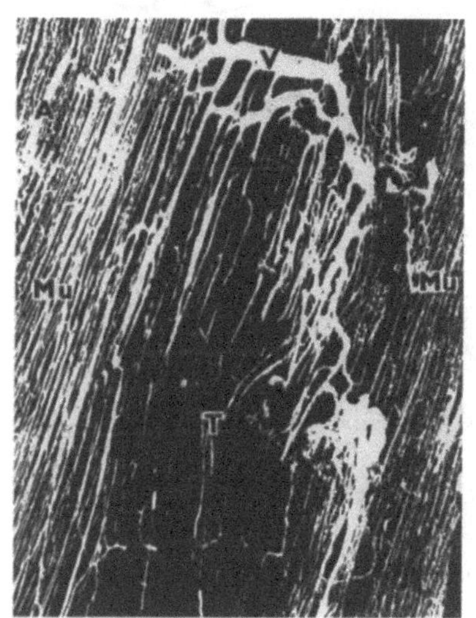

Fig. 8.14. Oblique section through a rat tibia to show confluence of cortical capillaries (T) with periosteal venule (V). Arterioles (A) are seen breaking up in muscle (Mu). (India ink; Original magnification ×33)

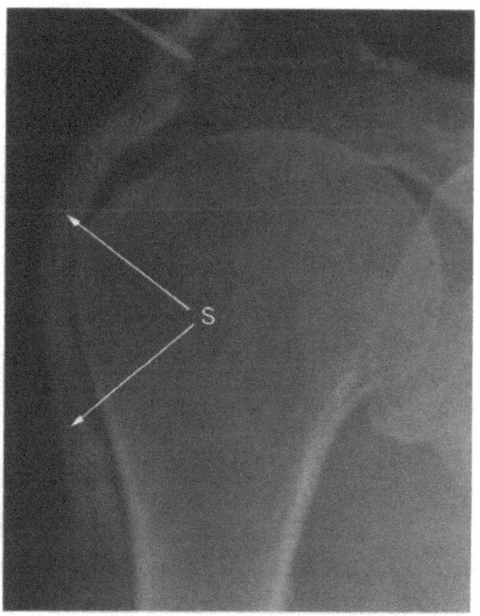

Fig. 8.15. Contrast medium injected *in vivo* into the human acromion process passes readily into the attached deltoid muscle (S).

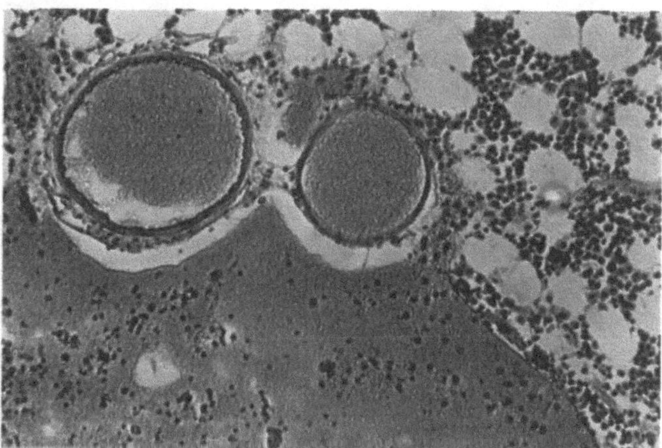

Fig. 8.16. Photomicrograph of two thick-walled medullary arteries close to a thin-walled sinus. (Thorotrast perfused rabbit femur; Original magnification ×120)

arteriolar wall (Fig. 8.22). Hence, in the rat or mouse, nerve fibres are difficult to detect because large neural networks are associated with the nutrient arteries of bone marrow; in a rat the characteristic medullary artery is the arteriole, carrying but a few isolated fibres. Nerve fibres are also difficult to find in cancellous bone, but when found are generally perivascular in location (Fig. 8.21).

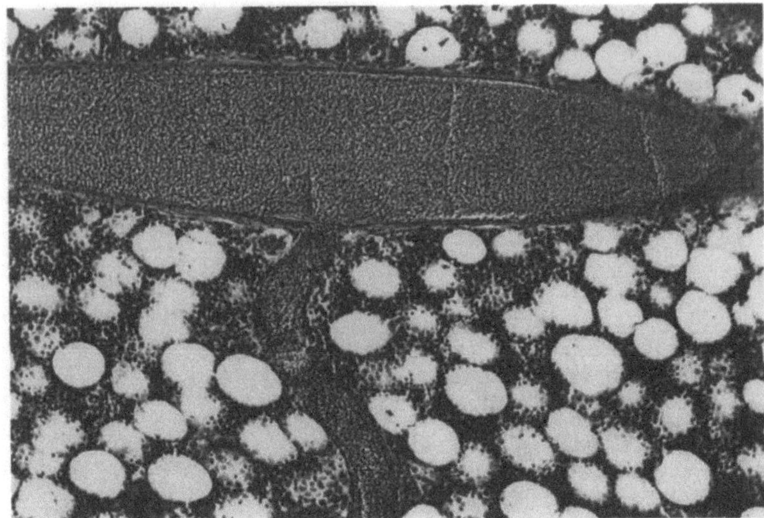

Fig. 8.17. A large medullary artery giving off a thin-walled arterial channel of only two cell layers. (Original magnification ×90)

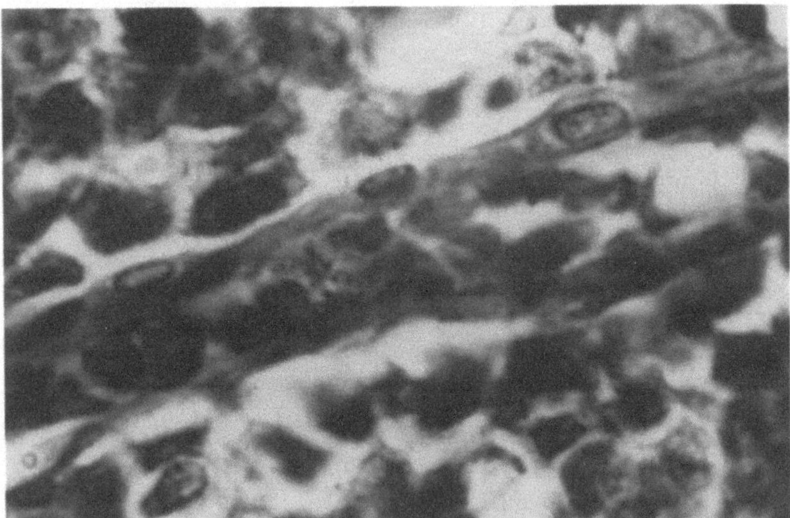

Fig. 8.18. Photomicrograph of a fine arteriolar channel in rat bone marrow. (Original magnification ×480)

No nerve fibres are to be seen passing on to marrow capillaries, but nerve bundles and isolated fibres are easy to detect on the central venous sinus and can be traced onto the walls of the lesser sinuses which it drains (Thurston 1982). Nerve fibres are sparse in the marrow parenchyma, breaking away from an arterial bundle to pass independently through the medullary cell masses (Fig. 8.23). Branching and small irregular plexuses develop here and there, but no nerve endings or boutons have been observed terminating on parenchymal cells (Duncan & Shim 1977; Thurston 1982).

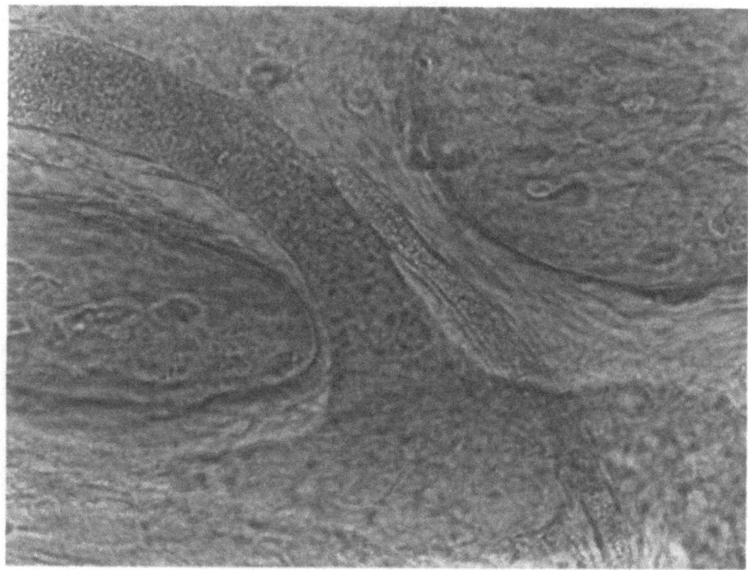

Fig. 8.19. Fine arterial channel (double-layered wall) emptying into a wide sinusoid (single-layered wall) in fetal bone cortex. (Original magnification ×175)

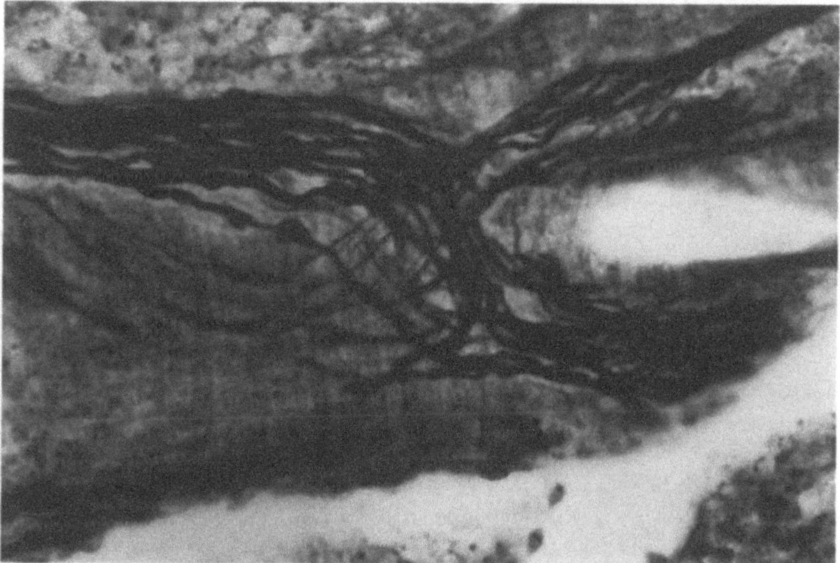

Fig. 8.20. (*see also Colour Plate section*) A large nerve bundle dividing at the bifurcation of a medullary artery. (Dog; Linder's silver impregnation; Original magnification ×450)

Experimental blood perfusion of an isolated tibia is directly affected by stimulation of its nerve supply, and the pattern of response is "characteristically vasomotor" (Drinker & Drinker 1916). Stimulation of the sympathetic nerves to the femur decreases blood flow in bone marrow (Lowenstein *et al.* 1958; Brookes 1974a), but the mechanism is now known to be complex. Reduced marrow flow

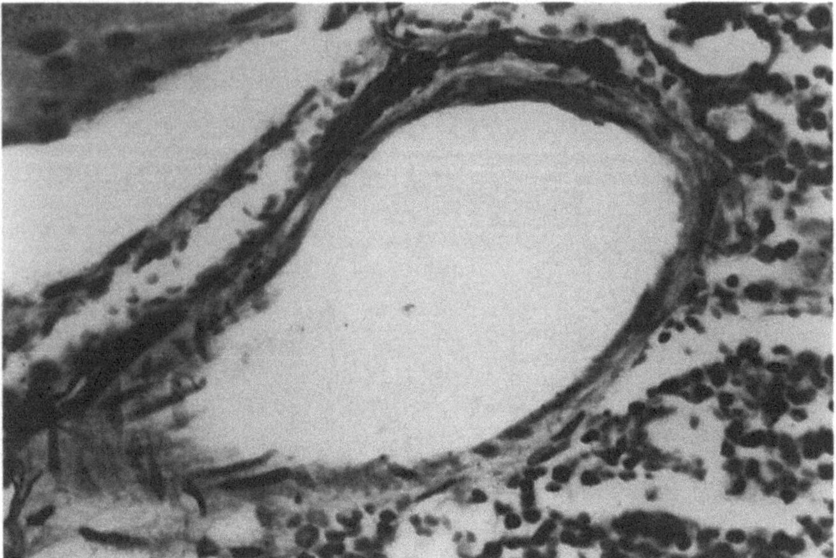

Fig. 8.21. (*see also Colour Plate section*) Perivascular fibres in contact with a small epiphyseal artery. (Dog, Linder's silver impregnation; Original magnification ×420)

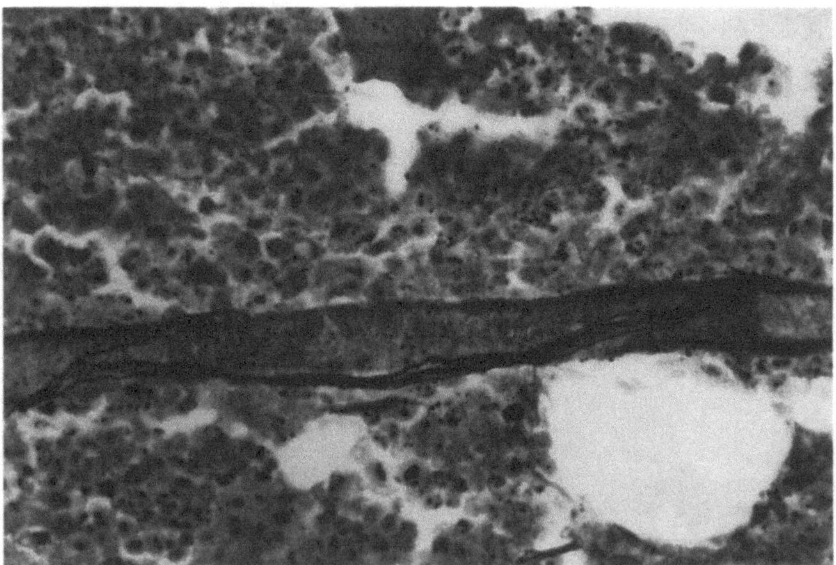

Fig. 8.22. (*see also Colour Plate section*) Straight arteriole in bone marrow with its sympathetic fibres. (Dog, Linder's silver impregnation; Original magnification ×420)

may result from sinus constriction and/or arteriolar constriction. The anatomical distribution of sympathetic nerves in bone marrow can activate constriction in both afferent and efferent sites.

Experimental surgical sympathectomy of a hind limb in animals has no immediate effect on blood flow in the femur (Davies *et al.* 1984). However, Wijeratne

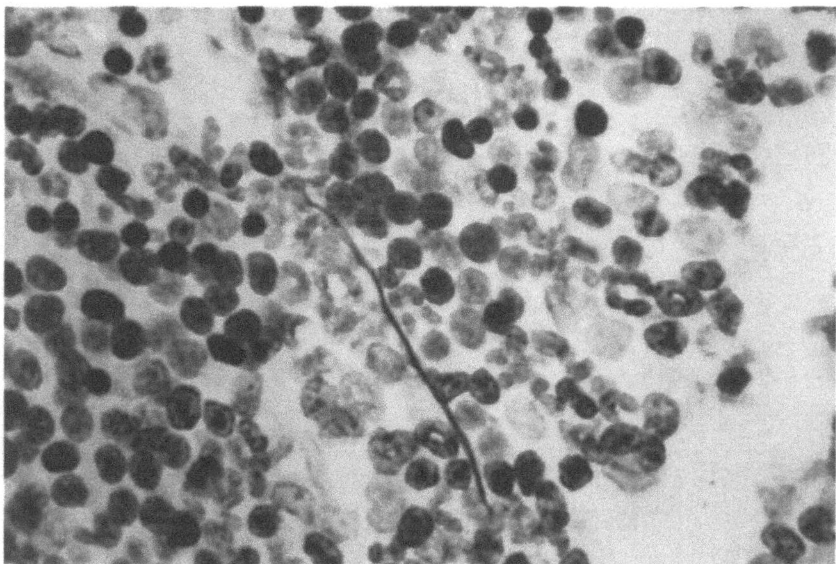

Fig. 8.23. (*see also Colour Plate section*) A solitary nerve fibre running between parenchymal cells. (Dog, Linder's silver impregnation; Original magnification ×420)

(1973) found in rabbits that there was a massive doubling of the blood flow rate in the femur, tibiofibula and metatarsal III 4 weeks after lumbar sympathectomy. By 12 weeks the effect had been abolished. After sciatic and femoral nerve section (which includes section of sympathetic fibres in the nerves) a massive rise in flow rate in the bones was immediate, which was abolished at 1 week and was double the normal at 12 weeks. The circulating red cell volume in the rat bones showed a modest increase rising up to 12 weeks. Wijeratne's results indicate profound vascular disturbances take place in bones after the abolition of the sympathetic or spinal nerve supply (Fig. 8.24, *overleaf*).

Vascular patterns

There are three major territories in the marrow of long bones, diaphyseal, metaphyseal and epiphyseal, and each is characterized by a distinctive vascular pattern. Differences in structure are usually an indication of differences in function, and the vascular patterns of bone marrow are no exception in this respect. As will be shown later, the various parts of the osseous circulation are characterized by distinctive haemodynamic features. Hence the account given below of the vascular patterns of bone marrow is not to be taken as merely descriptive, but rather as a step in the search for functional correlates.

Diaphysis

In small mammals, the larger arteries in diaphyseal marrow are highly tortuous close to their origin from the nutrient vessel (Fig. 8.2). In rabbits, monkeys and

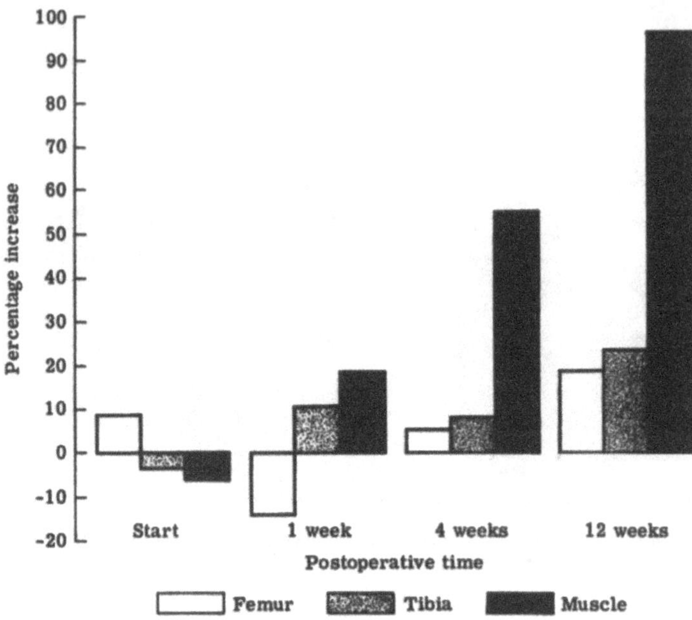

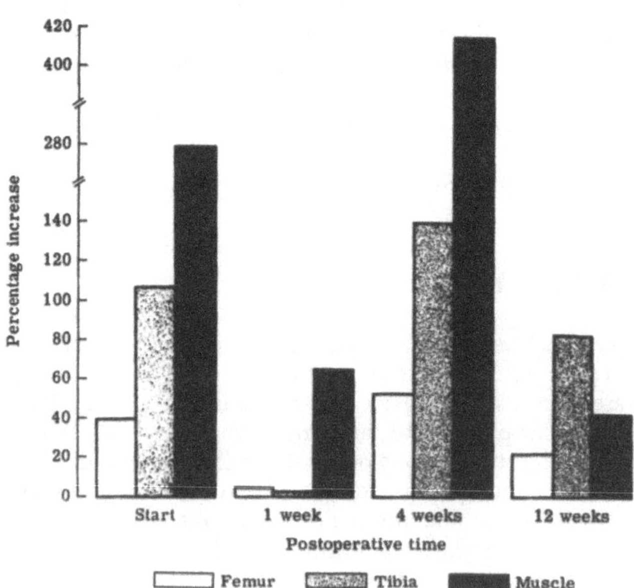

Fig. 8.24. **a** Bar graph showing the effect of sciatic and femoral nerve section on the CRCV of bone and muscle from start to 12 weeks postoperatively. **b** Blood flow rates after nerve section as above showing an immediate rise abolished at 1 week, and a subsequent increased flow at 4 and 12 weeks.

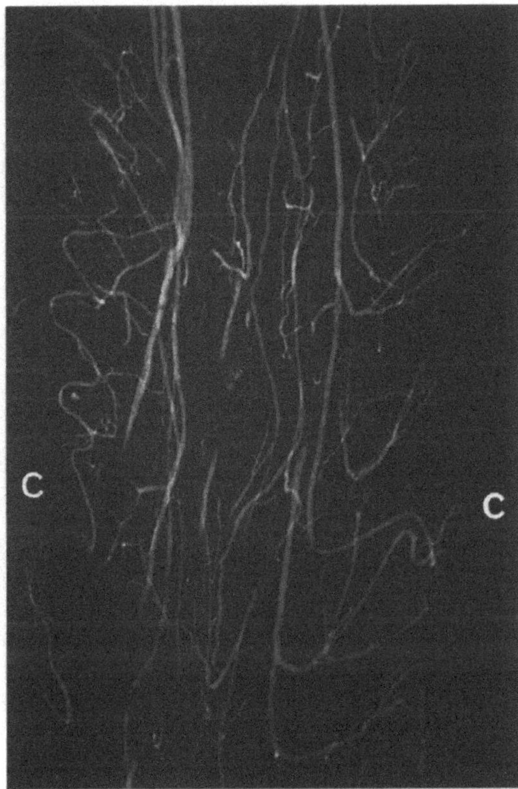

Fig. 8.25. Medullary arteries and their subcortical branches: microarteriograph of a longitudinal section through a rat femur. CC, cortex. (Original magnification ×20)

man they have more of an open corkscrew course (Figs 2.9, 2.10). They then run longitudinally and their subdivisions lie chiefly in the subcortical, that is, the peripheral zone of marrow (Fig. 8.25). The finer medullary arteries can usually be recognized by their straightness (Figs 8.18, 8.22).

The straight arterioles do not anastomose, and supply the cortex and the marrow (Figs 8.26–8.29, *overleaf*). The length of the straight arterioles suggest that they are end-arteries. It seems likely from the radiographic evidence that the delivery of blood to cortical capillaries and marrow sinusoids results in the presence of discrete, circumscribed vascular regions with little functional overlap because of their end-arterial supply. This conclusion is supported by the findings of Eletto (1933) and Rubascheva & Prives (1932), who remarked on the lack of anastomoses between branches of the principal nutrient artery in the medulla. It might help to explain the occurrence of irregular necrosis of bone cells in the cortex after intravascular injection of particulate suspensions (Bergmann 1927; Kistler 1934,1935) or interruption of the principal nutrient artery (Huggins & Wiege 1939; Bragdon *et al.* 1949). The subcortical site of straight arterioles to cortical capillaries is a considerable one. The arteriolar supply to medullary sinusoids comes from the inner, central small arteries in bone marrow, and not only those in a subcortical situation.

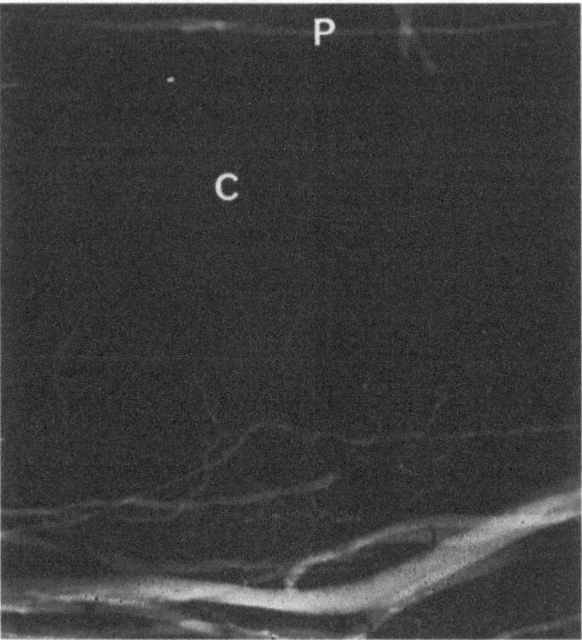

Fig. 8.26. Arteriograph (Micropaque perfusion) of rat bone cortex, showing subcortical marrow arteries giving centrifugal arterioles to the cortex (C). Overlying periosteal arteries (P) do not supply cortex in the young. (Original magnification ×30)

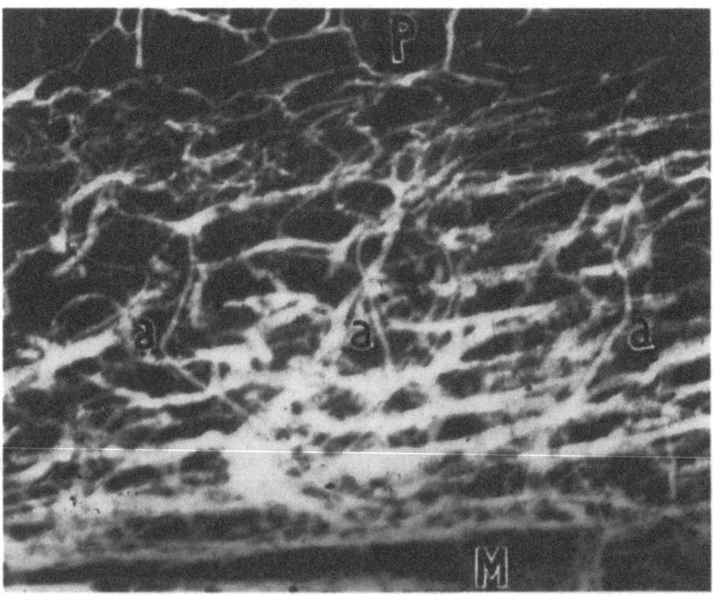

Fig. 8.27. Microangiograph of a longitudinal section through human fetal tibial cortex. Fine centrifugal arterioles (a,a,a) emanate from the marrow (M) and empty into the cortical capillaries. These then join periosteal venules (P). (Original magnification ×20)

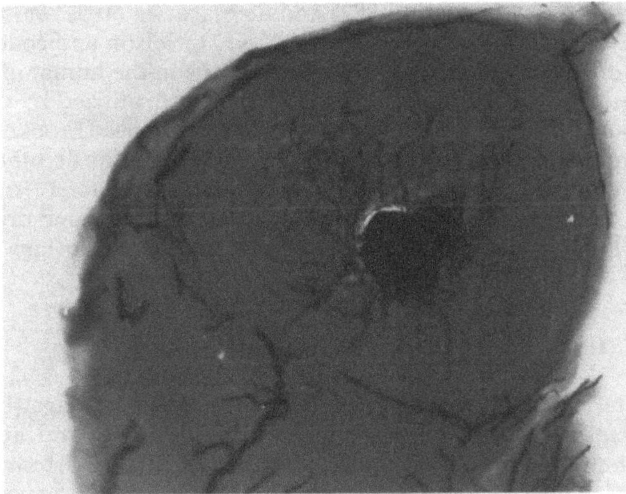

Fig. 8.28. Microangiograph of cross-section through human fetal tibia, showing that medullary centrifugal arterioles supply the cortex, not periosteal arteries. (Original magnification ×4.6)

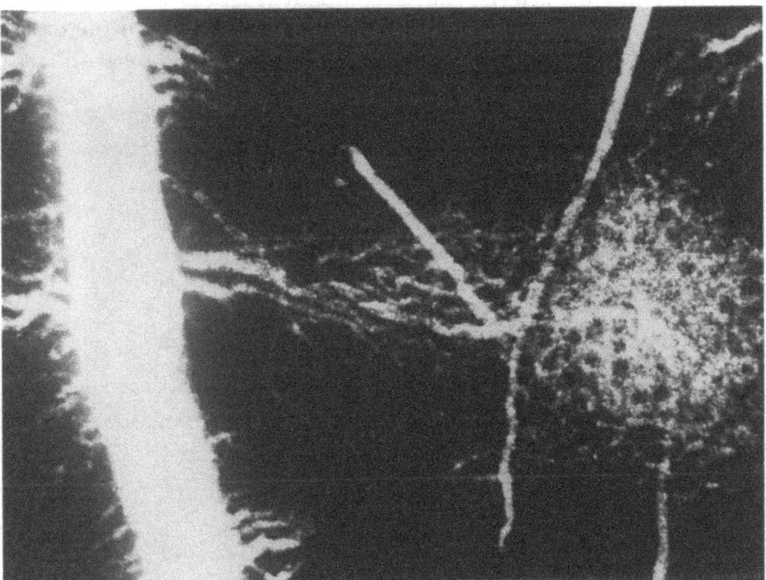

Fig. 8.29. Terminal arterioles passing into a sinusoid clump drained by a collecting sinus. The above arrangements possibly also conceal an arteriovenous anastomosis. (Original magnification ×80)

The venous arrangements in diaphyseal marrow differ considerably from the arterial. A central venous sinus, some four times wider that the nutrient artery but with a very much thinner wall, extends the length of the diaphysis, keeping to a central position (Figs 8.11–8.13). Piney (1922) described this structure in rabbits as a central artery, but its venous nature has been established beyond doubt by von Rustizky (1872), Bizzozero (1872) and de Marneffe (1951) in mammals and man by many recent workers (Figs 8.9, 8.11, 8.12). Nelson and colleagues (1960) signally failed to distinguish a central venous sinus in the human tibia, although it does seem to be present in material similar to that utilized by these authors, namely amputated limbs, as well as in human fetal bones (Brookes 1958a). The nutrient vein branches off from the central venous sinus, as do other large emissary veins which can occasionally be found traversing the cortex (Brookes 1958b). Collecting sinuses lie in the transverse plane of the diaphysis and drain a plethora of sinusoids in the marrow, which viewed *en masse*, lie in tiers (Figs 8.5, 8.9, 8.11).

Metaphysis

Here, the arteries are arranged vertically to the growth cartilage (Figs 8.3, 8.30). They are dispersed uniformly through cancellous bone, and are not chiefly located in the periphery, as in the diaphyseal marrow. Anastomoses are altogether absent in the metaphyseal region. The arteries pass to a specialized metaphyseal subchondral circulation next to the growth cartilage. They are end-arteries, as shown by metaphyseal ablation experiments. The venous sinuses and sinusoids of the metaphysis are also chiefly longitudinal in layout, but are far more numerous than the arteries they accompany (Figs 8.6, 8.30). They are coarse and irregular in calibre. The central collecting sinuses pass to the extremity of

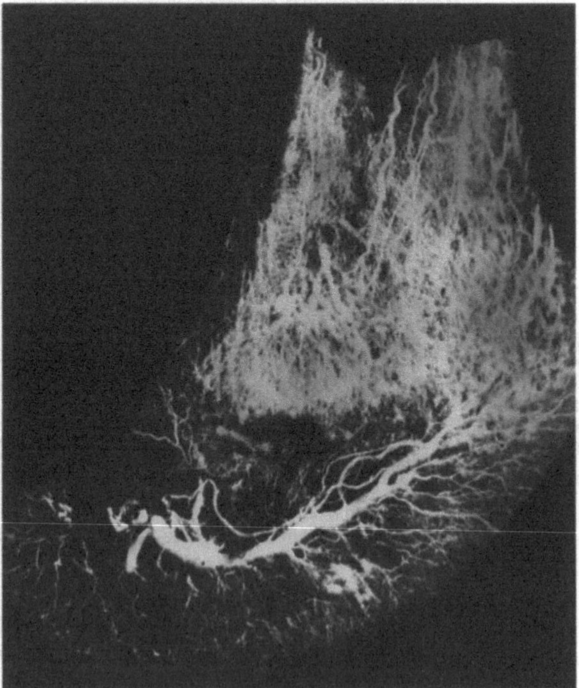

Fig. 8.30. Dense vertical metaphyseal vessels; below it, transverse venous sinus and radiating epiphyseal vessels. (Angiograph, rat femur; Original magnification ×7.5)

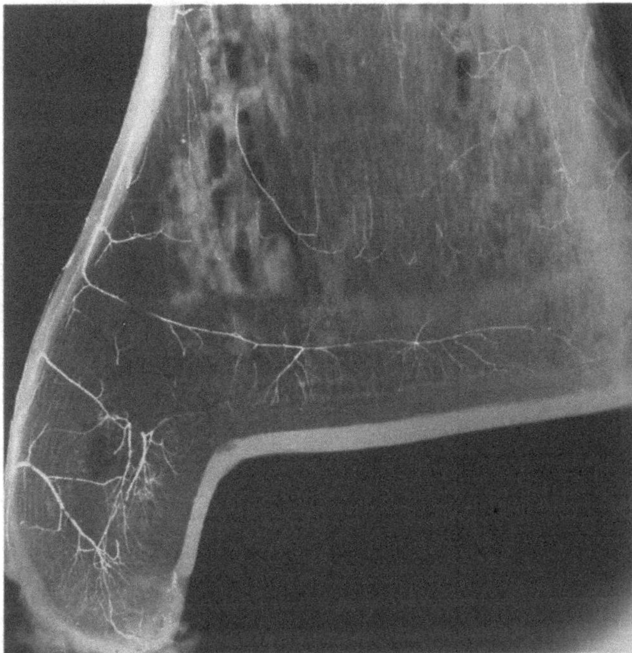

Fig. 8.31. Arteriograph of lower end of a mature human tibia, showing transverse epiphyseal arteries. Metaphyseal arteries do not communicate across the line of union. See also Fig. 8.39. (Original: Natural size)

the central venous sinus. The peripheral ones are continuous, extra-osseously, with metaphyseal veins.

Epiphysis

In the epiphysis, before or after fusion with the shaft has occurred, the arterial pattern differs from that found in the diaphysis or metaphysis in that they anastomose across its whole transverse extent (Figs 8.30, 8.31). Branches then pass radially, either to the articular cartilage or to the growth cartilage (or synostosis if fusion has occurred). Intra-osseous arcades are formed between epiphyseal arteries in human femoral and tibial condyles (Nussbaum 1923). Terminal branches supply the juxta-articular circulation (Figs 8.7, 8.32, *overleaf*) and in young animals a specialized subchondral circulation as well, on the epiphyseal side of the growth cartilage (Fig. 8.33, *overleaf*). The venous radicles are again extraordinarily profuse and tend, by confluence, to form a distinct transverse sinus in the epiphyses of long bones (Figs 8.30, 8.34, *overleaf*). Its horizontal disposition contrasts with the vertical orientation of the central venous sinus.

Epiphyseal sinusoids can be distinguished on sight from the sinusoids in the rest of the bone (Fig. 8.7). They are particularly uneven in calibre and irregular in distribution, contrasting with the longitudinal sinusoid pattern in the metaphysis (Fig. 8.6) or the tiered arrangement in the diaphysis (Fig. 8.5).

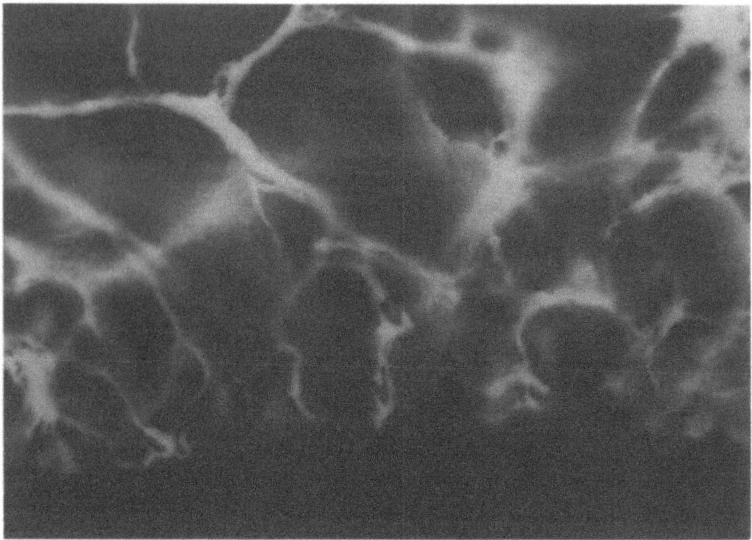

Fig. 8.32. Articular vessels. (Original magnification ×130)

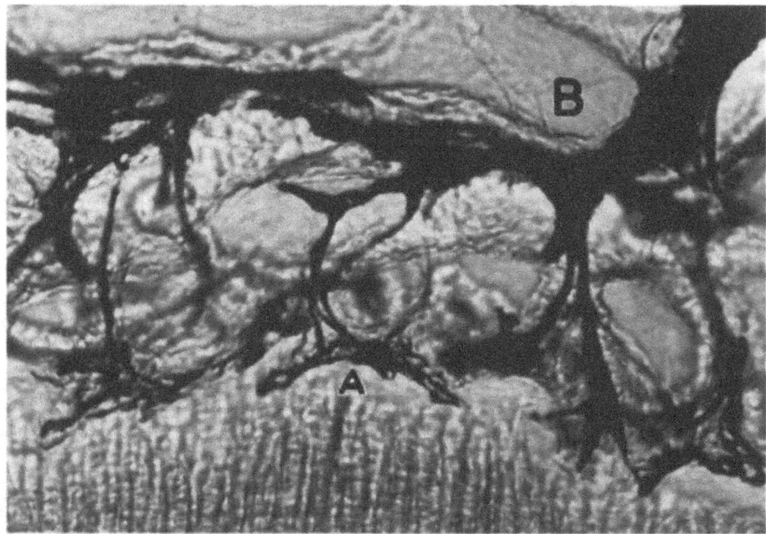

Fig. 8.33. Subchondral blood vessels on the epiphyseal side of the growth cartilage. **B**, Bone plate; A, amorphous zone of growth cartilage. (Original magnification ×120)

Sinusoids in bone marrow

Pulsation

The sinusoids in the diaphyseal marrow have been shown by direct vital microscopy, in the case of the rabbit fibula (Brånemark 1959), to dilate and

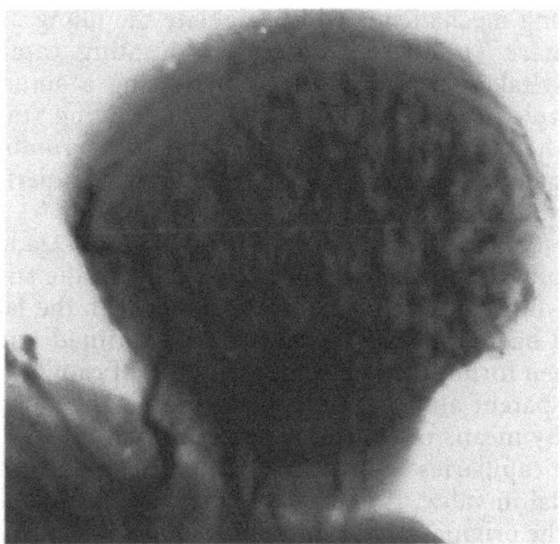

Fig. 8.34. Transverse sinuses in the superior epiphysis of the rat femur, surmounting vertically orientated metaphyseal vessels. (Venogram; Original magnification ×9)

contract rhythmically. Presumably this is a passive response to a pulsatile flow of blood in medullary arteries.

In the cardiovascular system generally, a pulse pressure is measurable only as far as the small arteries. In bone marrow, the straight arterioles are given off abruptly from arteries possessing muscular coats. It is improbable that a pulse pressure is transmitted to them. However the marrow in bone is also encased in a rigid and unyielding bony cylinder. The afferent stem vessels register a pulse pressure before they break up into their finer ramifications, which could be transmitted directly to the sinusoids and venules across the extravascular fluid.

Pulsatile changes in the tissue pressure of marrow have in fact been demonstrated by Stein *et al.* (1957) by means of electromanometers inserted into the bones of dogs. Their results do not only show the existence of a pulse pressure in the marrow parenchyma, they also reveal that it differs in diaphyseal and epiphyseal marrow. In the case of the dog, the pulse pressures are 6 mmHg and 1 mmHg respectively. These results may be correlated with the relative size of the arteries entering the medulla. The principal nutrient is the largest, and the epiphyseal vessels are the smallest. Medullary pulsation serves to promote the circulation in the bone as a whole.

Lobulation and vascular shunts

Some of the results, obtained by microradiography, of progressive filling of marrow sinusoids have been recorded (Brookes 1960b). It was noted that clumps of sinusoids at first fill up, and that with injection of increasing amounts of perfusate these areas enlarged and finally coalesced (Fig. 8.10). The evidence is suggestive of an ill-defined lobular arrangement of marrow sinusoids, each lobule being supplied by its own arteriole (Fig. 8.29). There is also some evidence in the literature of shunting mechanisms which regulate the filling of small lobules of sinusoids. Brånemark (1959) has described shunting capillaries which he observed by intravital microscopy, blood bypassing a sinusoid and flowing directly into a venule. Yet, in order to display the living sinusoid bed in the rabbit, Brånemark had to remove the fibular cortex with a rotating burr. It is possible that the heat generated may have caused collapse of superficial sinusoids, or otherwise disturbed their normal activity.

Brånemark's observation recalls the work of Doan (1922a,b), who described intersinusoidal capillaries in the hypoplastic marrow of the starving pigeon,and in the ribs of the white rat. According to Doan, between the fat spaces which in starvation replace haemopoietic cell nests, well-outlined and clearly defined channels can be seen forming an extensive network of capillaries. Many of these appear to be non-patent and functionally dormant. They are continuous with venous sinusoids by means of conical junctions. Doan himself thought they did not represent true capillaries interposed between arteries and veins, but rather were intersinusoidal in value. It is probable that the shrunken capillaries which he observed were the original sinusoids of a haemopoietic marrow, now collapsed in the presence of an inactive fatty marrow.

Open or closed circulation

In the light microscope, the endothelial cells ("littoral cells") which form the sinusoid wall show featureless cytoplasm and oval nuclei with a fine chromatin network. The endothelium appears to lack a basement membrane, although silver impregnation shows a reticulin network closely associated with the vessels.

Whether these vessels are open (Hoyer 1869) or closed (Bizzozero 1868) is an old controversy. According to the latter view, the endothelial cells of the marrow sinusoid form a complete layer, no intercellular gaps being present. Although it may be possible for colloidal dyes, bacteria and particulate matter to leave the vascular lumen either by diapedesis (that is, by passage through endothelial cytoplasm) or between the endothelial cells, no extravasations of whole blood, even as microhaemorrhages into haemopoietic spaces, are held to occur. On the other hand, the "open" school does envisage gross deficiencies in the wall, allowing circulating blood direct access to extravascular tissue.

Rindfleisch (1879) represents an extreme example of this latter point of view. He considered that marrow sinusoids hardly possessed a wall at all and that the blood-forming elements of the marrow were in free and open communication with the circulating blood. Few would accept this opinion today, in spite of the EM observations of Yoffey *et al.* (1965) which show extensive deficiencies in the sinusoid wall. Osmic fixation took place at least 10 minutes after death in their material, which gave ample time for the development of artefacts.

Bunting (1919) represents a more moderate viewpoint. His illustrations purport to show that the sinusoids in general have an endothelial coat, but that here and there, gaps occur in the wall. Nevertheless, modern histological investigations of marrow sinusoids show what appear to be an unbroken and continuous endothelial coat. Endothelial enclosures in which, according to Sabin (1932), intravascular erythropoiesis occurs are now no longer recognized. On the contrary, it is generally accepted that haemopoietic tissue is extravascular, filling in the interstices between the sinusoids so readily demonstrated by perfusion methods.

However beaded or varicose the sinusoids may appear when filled with India ink or Thorotrast, they remain sharply defined structures. It is probably true to state that nearly all those workers who in recent years have used injection methods to reveal vessels in bone marrow have been impressed by the clear-cut definition of vascular boundaries thus obtained. Extravasations are easily recognized when injection pressures are non-physiological (Reichel 1947), or vessels are damaged by injected noxious agents, such as saponin (Omura & Osogoe 1951), which destroy the cement substance uniting the endothelial cells. The resulting histological picture of red cell aggregations far removed from vascular endothelium is easily detected. Nevertheless, the walls of the marrow sinusoids are tenuous, and the possible occurrence of generalized minute fenestrae in the marrow sinusoids cannot be ruled out by LM alone.

Phagocytosis

Sinus endothelial cells take up intravital dyes such as Janus green or Congo red. Because of this property, they are counted in the reticulo-endothelial system of Aschoff (1906, 1924). This implies that apart from forming the vascular pathways for the medullary circulation, sinusoid endothelium can be mobilized for the ingestion of bacteria and foreign particles, and participate in the immune system generally.

The phagocytic property of sinus endothelium is considerable. Particulate titanium dioxide injected intravenously was rapidly incorporated into bone marrow (Huggins 1939). Intravenous Thorotrast is likewise concentrated after a few hours almost entirely in the spleen and bone marrow, and can be used as a means of visualizing these organs in the experimental animal (Foxon 1961). India ink particles can also be used to mark medullary sinusoids, because the reticulo-endothelial cells concentrate circulating particulate matter in their cytoplasm. The endothelial cells in such circumstances round off and become free wandering cells (macrophages) in the marrow parenchyma (Bloom & Fawcett 1962).

It is important in haemodynamic studies of bone marrow to bear in mind the phagocytic property of sinus endothelial cells, because they take up effete red corpuscles as well as bacteria. Red cells tagged with a radioactive isotope should be used fresh on the day of labelling for volumetric studies. The calculated red cell volume of bone marrow can be double the normal if cells are used that have been stored overnight. The values for marrow red cell volume also steadily rise the longer the "mixing time" allowed, the effect being observable once this is greater than half an hour (see Chapter 16). How the sinus endothelium distinguishes between a normal and a radioactive red cell is uncertain. Presumably damage to the red cell membrane by radioactivity is sufficient to excite the reticulo-endothelial cells into phagocytic activity.

Marrow endothelium

Medullary endothelial cells in the EM show nuclei which are somewhat flattened and angulated in outline (Figs 8.35, 8.36, *overleaf*). Two nucleoli are often present. The cytoplasm is comparatively electron transparent but exhibits small

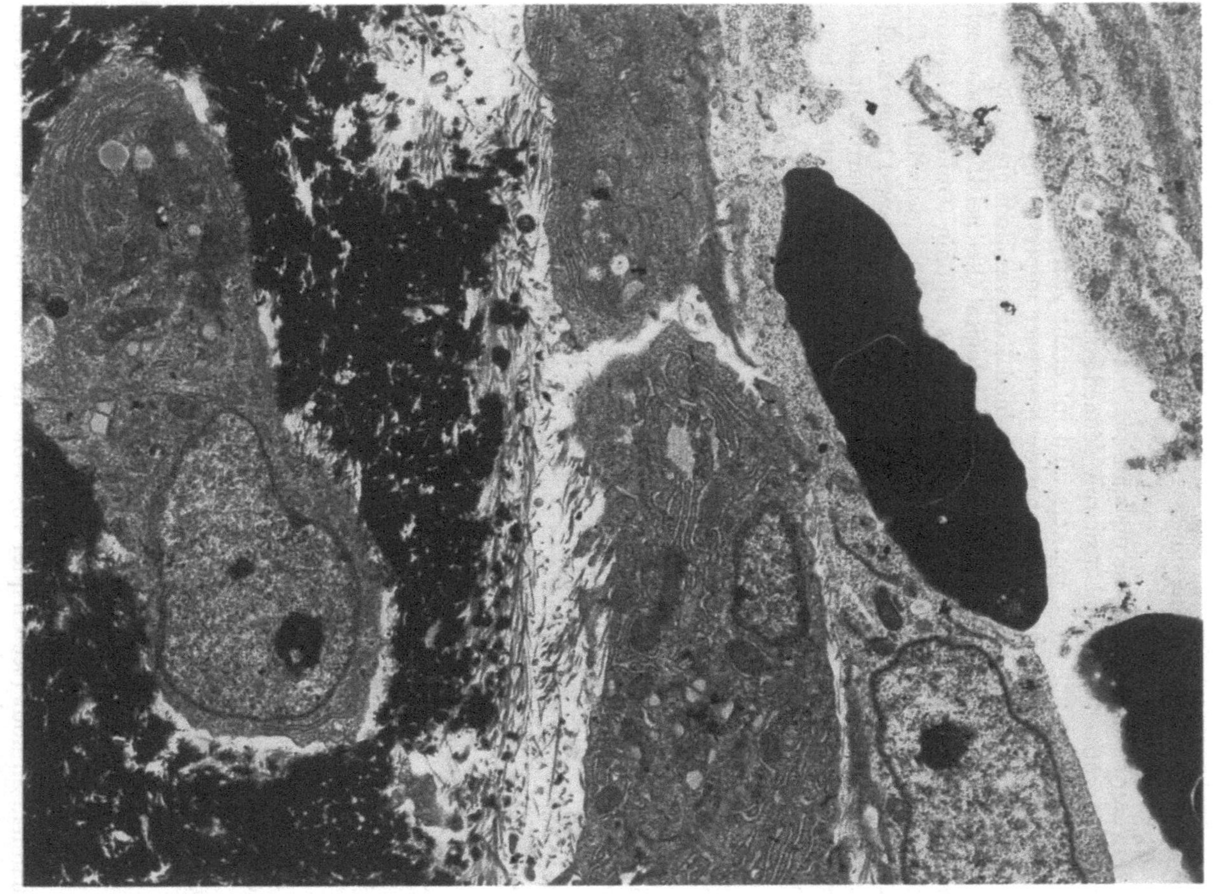

Fig. 8.35. EM of an ossifying chick tibia; 10 days' incubation. The intimate relationship of bone blood vessels to osteogenesis is evident. Note, from right to left, chick nucleated red blood corpuscles; capillary endothelial cell; two osteoblasts with dense cytoplasm and endoplasmic reticulum; calcified matrix and an osteocyte. (Original magnification ×3250)

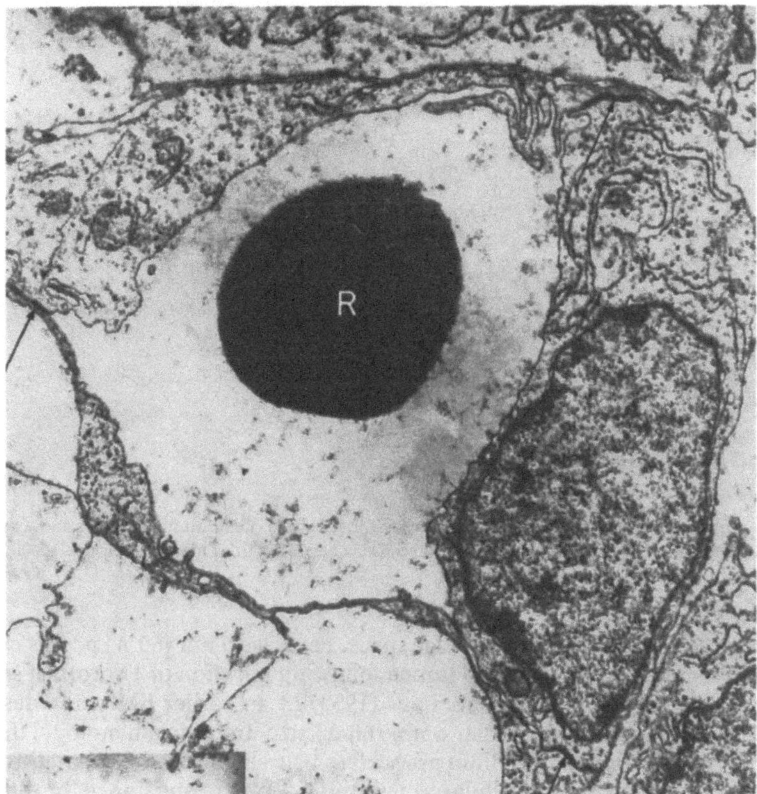

Fig. 8.36. Marrow capillary in transverse section, showing rat red blood corpuscle (R) and endothelial cells. Note angulated nucleus, and two junctional complexes (arrows). (EM: Original magnification ×3250)

mitochondria, numerous small vesicular profiles, and a sparse granular endoplasmic reticulum of the cisternal type. A Golgi apparatus is not conspicuous and does not achieve the same prominence of this organelle as in glandular or secreting cells. In addition, the cytoplasm contains scattered free ribosomes. All these appearances are non-specific and characteristic of undifferentiated mesenchyme cells which are not synthesizing protein to any marked extent. Endothelial cells can be distinguished from other primitive mesenchyme cells in bone marrow by the presence of terminal bars (Fig. 8.36), that is, points of junction between adjacent endothelial cells (Farquhar and Palade 1963). These are specialized regions of increased electron density of the apposed cell plasma membranes, which occur with obliteration of the normal 20 nm (200 Å) intercellular gap (Fig. 8.37, *overleaf*). A basement membrane is absent.

Weiss (1959, 1960, 1961) has described the EM appearances of marrow sinusoid endothelium and refers to it as made up of reticulo-endothelial cells. According to Weiss, ultrastructural wall deficiencies do occur in marrow endothelium, and these arise because of the highly labile nature of the reticulo-endothelial cells which wall off the vascular spaces. Certainly, large protein molecules can undoubtedly pass through into the parenchyma. ^{131}I-labelled serum albumin, for example, is unsuitable for blood volume estimations in bone marrow because it does not stay inside

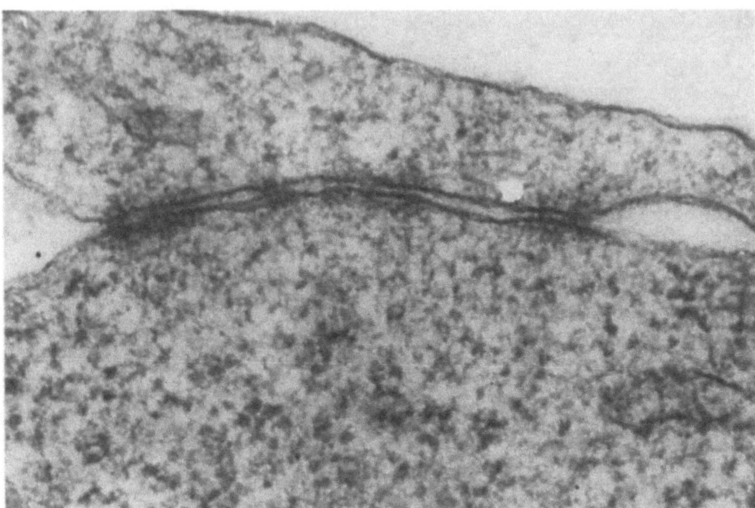

Fig. 8.37. Junctional complex between two chick endothelial cells. The unit membranes show increased electron density; microtubules straddle the intercellular gap. (Original magnification ×105 000)

the vessels but enters the extravascular space. Particles 6 nm (60 Å) or less can also be found lying outside the sinusoid lumen following injection of Thorotrast solution (Zamboni & Pease 1961). Pappenheimer (1953) in an earlier EM study described interendothelial spaces of a similar 6 nm (60 Å) size. In optical histology, the individual cells of vascular endothelium are seen to be welded together at their borders, as in a floor mosaic, by intercellular argentophilic cement substance. In the EM of marrow sinusoids, cement substance is not visualized: a 6 nm (60 Å) amorphous space separates the adjacent cell borders except where these are united at isolated points, the terminal bars. What is amorphous may nevertheless be substantial, albeit permeable.

It would seem, therefore, that sinus endothelium is open at the ultrastructural level. It is also open in a functional sense. Zamboni & Pease (1961) have shown how the sinusoid wall seen in cross-section is sometimes completed by an erythrocyte or a metamyelocyte, suggesting an open marrow circulation. Their results demonstrate the passage of blood cells from the marrow parenchyma, between the sinus endothelial cells, and then into the lumen. The older cells are pushed from behind by the tissue pressure of the younger, the wall of the sinusoid being at no time open, certainly not in the sense of having permanent fenestrae of 5 μm or more in diameter, allowing extravasation of whole blood to take place into the medullary stroma.

Origin of angioblasts

Embryonic blood vessels develop by two processes. *Angiogenesis* implies growth by budding off from existing vessels and by branching, a process which is held to be more prevalent. A second process is well documented in early embryogenesis and takes place in mesoderm close to yolk sac endoderm. In this situation it gives

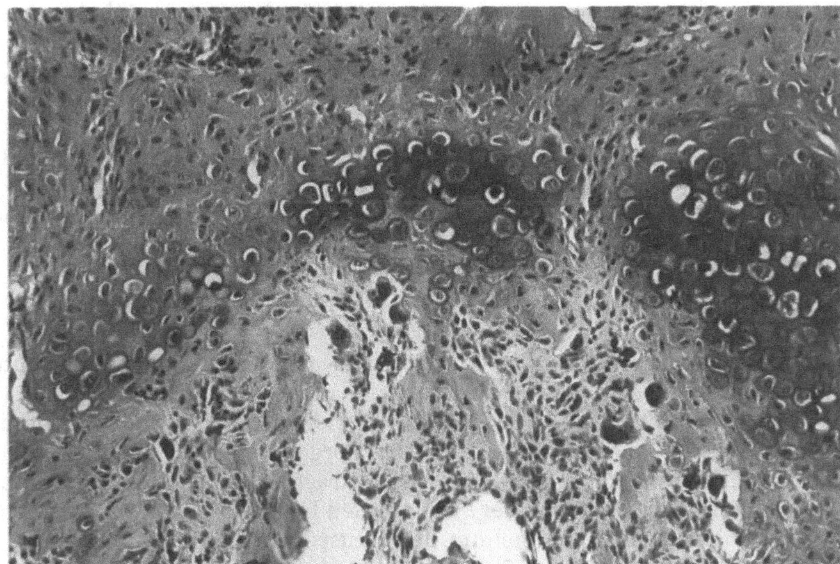

Fig. 8.38. (*see also Colour Plate section*) Photomicrograph of a section through the site of a rat fibular fracture (4 days postoperation), stained with Elbadawi's (1976) hexachrome modification of Movat's stain. The purple "giant cells" close to the blue cartilage, are primitive angioblastic islands in the EM.

rise to the vitelline and umbilical veins and chorionic vessels, by the formation of islands of *angioblasts*. The blood islands differentiate into blood vesicles comprising an endothelial wall containing blood plasma and haemocytoblasts. By coalescence primitive blood vessels arise.

Hudlicka & Tyler (1986) pointed out that both reparative and developing vascular endothelium have similar ultrastructural appearances. Angioblast islands were shown to occur in fracture repair (Fig. 8.38) for the first time by Hasán & Brookes (1990), who noted the similarity of fracture angioblasts in the EM 3–7 days postfracture, with those in the human yolk sac. Noden (1990) transplanted precursor populations from quail embryos into chick embryos and applied antibodies to quail endothelial cells in sections of chimaeric embryos fixed 2–5 days after surgery. He found that all intra-embryonic mesoderm except that of the notochord and prechordal plate contain angioblast precursors, which spread invasively and contribute to the formation of arteries, veins and capillaries; a third process for endothelial production. Angioblasts excised from quail trunk regions and transplanted to the embryonic head form locally appropriate blood vessels and cardiac outflow tract, conforming with Positional Information doctrine. Blood vascular development is controlled by the local mesenchyme and does not reside in the angioblasts themselves.

Regulators and mediators

In bone tissues, systemic regulators of bone metabolism and local mediators, including matrix molecules, cytokines, leukotrienes, prostaglandins and many other autocrine or paracrine factors, are involved in the control of the cells participating in bone formation and removal. New findings suggest that vascular endothelium may be part of a communication network operating between endothelial cells and a range of bone cell types. It seems that the endothelial cell and the microvasculature may make a central contribution to the regulation of bone physiology (Collin-Osdoby 1994).

For example, endothelin-1 is a vasoactive peptide produced by vascular endothelium, and is a potent endogenous vascular smooth muscle constrictor. Two subtypes of endothelin receptor have been cloned, sequenced and named endothelin-A and -B. Coessens *et al.* (1995) have used an *in vitro* bone perfusion model isolating the vascular endothelium from blood components. They found that endothelin-1 production by the bone vasculature was not altered after 24 hours of cold ischaemia. The response of endothelin-A receptor (but not the -B receptor) was significantly increased, the only change detected in vascular function at the end of the cold period. This mediated response may be involved in the pathogenesis of vasospasm. Coessens *et al.* (1996) have used two different models, the isolated nutrient tibial artery in an organ bath, and *in vitro* perfused canine tibial bones. Endothelin-1 caused contraction rings with and without endothelium, and its responses were not affected by L-arginine acetate complex, or by the removal of the endothelium. In perfused tibial bones it did not cause vascular relaxation. Other concordant data were gathered indicating the constrictor function of endothelin in the bone vasculature, an effect mediated only through endothelin-A receptors.

Moran & Wood (1992) have used an *ex vivo* canine tibia preparation perfused at constant rate with a Krebs–Ringer solution aerated with 95% O_2–5% CO_2 gas. Bolus injections of noradrenaline followed by acetylcholine were used to stimulate release of relaxing factors from endothelial smooth muscle. Acetylcholine significantly attenuated the response to the constrictor molecule, but faded after 4 hours of perfusion. Adding L-arginine (the precursor of endothelial-derived relaxing factor) restored attenuation of noradrenaline by acetylcholine. No attenuation was found after 6 hours of perfusion. Endothelial eccrine function can be demonstrated up to 4 hours, but not thereafter on account of substrate depletion. Similarly, Davis & Wood (1992) have shown that EDRF (endothelium-derived relaxing factor) and vasodilator prostaglandin are synthesized by intraosseous endothelial cells. Hence, these can modify vascular resistance in long bones and provide an autoregulatory mechanism responding to vasodilator stimuli.

Davis & Wood (1993) have also studied the effects of acidosis and alkalosis on vascular resistance in bone, employing noradrenaline and periarterial sympathetic nerve stimulation. They find that alkalosis increased baseline vascular resistance by 56% ($P<0.0001$), i.e. vascular constriction. Acidosis reduced resistance by 18% (vascular relaxation), and alkalosis enhanced by 66% the vasoconstrictor action of noradrenaline. Acidosis also reduced by 11% the effect of nerve stimulation (vascular relaxation). It is clear that the pH, i.e. the hydrogen ion concentration of locally perfusing blood, has a marked influence on the sensitivity of bone resistance vessels to circulating noradrenaline, or sympathetic nerve stimulation.

Endogenous nitric oxide (NO) has been shown to be a potent vasodilator in many tissue vascular beds. Blood flow to bone marrow, bone and spleen has now been measured in rats (Iversen *et al.* 1994) by the microsphere method (see Chapter 19). Marrow vascular resistance was reduced by about 30% of the baseline control, 10 hours after haemopoietic stimulation by either bleeding or rhG-CSF (recombinant human granulocyte colony-stimulating factor). Marrow blood flow increased to 260% of the baseline in bled rats, and nearly tripled after rhG-CSF. Nitric oxide synthase blockade brought about an increase in the vascular resistance and a reduction in marrow flow to 50% in bled rats, and 75% in those given rhG-CSF. There can be no doubt that NO regulates bone vascular tone, tending to increase blood flow rate in the marrow.

Osteoblasts produce prostaglandins E_2 and $F_{2\alpha}$. Ida *et al.* (1994) have demonstrated that bone-derived endothelial cells respond to these molecules and to human PTH, but not to bovine bPTH by an increase in calcium ions. cAMP and Ca^{2+} second messenger responses in bone-derived endothelium are nevertheless dependent on the cells being confluent.

As examples of hormonal bone regulatory factors, Kapitola *et al.* (1993) gave or withheld testosterone and oestradiol in large numbers of male and female rats, flow rates were measured by microspheres. They found that after gonadectomy blood flow rate in the tibia and distal femur was increased. Oestradiol depressed bone blood flow rate in both sexes. Testosterone in castrated rats depressed bone blood flow and similarly in spayed females. Unit bone density and ash weight fell after gonadectomy, but rose with oestradiol. Zallone & Teti (1993) in their review paper emphasized the protective effect of oestradiol against bone resorption.

The effect of exercise in increasing bone mass may be related to the inositol cascade, an intracellular transduction pathway for mechanical stimuli.

Conjunction of vascular territories in bone marrow

The vascular level at which union occurs between the various regions of bone marrow is debatable. Diaphyseal, metaphyseal and epiphyseal arteries appear to be discrete and quite separate when viscous suspensions are utilized for intra-arterial perfusion. In some of his studies on bone vascularization, de Marneffe (1951) used Neoprene latex as an injection mass, a particularly viscous medium to work with, and one not calculated to perfuse capillary beds. He showed that in these circumstances, corrosion specimens could be prepared of isolated metaphyseal or epiphyseal arterial subgroups lying in cancellous tissue.

Brookes and Harrison (1957) in their early work used a 70% Micropaque barium sulphate suspension for arterial perfusion of the rabbit, and showed radiographically the discrete occurrence of epiphyseal and metaphyseal arteries. The arterial packets were connected neither with each other nor with the branches of the nutrient artery. Hence, it seems that medullary arteries do not anastomose above the small artery level, and that normally the major nutrient groups, diaphyseal, metaphyseal and epiphyseal, largely supply their own territories.

When more fluid suspensions such as 50% Micropaque are used which can fill vessels down to the capillary bed, again there is little doubt that diaphyseal and metaphyseal arterial networks are linked only at the capillary or precapillary level. Fyfe (1964) found that ablation of the principal nutrient artery of the tibia in growing rabbits resulted in a central area of marrow ischaemia extending up to the growth cartilage at the knee. This was sharply demarcated at the metaphysis from a surrounding annular zone of vascular cancellous bone. In long-term rabbit experiments, however, Brookes (1957, 1960b) showed that metaphyseal arteries can take over the territory of the principal nutrient vessels (Figs 2.24–2.27). On the other hand, the extent to which epiphyseal arteries anastomose with metaphyseal ones is still not entirely resolved.

In the human fetus there is an interval in the last 5 months of intra-uterine life when the forerunners of the epiphyseal arteries in the cartilage canals make some anastomotic union across the growth cartilage with vessels in the metaphysis (Figs 8.39, 10.5, 10.6). However, it is generally conceded that in infancy and after, the presence of a growth cartilage isolates the arteries of the epiphysis. This of course does not gainsay the existence of an extra-osseous vascular union between epiphyseal and metaphyseal arteries, brought about through their common stems of origin.

Even in an adult bone after the epiphysis has fused with the shaft, it is uncertain whether any considerable arterial connection exists across the synostosis (Fig. 8.31). The perfusion results obtained by some authors indicate that union occurs here principally at the capillary level (Brookes and Harrison 1957) or at the small artery level (Trueta 1957, in the case of the head and neck of the human femur). On the other hand, Cretin (1952) and Courbil (1954) insist that arterial penetration of the synostosis is negligible. In their view, arteries in adult epiphyses are isolated by the presence of the epiphyseal scar. More recently, Watermann (1961) examined histologically the synostosis in adult human knee joints. He found no vascular passage at all of the epiphyseal scar in a 19 year old. In another subject 30 years of age, many holes were present in the bone plate separating epiphysis from metaphysis, but they were largely full of fat and only rare vessels traversing them were observed. Crock (1967), in his perfusion study on human bones, supplies evidence suggesting that small arteries cross the scar line in abundance in senescent material. It seems that arterial union across the epiphyseal scar is related to senescence; in youth, the synostotic scar prevents arterial union of the two circulations.

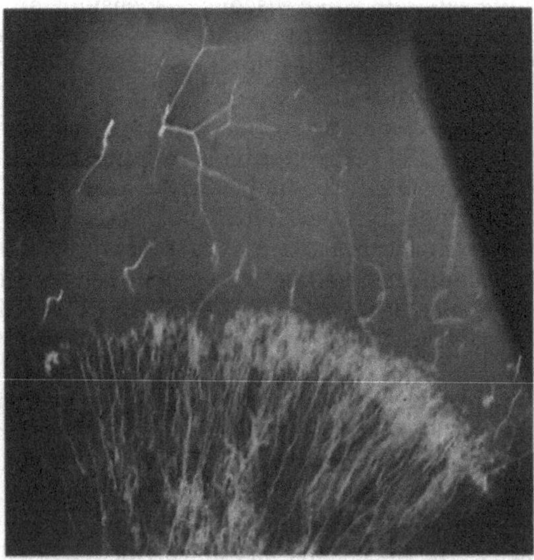

Fig. 8.39. Coronal section at upper end of human fetal femur (22 cm CR length), showing metaphyseal arteries and occasional communicating cartilage canals. (Original magnification ×5)

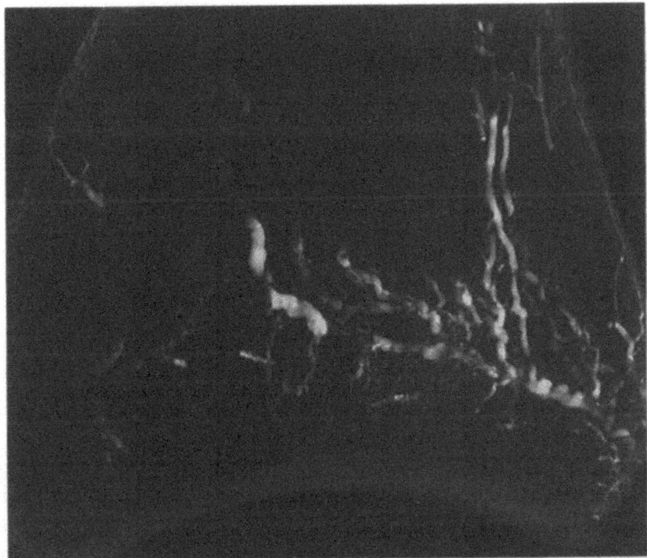

Fig. 8.40. Venogram of coronal section of the lower end of a human tibia. Note free venous connection between metaphysis and epiphysis after the demise of the growth cartilage (Original magnification ×2)

It also seems probable that wide venous connections normally occur between the two cancellous territories in adult bones. Retrograde venography of mature long bones usually shows capacious venous sinuses which arise in the epiphysis and traverse the epiphyseal scar to join the central venous sinus (Fig. 8.40).

On balance, it seems that the epiphyseal, metaphyseal and diaphyseal regions of bone marrow are not normally united at an arterial level. Ligation of the principal nutrient artery (Huggins & Wiege 1939; Bragdon *et al.* 1949; Brookes 1960b), disruption of metaphyseal nutrients (Harris 1933; Trueta & Amato 1960) and damage to epiphyseal arteries, for example, the middle genicular (Nussbaum 1923), all lead to profound structural changes in bone marrow, usually temporary in nature. Such evidence is a further indication that disparate vascular territories exist within the marrow and that the arteries supplying them are end-arteries. Given sufficient time, however, new channels are formed (Brookes 1957, 1960b), vascular patterns are restored, and medullary structure is re-established.

Chapter 9
Cortex and periosteum

Although it has been known for three centuries that compact bone is irrigated by numerous small vessels, it is only in recent times that it has become possible to investigate with any precision the anatomical character and distribution of these vessels in long bones. Histology, microradiography, and, recently molecular biological techniques have all helped to elucidate new facts on the vascular anatomy of bone cortex, and serve to focus attention on the microcirculation as an indispensable factor in the production of bone substance, and the regulation of bone metabolism.

Bone structure

The internal structure of bone cortex is very variable (Amprino 1968). In man, fetal cortex is made up of layers of bone *trabeculae* separated by vascular tissue; in early childhood the trabecular spaces become filled with *primary osteones* (Gebhardt 1901), that is, tiny cylinders of concentric lamellae, formed around a central vascular space. *Circumferential lamellae* are deposited at the periosteal and endosteal surfaces and have been designated surface bone by Smith (1960). Later, secondary, tertiary and quaternary osteones, otherwise called *Haversian systems*, are formed by the substitution of new concentric lamellae in sites prepared by the local removal of older bone cortex. As for the blood vessels, multiple vessels occur in the intertrabecular spaces of *fetal cortex*; two or three vessels occur in a toddler's *primary osteones*; but the vascular canals of Haversian systems generally contain only a single vessel in skeletally mature cortex (Brookes & Harrison 1957; Peterson *et al.* 1959).

Blood vessels in the diaphysis

Less than 40 years ago, the vessels in compact bone were generally conceived of along conventional lines (Fig. 9.1) in terms of a plexus of arteries, veins and capillaries, with the arterial blood coming from periosteal and medullary vessels, and venous blood passing predominantly into the medulla (Testut & Latarjet 1948). Nowadays it is recognized that the branches of the nutrient artery in bone marrow are *distributive* in function. Medullary arterioles, however, control the

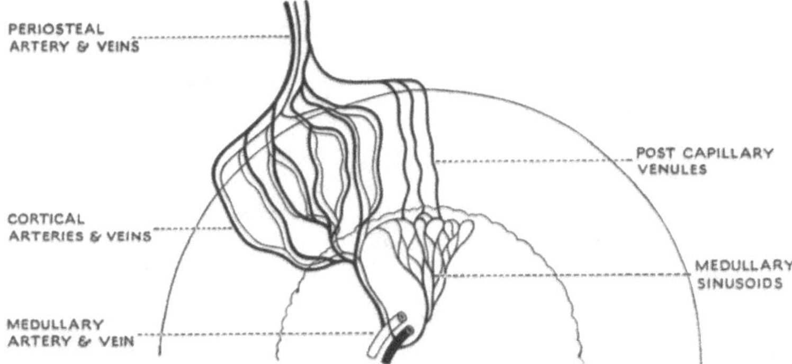

Fig. 9.1. Drawing to illustrate a dated view of the blood supply to bone cortex, according to which an artery and a vein, at least, are present in every vascular canal.

blood flow rate and are the *resistance* vessels of the osseous circulation. They diminish in calibre from 100 μm to the 5 μm metarterioles. The latter are equipped with *precapillary sphincters*, and feed into the cortical capillaries and marrow sinusoids, the *capacitance* or reservoir vessels of the cortex and marrow. They regulate the volume of blood in bone.

From the investigations of Testut (1880), Weidenreich (1923), Marneffe (1951), Brookes & Harrison (1957), Ham & Leeson (1964), Brookes (1971), Rhinelander (1980), Dillaman (1984) and Bridgeman & Brookes (1996) and many others, the characteristic capacitance vessel to be found in compact bone is a simple endothelial tube of unusual diameter, about 15–30 μm, and can be of unusual length, possibly 2 cm or more in large mammals (Figs 9.2, 9.3, *overleaf*). Cortical capillaries situated near the endosteal surface of the bone, where they are continuous with marrow sinusoids, tend to have a wider calibre than the capillaries in the cortex generally.

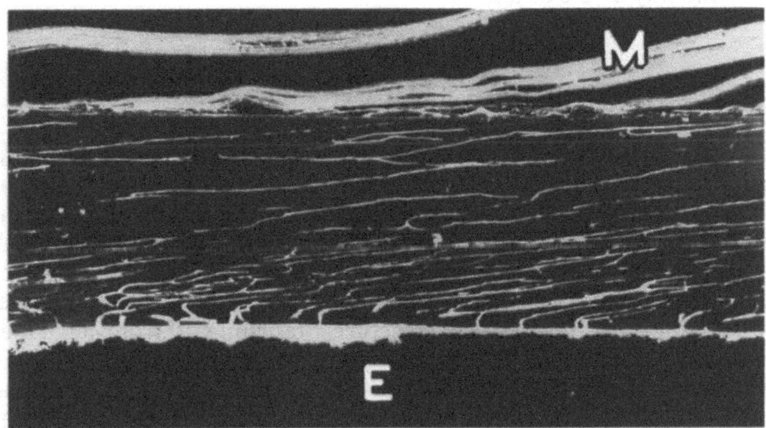

Fig. 9.2. These capillaries in monkey bone cortex largely belong to the periosteal vascular radiation. Those in a thin bony layer close to the marrow cavity (E) belong to the endosteal group of cortical vessels. M, Muscle fasciculi. (Original magnification ×17)

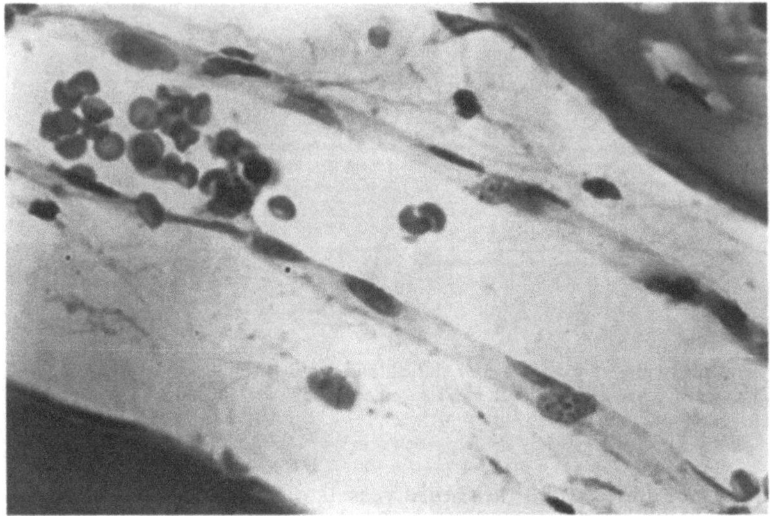

Fig. 9.3. A capillary in the cortex of a human fetal tibia. Its calibre is about 30 μm.

This does not permit the conclusion that blood flows in the cortical capillaries from the periosteal surface into the marrow sinusoids, on the analogy of capillaries widening into venules as in other tissues (Cohen & Harris 1958; Heřt & Hladíková 1961). The continuity of marrow sinusoids with cortical capillaries can give no indication of the direction of blood flow in the cortex. It does, however, draw attention to some basic problems in the cortical microcirculation: namely, what is the afferent source of the blood to compact bone, and how is venous drainage effected? What is the direction of blood flow in cortex? From the periosteum inwards or from the marrow outwards, or both? This elementary description of cortical vessels in young bone suggests that the direction of flow is uniform, one way or the other.

Young cortex: medullary supply

Thick-section histology shows that not all vessels in the cortex are endothelial tubes. In the endosteal region, sparse vessels occur whose endothelial lining is associated with a coat of pericytes, possibly contractile (Fig. 8.19). At the junction of these vessels with the general cortical vascular network, they are actually narrower than the cortical capillaries. Microradiographic methods show that they belong to the arterial side of the circulation (Figs 9.4, 9.5, 9.7, 9.9) and are arterioles, possessing a two-layered wall structure, branching off from small medullary arteries.

In the long bones of rats, rabbits and dogs (Brookes 1971, 1986; Rhinelander 1980), as well as human fetal and adolescent material (Brookes 1990b), intra-arterial perfusion of barium sulphate shows that the larger branches of the nutrient artery lie generally in a subcortical location and supply both cortex and marrow *in parallel*, and not in series. Histologically these are “small arteries”

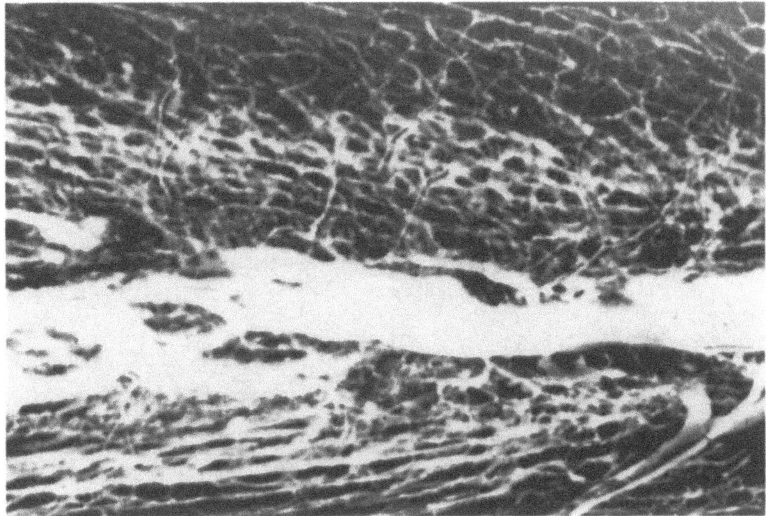

Fig. 9.4. Microangiograph of a human fetal tibia, showing nutrient arteries giving off straight arterioles at right angles to the bone axis. (Original magnification ×13)

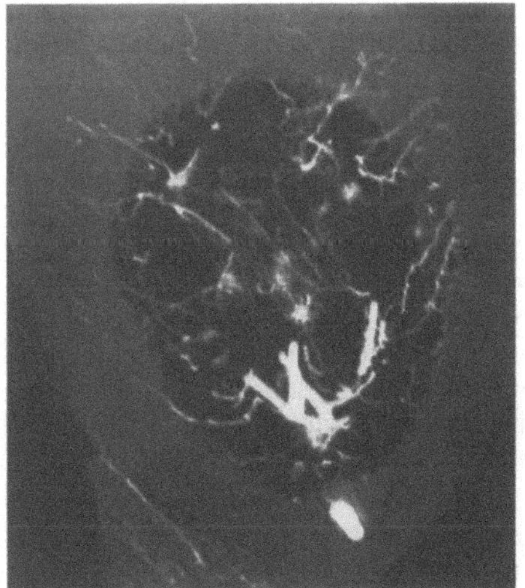

Fig. 9.5. Cross-sectional arteriogram of a normal rabbit tibia, the contralateral to that shown in Fig. 9.6. The cortex has a medullary arterial supply. (Original magnification ×8)

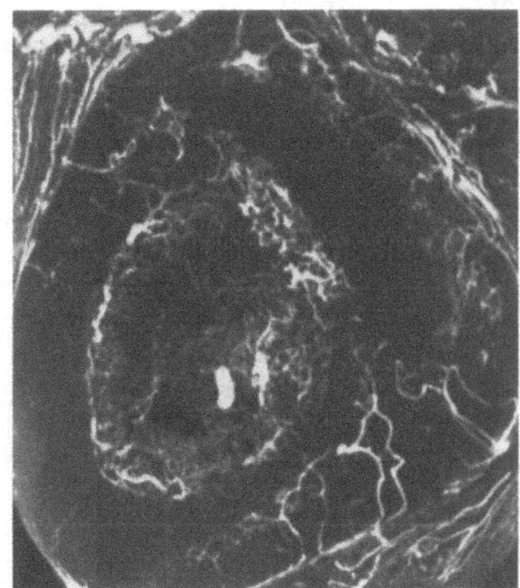

Fig. 9.6 . A periosteal arterial supply to the cortex is present after ligation of the nutrient artery. (Original magnification ×8)

with much elastic tissue in the tunica media. They give rise to arterioles whose finest branches, the metarterioles, terminate in the marrow sinusoids, or penetrate the bone endosteally to end in the cortical capillary reservoir.

Arterioles and precapillaries have been observed by many workers (Brookes & Harrison 1957; Brookes 1960a,b; Nelson *et al.* 1960; Rhinelander & Baragry 1962;

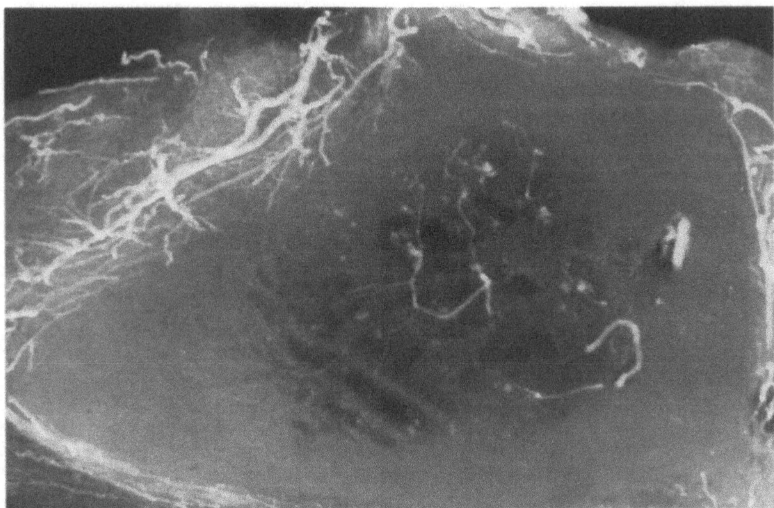

Fig. 9.7. Cross-sectional arteriogram of a human tibia removed because of femoral sarcoma. A periosteal arterial supply to the cortex is absent. (Original magnification ×2.7)

Rhinelander 1968), passing through the cortex towards the periosteal surface. It must be emphasized that they amount to but a small fraction of the simple capillaries present everywhere in bone cortex, the functional vascular lattice permitting chemical exchange between blood and bone (Fig. 9.4).

When periosteum and surrounding muscle are well perfused, a similar penetration of the external surface of the cortex by periosteal arterioles is not seen. A minor exception to this is that diaphyseal zygapophyses such as the linea aspera, gluteal tuberosity and soleal line, are pierced by a few periosteal arterioles. Hence, bone angiography suggests that the arterial blood input to the cortex of long bones, *in youth*, comes overwhelmingly from the marrow, a principle first emphasized by Brookes and Harrison (1957). It is interesting to note that shortly after Wilhelm von Roentgen's discovery of X-rays (1895), Soulié (1904) used bone angiography in dogs, and pointed out the absence of an anastomosis between medullary arteries in bone cortex and the periosteum.

Centrifugal flow in young bone cortex

The Haversian cortical capillaries freely communicate with medullary sinusoids internally, and with periosteal capillaries externally. Cortical capillaries pass directly into the periosteal capillary network in regions lacking muscle attachment and are continuous with intramuscular venules, where muscles have a fleshy attachment. Hence, the anatomical evidence suggests that there is a centrifugal flow of blood from the endosteal to the periosteal surface of the cortex (Brookes 1971), the blood current draining ultimately into periosteal and intramuscular veins. These provide a mechanism for cortical venous escape.

Centrifugal blood flow has been directly observed in living human femoral bone cortex after the injection of Evans Blue during amputation (Lamas

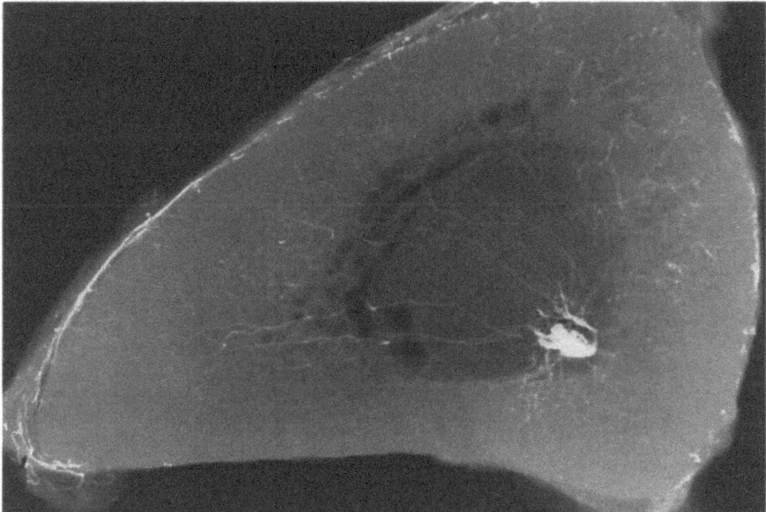

Fig. 9.8. Cross-sectional arteriogram of a human tibia, from a limb amputated because of peripheral occlusive vascular disease. A periosteal arterial supply is present. (Original magnification ×2.7)

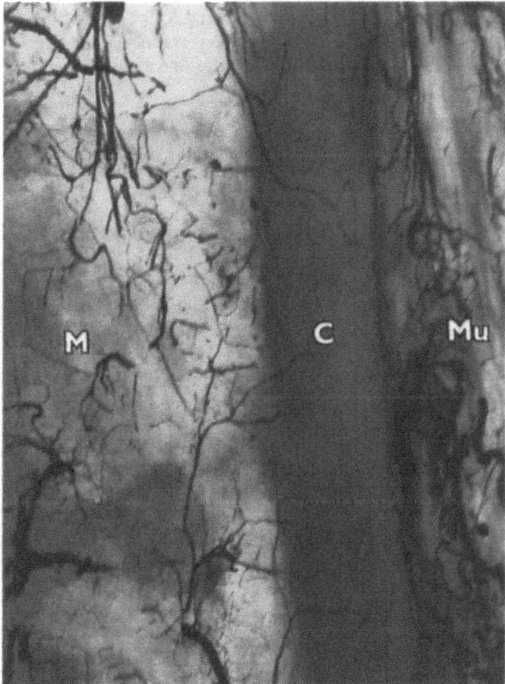

Fig. 9.9. Arteriogram of a longitudinal section of a normal human tibia. Subcortical branches of medullary arteries (M) pass centrifugally into the cortex (C). Arteries in attached muscle (Mu) do not penetrate the underlying bone. (Original magnification ×2.7)

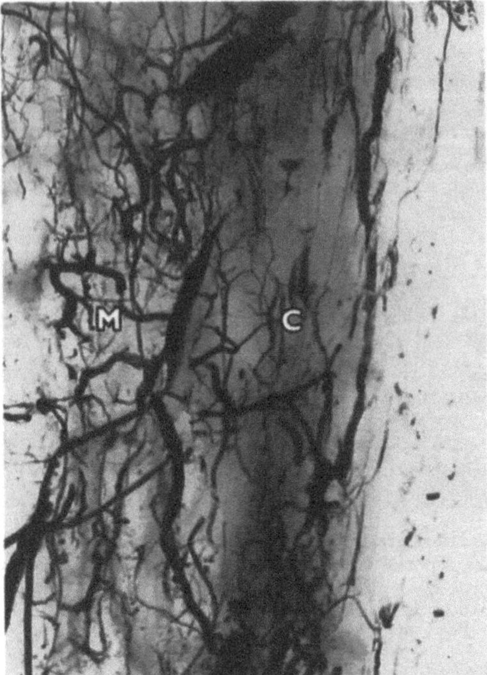

Fig. 9.10. Arteriogram of a longitudinal section of a human tibia, amputated for peripheral occlusive vascular disease. The cortical vessels (C) and medullary vessels (M) are grossly irregular. Periosteal arteries penetrate the ischaemic and porotic bone. (Original magnification ×2.7)

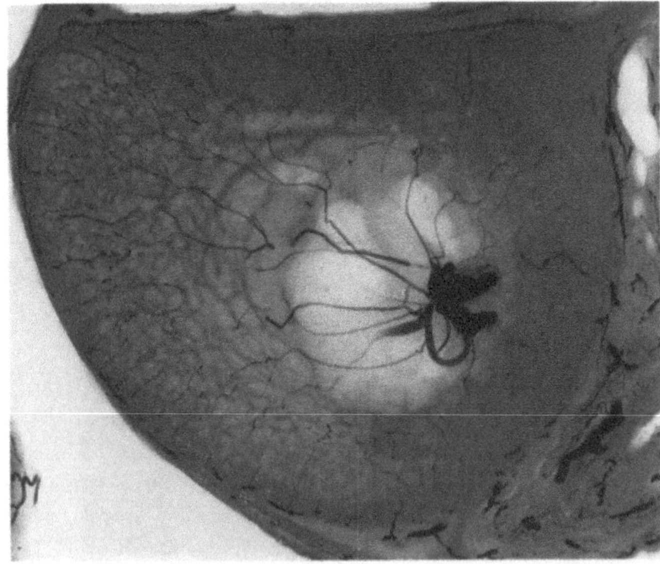

Fig. 9.11. Cross-sectional arteriogram of the tibia from an individual aged 59 years (leg amputated because of pyarthrosis of the knee joint), showing periosteal and medullary arterioles in the cortex. A few periosteo-medullary anastomoses are also present. (Original magnification ×2)

et al. 1946). Centrifugal uptake of Disulphine Blue has also been demonstrated in the cortex of rabbit long bones (Gunst 1980). The use of ferritin has confirmed the presence of centrifugal flow in intact chick bone; and not only of blood, but also of extravascular bone water in the tibial cortex (Dillaman 1984; Montgomery *et al.* 1988; Dillaman *et al.* 1991).

A small proportion of adult vascular canals in histological sections contain two fine vessels (Bloom & Fawcett 1962). However, it seems hardly valid to distinguish between the two on the basis of calibre alone as was done by Ham and Leeson (1964), who suggested that in these instances the larger vessel was a venule. High power microscopy of barium-perfused material, on the other hand, might well confirm that the smaller of the two was a precapillary, the larger vessel belonging to the general vascular lattice. Precapillary pericytes do not form a tightly packed layer around the endothelial coat, but are loosely arranged and are best seen in the light microscope not in transverse but longitudinal sections (Fig. 8.19).

Biomechanics of the osseous circulation

The following haemodynamic factors operate in the cortex.

Muscle pump

Systemic venous valves are plentiful in the veins lying in intermuscular spaces. Muscle contraction empties the veins. The venous valves, however, prevent retrograde flow. It follows that muscle activity pumps the blood from the bone towards the heart (Langer 1876). In youthful bone, the flow of blood in the cortical capillaries is centrifugal, from the marrow to the periosteum. In a venous sense, this might well apply to ageing bone; even with the marrow cavity packed with cement, and the cortex supplied wholly by periosteal arterioles, blood flow in the cortical capillaries is still centrifugal allowing venous escape at the periosteal surface. With an extant marrow, venous escape presumably has an ebb and flow action, fluctuating between periosteum and marrow in response to intermittent muscle contractions.

Driving pressure

Pressure within the marrow cavity is considerably higher (45–60 mmHg) than the 12–15 mmHg in extraosseous capillaries. The vascular driving pressure is therefore centrifugal across the cortex, from marrow to periosteum.

Pulse pressure

This is of the order of 8–10 mmHg in bone marrow, confined in an unyielding cortical container (P.W.T. Stolk, 1987, personal communication). Thus the pulse pressure promotes centrifugal flow at each heart beat.

Impact forces

These have been demonstrated photographically during human locomotion as a wave of deformation passing up the limb (H. Light, 1987, personal communication). In a simulated laboratory exercise utilizing rabbits, impact forces have been demonstrated manometrically to pass along the bone marrow. These add to the pre-existing medullary pressures, and wring out the blood from the marrow as if it were a sponge.

Blood flow rate

In round figures, 17% of the cardiac output is delivered to the skeleton in the resting adult human; skeletal perfusion rate as an overall average is 12 ml 100 g^{-1} min^{-1} (Charkes *et al.* 1979a). In rats the corresponding values are 10% of the cardiac output and 20 ml 100 g/min^{-1} for skeletal flow (Brookes 1970; Charkes *et al.* 1979b, and many others).

Flow partition

Kelly (1973) using hydrogen washout flow measurement in the canine tibia found that 71% of the nutrient flow went to the cortex; 30% went to the marrow. His dogs were of unstated age. Brookes (1971) supplied volumetric data in rat femora, from which it can be calculated that the marrow accounts for 90% of the diaphyseal blood volume in 24-month-old rats, and the cortex received 10%. Similarly, M. Okubo (1977, personal communication) using microspheres for blood flow measurement in dogs, found that 88% of the femoral diaphyseal flow went to the marrow, and 12% to the cortex.

Evidence for blood supply to young bone

Drinker *et al.* (1922) injected India ink *in vivo* in dogs and found that ink did not penetrate from the periosteum into the underlying cortex. This justified their isolated canine tibia model for venous collection flow studies. In their view a periosteal arterial supply to the canine tibia was negligible. Johnson (1927), often misquoted, failed to stain dog diaphyseal cortex with India ink, injected solely through the periosteal system, and therefore chose to neglect it. Using barium sulphate perfusion and microangiography, Brookes & Harrison (1957 (rabbit)) and Brookes (1958a (fetus); 1958b (rat); 1963; 1986 (dog)) showed that diaphyseal nutrient arteries give off arterioles which join the cortical capillaries and also the marrow sinusoids; i.e. the two arterial supplies to bone marrow and to cortex are in parallel. Furthermore, periosteal capillaries communicate freely with cortical capillaries, and they in turn with the sinusoids of bone marrow in young material. The above results have recently been confirmed by Skawina *et al.* (1994a), by means of microvascular corrosion casts, who found that "the medullary arteries supplied both bone cortex and marrow", and "there was no arterial supply to the (fetal) shaft cortex from the periosteal side".

Contrary opinion

De Bruyn *et al.* (1970) in a wholly India ink study believed that nutrient artery blood normally feeds into the cortical capillaries, but then exits into the marrow sinusoids. Trias & Fery (1979) concluded in their adult mongrel dogs that "The direction of arterial blood flow.... is predominantly centrifugal while the venous drainage is centripetal". Their finding that "in an Haversian canal there is usually only one vessel, and this has the structure of a capillary", suggests their dogs were young. de Saint-Georges & Miller (1992) injected India ink into 3-month-old rats. They report that "most of the vascular flow appears to be centripetally through the diaphyseal cortex, and this appears to be the primary blood supply for the adjacent bone marrow". The authors state that most of their results are based on inadequately filled preparations. One fully filled specimen (their Fig. 2), shows the cortical vessels, sparse in relation to the marrow sinusoids, passing obliquely to the external surface, and manifestly bifurcating towards the periosteal surface, becoming thinner as they go. In any other tissue, such a vascular layout would coincide with a blood current from stem vessel to branches; from thicker to thinner; and here in bone cortex, from within outwards.

Regardless of the above contrary opinions, centrifugal blood flow in the cortex of young long bones has also been demonstrated after the injection of intravital dyes in the living human femoral cortex during amputation (Lamas *et al.* 1946 (Evans Blue)), and in the rabbit (Gunst 1980 (Disulphine Blue)). In young rats, Dillaman (1984) has shown a transcortical passage of ferritin from marrow to periosteum. The passage of horseradish peroxidase has been similarly tracked, suggesting that not only is the blood flow centrifugal in young material, but also the movement of bone water across the entire cortex (Montgomery *et al.* 1988; Dillaman *et al.* 1991).

The cortex of long bones is permeated overwhelmingly by simple capillaries. The principal features of the cortical vascular lattice are the great length of the capillaries, and the fact that it is sandwiched between an external periosteal and an internal medullary circulation. In addition, terminal branches of medullary arteries course centrifugally into the cortex as far as the intermediate zone of the transverse cortical profile (Figs 9.26, 9.35–9.37).

Concept of a dual blood supply

The general presence of a single vessel in an Haversian canal was denied by Trueta (1968) and Crock (1967), both of whom supported the concept of a dual arterial supply to bone cortex; that is, from the periosteum and the marrow. Crock worked on aged post-mortem human material, but did not take into account that osteone formation increases with age (Amprino & Bairatti 1936; Amprino 1968). Resorption cavities are frequent in senescent bone, even in aged rats, whose bone cortex in maturity, unlike the human, shows very few osteones. Such cavities, the preliminary phase of osteonic substitution, may contain several capillaries and sometimes, in aged material, even medullary tissue (Figs 9.12, 9.13). Crock (1967) showed a perfusion preparation in which two vessels are present in one large vascular space, and writes that this "merits close examination as it shows arteries and veins together in the osteones". From its size, this vascular space appeared to be a resorption cavity. No histological control was offered of what at the time was an important piece of evidence for the dual supply concept.

Trueta (1968) believed that there are two or three vessels in Haversian canals and two blood currents, one counter to the other. He conjectured that the current from the marrow is largely concerned with haemopoiesis. It would appear to be inconsiderable because of "the large vein or veins leaving the bone with the nutrient artery, thus indicating that a large outflow of blood was not taking place through the cortex". He goes on to surmise that the blood flowing from the periosteum into the bone is mainly responsible for osteogenesis in the cortex (page 167 of his treatise). How the bone cells in the cortex recognize blood of periosteal origin and use it, and distinguish it from marrow blood which is rejected, was not explained.

De Bruyn *et al.* (1970) in rats, rabbits and guinea pigs, Trias & Fery (1979) in young dogs, and de Saint-Georges & Miller (1992) in rats, have reported findings in support of a dual blood supply to bone cortex. De Bruyn *et al.* (1970), regarded cortical capillaries as venous structures and assumed from the start that cortical blood flow is centripetal; and also that the major blood supply to the bone marrow is "transosteal" from the periosteal and cortical capillaries. Trias & Fery (1979) find it difficult to draw inferences on the direction of blood flow in bone from their studies on bone vasculature. de Saint-Georges & Miller (1992) are convinced centripetalists. The above three groups of investigators, however, all confirm the anatomical continuity of the fine vessels of the periosteum, cortex and bone marrow. On the other hand, Lopez-Curto *et al.* (1980) find in dogs that the "capillary beds of marrow and cortex are totally independent" and "no arteriolar or capillary anastomoses were observed linking these separate beds". However, even these workers agree that cortical venous drainage is centrifugal, but consider that periosteal and nutrient arteries supply the cortex irrespective of age.

It seems that the concept of a dual blood supply to young or mature bone (35–40 years of age) is ill-founded. On the other hand, it does apply to bone in senescence.

Old cortex: medullary and periosteal supply

Descriptions of canals as normally containing arteries, veins and capillaries (Steinbach *et al.* 1957; Johnston *et al.* 1958) are invariably lacking in supporting visual evidence and appear to stem from Langer's classical account in 1876. He described in detail how periosteal arteries and veins enter the cortex everywhere to participate, together with the medullary vascular system, in the vascularization of compact bone. He insisted that at least two vessels, an artery and a vein, are normally to be found in an Haversian canal, and that larger spaces often occur in the cortex which contain a leash of vessels. Stellate vascular figures ("Gefässsterne") were also commonly encountered by Langer in his diligent examination of human bone. The age and source of the material, tibiae in the main, used in Langer's work on adult bone cortex are not, however, given in his essay. His results correspond closely with the findings in ischaemic and ageing material (Figs 9.6, 9.8, 9.10–9.12, 9.30, 9.31). It follows that senescence and vascular decline are appropriately linked to those accounts of cortical vascularization which emphasize a periosteal arterial supply to bone cortex, with multiple vessels in vascular canals, and the frequent occurrence of large vascular spaces.

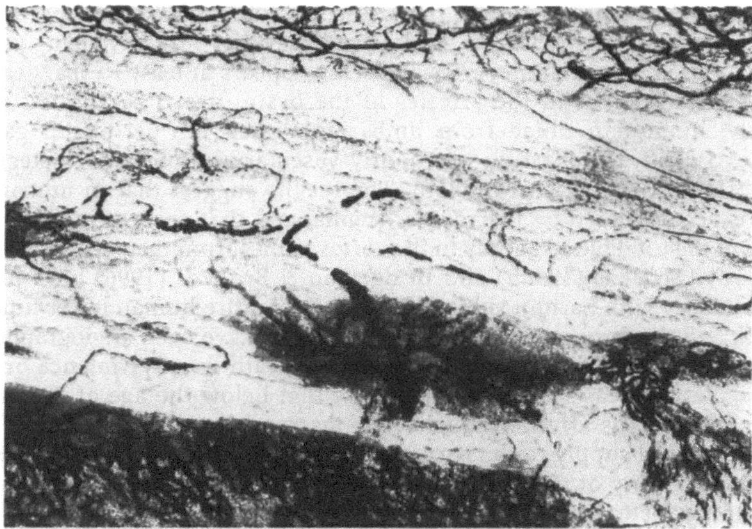

Fig. 9.12. India ink preparation of senescent rat bone cortex, showing the presence of irregular cortical vessels and areas of medullary substitution. (Original magnification ×53)

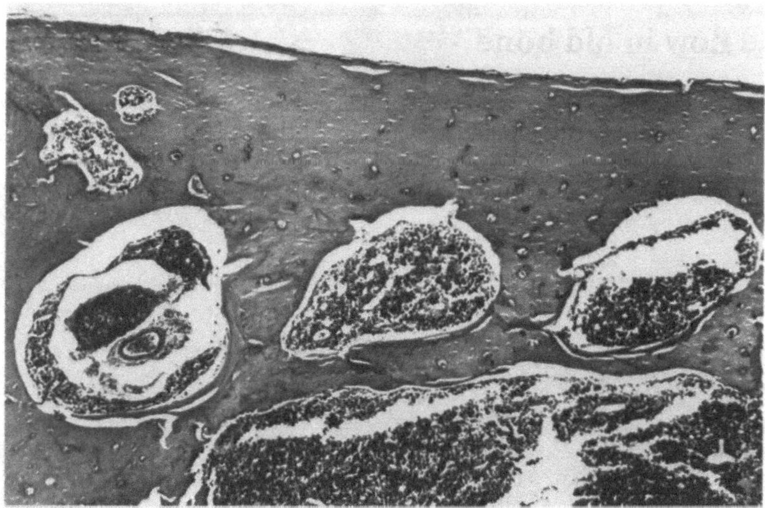

Fig. 9.13. Paraffin section of Fig. 9.12, showing osteoporotic cavities filled with marrow. (Original magnification ×37)

In the laboratory rat, cortical flow normally declines exponentially with age, so that bone vascularity in the aged rat is reduced to a tenth of what it was in youth (Brookes 1971). Experimentally, obstruction of the nutrient artery (Brookes 1960b) or extra-osseous systemic arteries (de Marneffe 1951) in rabbit long bones, causes osteoporosis and the development of a periosteal arterial supply to the now ischaemic bone.

According to Ramseier (1962), the arteries of human bone marrow are commonly subject to arteriosclerosis, increasing in severity with advancing years. He reported that grade for grade, arterial disease appears at least 10 years earlier in femoral marrow than in the arteries of the brain, heart, or striated muscle. Similarly, in human tibiae from limbs amputated for peripheral gangrene (Brookes 1960a), the marrow was poorly vascularized and a periosteal blood supply to the cortex was prominent. The results suggest that in human bone, ageing is accompanied by marrow ischaemia, and that an ever increasing proportion of the total blood supply to the cortex comes from the periosteal vessels.

Recently, Brookes (1990b) and Bridgeman & Brookes (1996) have perfused intravascularly with barium sulphate suspension entire human lower limbs post mortem, and the femoral diaphyses of 15 subjects have been angiographed. The age at death ranged from 21 to 91 years, and death was by violence or supradiaphragmatic disease. The results suggest that below the age of 35 years, the diaphyseal cortex is arterialized from the marrow alone (Fig. 9.14b). After this time, the arterial supply to the cortex is increasingly periosteal (Figs 9.15, 9.16), and the vascularity of the mid-shaft marrow diminishes. In advanced years (70 plus) the periosteal supply is dominant (Fig. 9.17, *overleaf*). In a male aged 56 years, the upper femur had been reamed and the stem of a hip prosthesis implanted in the marrow cavity using acrylic cement, 4 years before death. Angiography shows that the femoral cortex in life was wholly sustained by the periosteum (Figs 9.18, 9.19, *overleaf*).

Blood flow in old bone

Both Crock (1967) and Trueta (1968) illustrated a periosteal supply to human bone cortex, significantly in aged specimens of the seventh decade. Nelson *et al.*

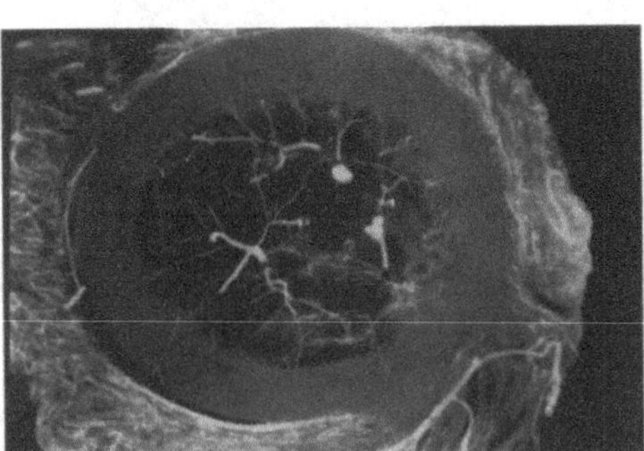

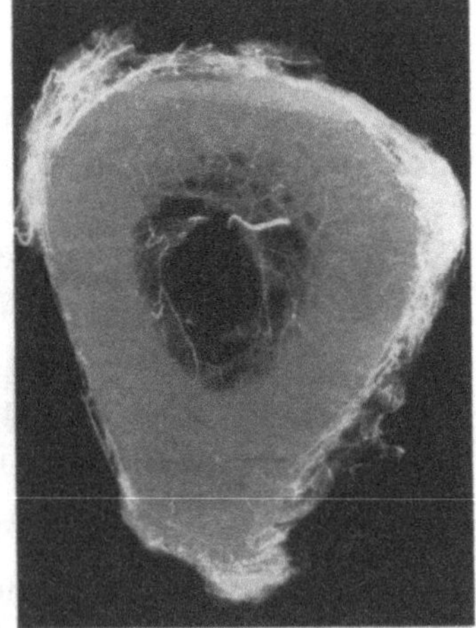

Fig. 9.14. **a** Angiograph of transverse section of a femur (2 years old), perfused *in vivo*. The arterial supply to the cortex is from the marrow only. The well-filled periosteum does not supply the cortex. (Original magnification ×3) **b** Angiograph of transverse section of a femur perfused 3 days post-mortem; youth aged 21 years who died by violence. Central necrosis of the marrow is present, but the peripheral arteries are numerous and robust. The arteries supply the entire cortex, except the linea aspera. (Original magnification ×3)

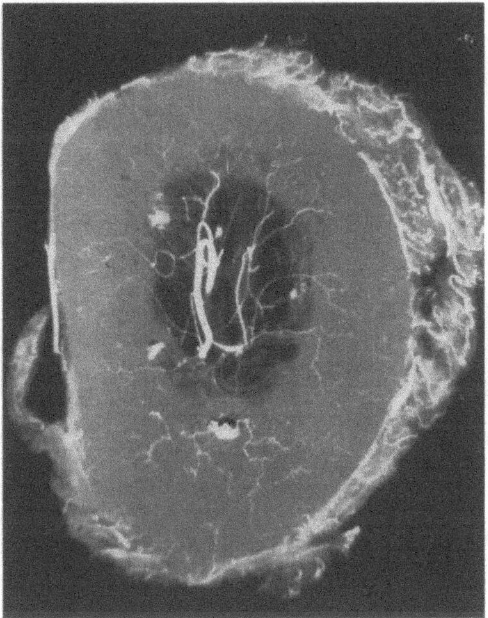

Fig. 9.15. Angiograph of transverse section of femur aged 42 years. The medullary arteries are robust, and supply the cortex entirely, except in the right posterior quadrant where periosteal arterial traces are detectable. (Original magnification ×3)

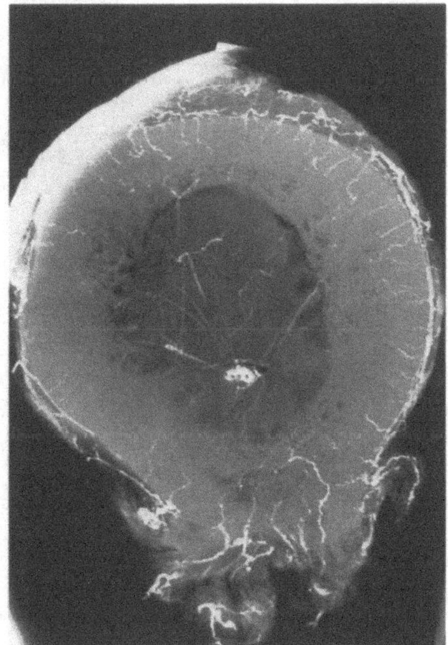

Fig. 9.16. Angiograph of transverse section of femur aged 65 years (linea aspera, below), showing a dominant periosteal arterial supply to the cortex. The barium traces represent arterioles. The marrow is ischaemic. (Original magnification ×4)

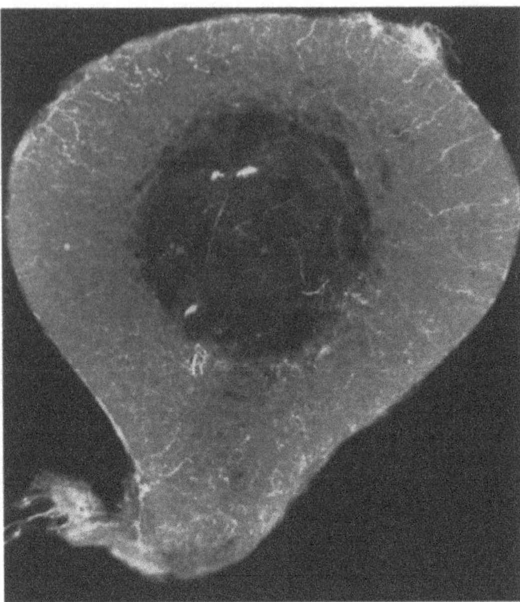

Fig. 9.17. Angiograph of transverse section of femur aged 72 years. The marrow is ischaemic. The cortex is supplied almost wholly from the periosteum. (Original magnification ×2.5)

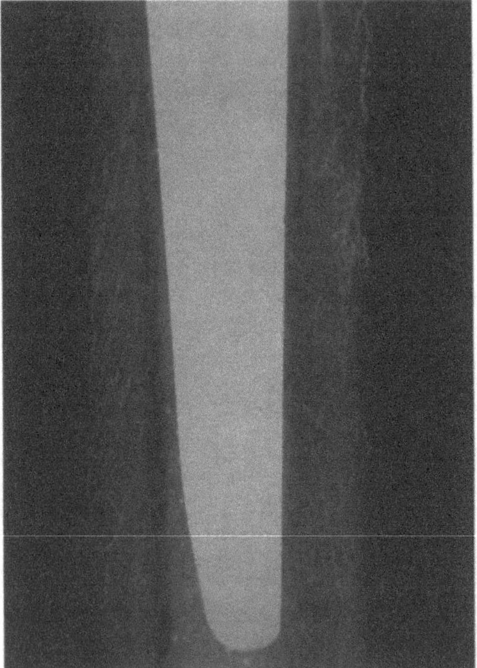

Fig. 9.18. Angiograph in longitudinal section showing the stem of a hip prosthesis held in the femoral diaphysis by acrylic cement; cadaver aged 56 years perfused 4 years after implantation. The cortex is entirely vascularized from the periosteum. (Original magnification ×2)

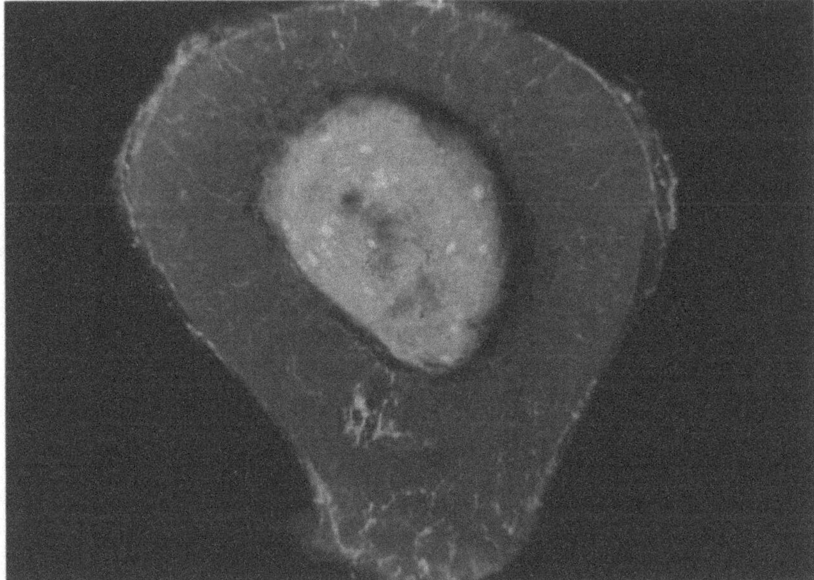

Fig. 9.19. Angiograph of transverse section of the femur below the prosthetic stem. The marrow cavity is blocked with acrylic cement. The entire cortex is vascularized from the periosteum. (Original magnification ×4)

(1960) examined 14 human tibiae amputated for femoral cancers. Regrettably the age range of this material, presumably old, was not supplied, but they did describe a periosteal arterial supply to the tibia, with multiple blood vessels in cortical canals, and periosteo-medullary anastomoses. An osteoporotic cortex and ischaemic bone marrow also illustrate their text, without comment. Lopez-Curto *et al.* (1980) pointed out that the diaphyseal nutrient arteries supplied the canine marrow and cortex *in parallel*, in the six adult dogs of unstated age that they examined; but for them, cortical and medullary vascular beds did not communicate. Transcortical periosteo-medullary anastomoses were also noted in their material. It is possible that their use of Microfil, a silicone elastomer, capable of filling the total vasculature of a tissue, failed for technical reasons to demonstrate the continuity between sinusoid and capillary at the osteomyeloid junction. The possibility must also be considered that the bone marrow was ischaemic on account of the age of the dogs.

Arterial periosteo-medullary anastomoses, demonstrated by the use of the more viscous Micropaque, were illustrated as a feature of 25 aged human tibiae aged 59–80 years, average 70, amputated for senile atherosclerosis (Brookes 1960a). A periosteal arterial supply to bone cortex was also prominent in this material, and contrasted with its *absence* in a perfused tibia of a 15-year-old youth (leg amputated for femoral sarcoma), which acted as a control. Vascular canals in the bone cortex of these aged specimens were irregular in size and contained a variable number of blood vessels. The above features and medullary ischaemia were taken to reflect the ageing process in long bones. This view was strengthened (Brookes 1960b) by the demonstration in rabbits that unilateral ligation of the nutrient artery of the femur provokes an abnormal centripetal blood flow into the compact bone from the vessels in the periosteum. This contrasts with the normal medullary blood supply and centrifugal vascular penetration of the cortex in the contralateral controls. Enlarged Haversian spaces in the ischaemic cortex contained multiple blood vessels (Figs 9.5, 9.6).

The circulating blood volume in rat bone declines semilogarithmically with age from 1 month to 24 months, when the blood volume reaches a tenth of what it was in youth (Brookes 1971). Kita *et al.* (1987) in rabbits, using hydrogen washout for blood flow measurement, demonstrated a falling blood flow in bone marrow of 50, 23, 15 and 12 ml min^{-1} 100 g^{-1} in immature, mature, middle-aged and advanced-aged rabbits, respectively.

Clinical considerations

Early detection of atherosclerosis

Medullary ischaemia in human long bones is not rare. Ramseier (1962) in more than 200 consecutive post-mortem examinations assessed histologically the grades of atherosclerosis in intra-osseous, muscular, coronary and cerebral arteries. He found that human bone marrow is generally subject to arterial disease, and that grade for grade, atherosclerotic disease appears at least 10 years earlier in femoral marrow than in the arteries of the brain, heart or thigh muscles. Ramseier's findings and those of Brookes (1960a,b; 1990a,b; 1993), Nelson *et al.* (1960), Crock (1967), Trueta (1968), Lopez-Curto *et al.* (1980) and Kita *et al.* (1987), indicate that ageing in long bones is accompanied by marrow ischaemia.

Problem of osteoporosis

With the known increasing severity of atherosclerosis in bone marrow with age, it is also likely that the normal high diaphyseal pressures in youthful bone marrow fall below those at the arterial end of the periosteal capillaries. This haemodynamic pressure change accounts for a centripetal blood flow from the periosteum into the senescent cortex. With the development of a combined, yet directionally contrary, dual blood supply to the cortex, the evidence also suggests that the amount of circulating blood, and its speed, in the cortex also fall (Brookes 1974b; Kita *et al.* 1987). This may be related to the osteoporosis of age. The incidence of this, the commonest metabolic bone disease, is much greater in women than in men, and is usually accounted for by hormonal and mineral imbalances. It is possible that bone vascular change in senescence supplies an aetiological background of reduced bone blood pH and disturbed $P\text{O}_2$ and $P\text{CO}_2$ (Brookes 1971; Arnett & Dempster 1990; Arnett *et al.* 1994) against which hormonal, nutritional and cellular factors operate in this disorder.

Assessment of general vasculature

Bone marrow biopsy and its histomorphometry might be added to aortic radiography and retinoscopy, to make a quantitative overall assessment of the degree of atherosclerosis in the vascular system. Marrow biopsy might also provide a predictive element with respect to other arterial territories.

Fracture treatment

A combined periosteal and medullary blood supply to bone cortex in senescent bones, contrasts with a purely medullary supply in youth, and may help to explain the success of intramedullary reaming and nailing of long bone fractures, particularly in the weight-bearing femur and tibia (Gahr *et al.* 1995). In old and young fractured bones the periosteum is conserved, thus keeping the cortex alive while the marrow regenerates. At the same time, the intramedullary nail maintains the bone fragments in mechanical reduction in a maximally advantageous site, the medullary axis. Medullary reaming in sheep is known to provoke a six-fold increase in the blood supply to the periosteum (Reichert *et al.* 1994). In rabbits, reaming of the marrow cavity followed by intramedullary nailing has been shown to promote an abundant callus deposition from the periosteum, essential for the rapid establishment of firm bony union (Brueton & Brookes 1995).

Cortical vascular patterns

The vessels of cortical bone form a network usually described by textbooks and investigators as longitudinally orientated (Petersen 1930; Schumacher 1935; Krompecher 1937; Vasciaveo & Bartoli 1961; Ham & Leeson 1964; Gray 1989). The horizontal short limbs of the mesh are said to lie in Volkmann's canals.

A considerable body of information has accumulated which is not wholly in agreement with this description. de Marneffe (1951) and Brookes (1958b) found that typically, cortical capillaries are oblique in disposition. Vascular obliquity in bone cortex has also been described by Koltze (1951) in the cortex of the adult human phalanx, and by Cohen & Harris (1958) in the canine femur.

Oliveira (1932) found that vessels of the human tibia in the upper part of the cortex pointed upwards and outwards; at mid-diaphyseal levels the vessels were transverse, while inferiorly they pointed downwards and outwards, i.e. the cortical vessels had a radiate, fan-shaped disposition when viewed as a whole. Fawcett (1942) and Bhaskar *et al.* (1950) described similar radiate trabecular patterns in the bones of the manatee and in the mutant *ai* strain of the rat respectively. In the case of the manatee and Sirenia generally, remodelling of bone cortex does not occur, so that early formed bone persists throughout the lifetime of the animal. The same applies to the mutant strain of rat investigated by Bhaskar and his co-workers.In both instances the trabeculae form in relation to blood vessels, and their arrangement gives a clear indication of the radiate cortical vascular pattern present in bone formed by periosteal apposition. A radiate pattern of vascular spaces in bone forming under a variety of pathological and experimental circumstances was also observed by Landauer (1927), Murray and Selby (1930), Studitsky (1936) and Murray & Kodiček (1949). Pinard (1952), in his valuable thesis, has described the vessels of normal human metatarsals as radiating outwards through the cortex, emanating as it were from a central marrow point.

As a follow up on these consistent observations, and at the time of writing still at variance with generally accepted opinion, Heřt (1960) and Brookes (1963, 1964) carefully investigated the layout of vessels in compact bone and described three fundamental vascular patterns present in the cortex of long bones in mammals.

Periosteal bone is permeated by vessels having a radiate, fan-shaped pattern. The centre point of the radiation corresponds to the site of primary ossification of the shaft. That considerable part of the cortex which forms endochondrally (Greulich & Leblond 1953; Pratt 1959) has a longitudinal pattern. Endosteal bone (Payton 1934) again shows a radiate pattern of vascularization, but the vessels converge on to a point outside the shaft (Figs 3.2, 9.2, 9.20–26). Communicating vessels (Jaffe, 1929) link the three groups together, but these are by no means wholly transverse, nor so numerous as to obliterate the three primary patterns, radiate periosteal, longitudinal endochondral and counter-radiate endosteal, observable in the cortex of long bones.

Vasciaveo and Bartoli's findings (1961) on the metacarpal bones of the ox appear partially to contradict the above findings. They insist on a total longitudinal pattern of vascular canals in the bones of this animal; some of their illustrations of fetal and yearling metacarpal patterns do, however, show characteristic vascular obliquity. A true longitudinal-transverse pattern is shown in their illustration taken at mid-shaft level, which might possibly be expected in the metacarpal bone of this animal. At all events, the total osseous vascular configuration in the cortex of the ox and in adult man is still to be elucidated, in order to gain a three-dimensional picture of cortical structure, and from that the precise manner of its development.

Pattern determinants in bone cortex

In a discussion of the genesis of cortical vascular patterns, Brookes (1963) discounted the role of muscle pull and extrinsic mechanical factors (Carey 1929; Landauer 1929, 1931; Oberdahlhoff 1946; Altmann 1950). In the femur, for example, the cortical vessels deep to the origin of vastus intermedius pass obliquely upwards

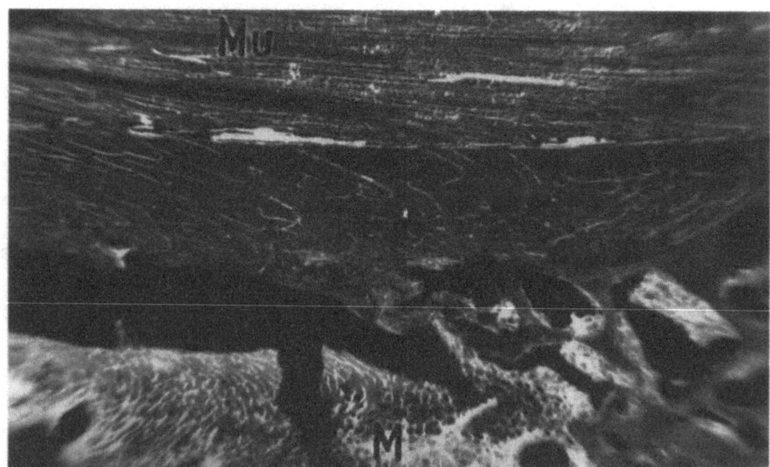

Fig. 9.20. India ink preparation of the shaft of a rat femur, to show the vascular radiation in cortical bone of periosteal origin. M, Marrow; Mu, muscle. (Original magnification ×25)

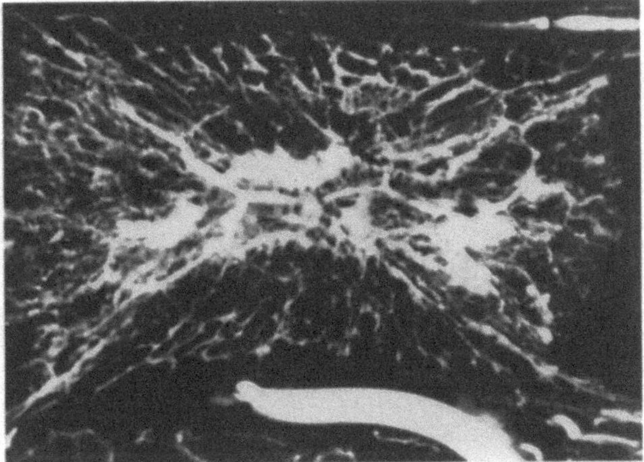

Fig. 9.21. Microangiogram of a first metatarsal bone from a human fetus, 16 cm CR length, showing the periosteal vascular radiation in the cortex. (Original magnification ×18)

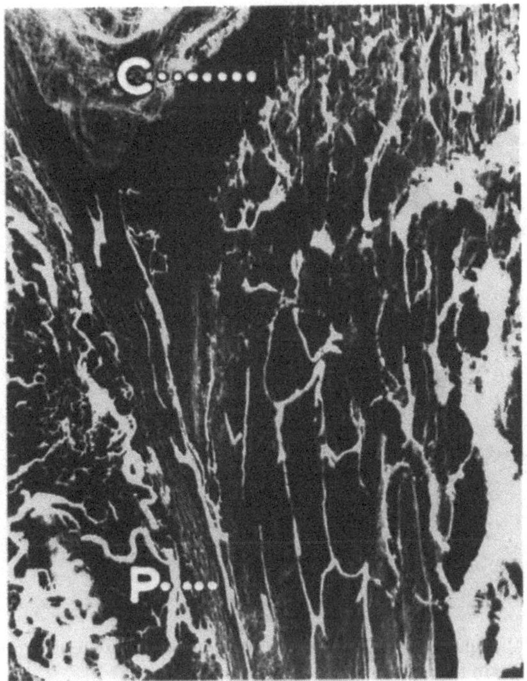

Fig. 9.22. Vertical orientation of capillaries in bone cortex of endochondral origin. C, Growth cartilage; P, periosteum. (Rat tibia; Original magnification ×50)

at the upper end of the muscle's attachment (Fig. 9.27) and obliquely downwards at the lower end. The line of pull of the muscle fibres themselves shows no such change. Moreover, the basic vascular patterns so clearly demonstrable in the cortex of young individuals are also foreshadowed in the fetal condition. Hence mechan-

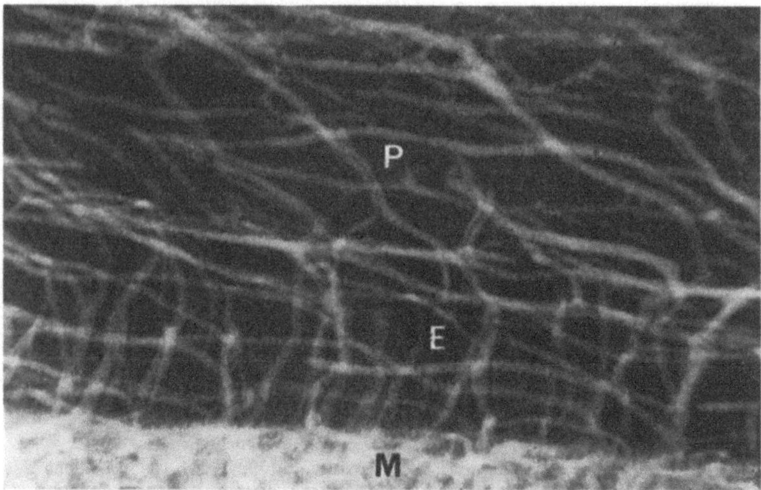

Fig. 9.23. Microangiograph of rat bone cortex showing oblique vessels in periosteal bone (P) and transverse vessels in endosteal bone (E), confluent with the sinusoids in marrow (M). (Original magnification ×70)

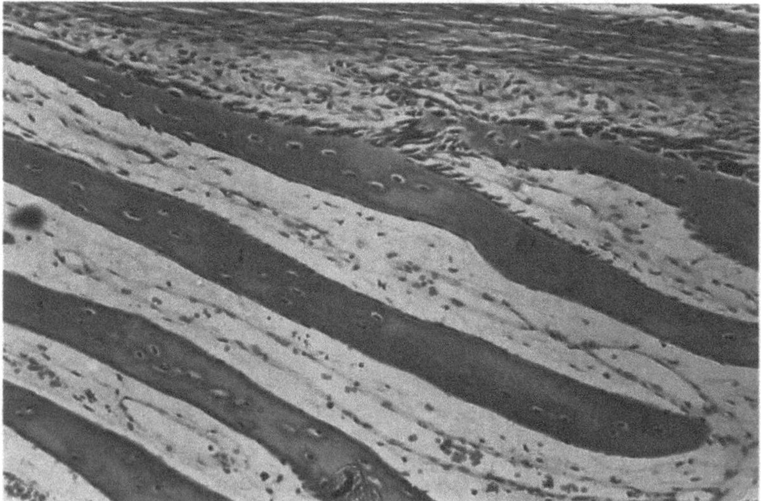

Fig. 9.24. Oblique trabeculae of periosteal bone and intervening vascular mesenchyme. Note high calibre capillaries. (Human fetal tibia; Original magnification ×125)

ical strains, such as those set up by the pull of muscles on newly forming trabeculae, play no important role in a bone's acquisition of its trabecular or vascular patterns. Vascular patterns in bone cortex are morphogenetically determined: the factors controlling their development are to be sought primarily in the bone tissue and bone cell systems within a whole bone organ.

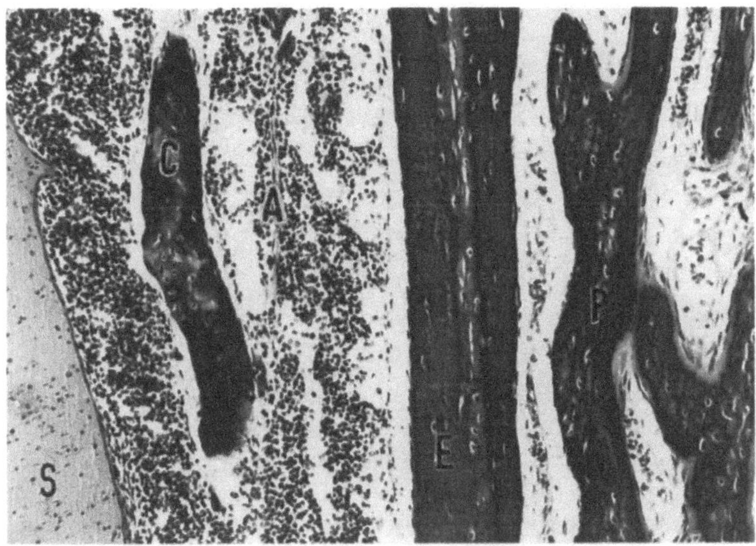

Fig. 9.25. Longitudinal section through a human fetal phalanx showing the three types of bone, periosteal (P), endosteal (E) and endochondral (C). A medullary sinus is indicated by S, and an arteriole by A. (Original magnfication ×185)

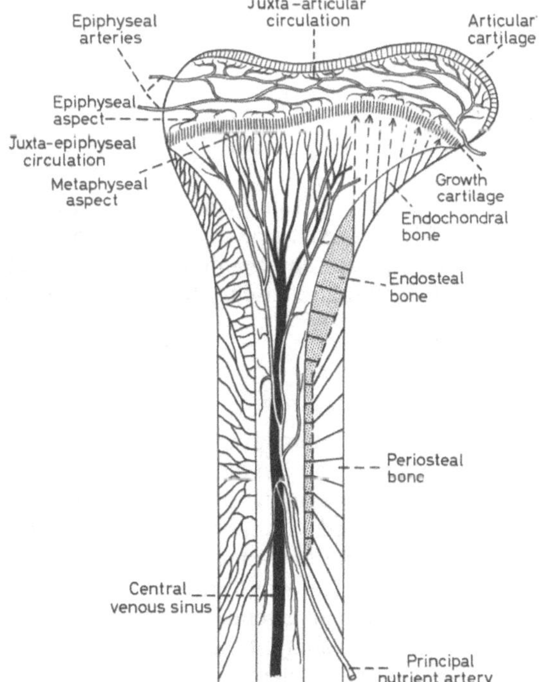

Fig. 9.26. The three vascular patterns in bone cortex, corresponding to the three types of bone present.

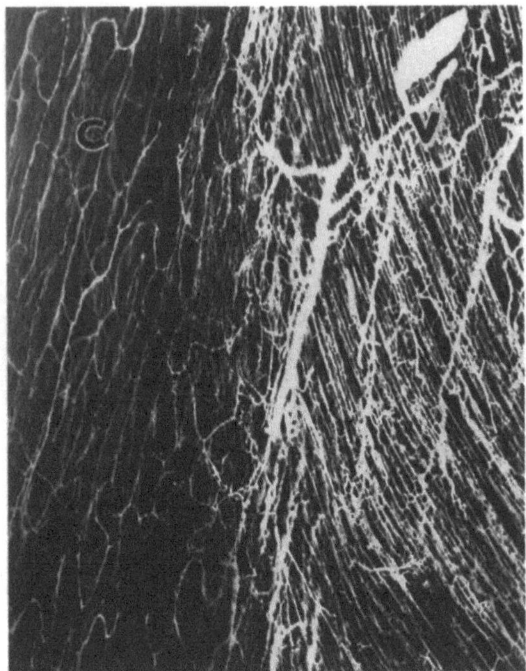

Fig. 9.27. Longitudinal section through the anterior surface of the upper part of an adult rabbit femur. The cortical capillaries (C) radiate upwards and outwards. The attached vastus intermedius (V) and its capillaries are orientated downwards and outwards. Cortical vascular pattern is independent of muscle pull. (India ink; Original magnification ×70)

Endochondral bone

Bone forms in relation to vascular mesenchyme. In the case of endochondrally formed bone (see Chapter 11), the axial orientation of trabeculae is the result of the way in which the growth cartilage and the metaphyseal vascular mesenchyme interact, the trabecular pattern being secondary to the vascular pattern.

Periosteal bone

The periosteal capillaries with their attendant mesenchyme are anchored both to the periosteum growing interstitially, and to the underlying bone growing by apposition at its extremities. Hence, the vessels continually incorporated into the shaft surface tend to be obliquely orientated with respect to the long axis of the bone; and the trabeculae forming from the mesenchyme around them likewise assume an oblique disposition. When account is taken of the two growth cartilages of a long bone, and the effect similar to that of an extending elastic membrane that periosteal growth exercises with respect to the shaft, it follows that vessels in bone cortex of periosteal origin exhibit the radiate, fan-shaped layout described by investigators in fetal and postnatal material. In particular, the gross trabecular pattern of periosteal bone is secondary to the primary vascular pattern.

When rates of growth are the same at proximal and distal cartilages as in fetal long bones (Bisgard & Bisgard 1935; Felts 1954; Brookes 1963), the vascular radiation is symmetrical and its centre corresponds to the primary ossification site at mid-shaft level (Fig. 9.21). With the accession of disparity in rates of elongation at the growing and non-growing ends in the postnatal period and their progressive divergence with age, the radiating pattern becomes lopsided, the centre of the fan being nearer to the non-growing end but still indicating the primary ossification site (Fig. 9.20).

Endosteal bone

Formation of endosteal bone was formerly considered to take place in the diaphysis of a long bone as an even deposition of circumferential cortical lamellae at maturity. Endosteal bone is now known to be localized to definitive sites (Tomlin *et al.* 1953; Smith 1960; Brookes 1963), making growth in girth eccentric (Fig. 9.28). The vessels of endosteal bone have their own characteristic pattern, tending to increasing obliquity towards the metaphysis (Fig. 9.26). For reasons analogous to periosteal vascularization and bony architecture, it seems that endosteal bone deposits have a pattern consequent on the interaction between endosteum and the inner face of the cortex.

Vascular neogenesis

The three vascular patterns of bone cortex are easy to detect in fetal and growing postnatal bones. Evidence is still wanting which would show with certainty whether they persist in man after maturity, or whether they are superseded by a longitudinally orientated mesh with transverse cross-connections. The latter process would, of course, entail vascular remodelling as well as internal structural alteration to the bone substance.

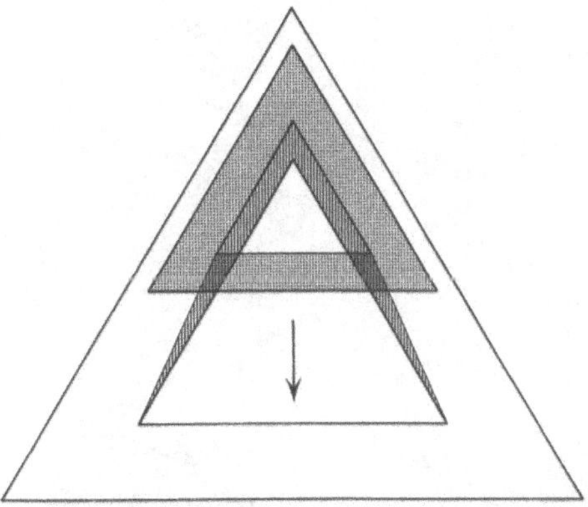

Fig. 9.28. Drawing in cross-section of a long bone to show eccentric growth in girth. Endosteal bone deposition (vertical hatching) is one-sided, so that the tibia, for example, grows backwards. Unshaded areas indicate periosteal bone deposition. Small dotted triangle shows cross-section of original young bone.

Cortical structure is undergoing continual internal modification, in the formation of new generations of osteones throughout the lifetime of an individual (Amprino & Bairatti 1936; Amprino & Sisto 1946; Amprino 1955). Because osteonic renewal requires the near presence of vascular mesenchyme, it seems likely that the cortical vessels, like the mesenchyme in which they are embedded, are not static elements congealed in compact bone substance but are reactive and capable of variation in size and number, an activity seen in exaggerated form in fracture repair (Nilsonne 1959; Rhinelander 1968; Richards & Brookes 1969; Brookes *et al.* 1970) (Fig. 9.29) or bone ischaemia (Brookes 1960a,b) (Figs 9.30, 9.31). In particular, osteonic renewal is a function of newly formed vascular mesenchyme, with the implication that new vessels can originate within bone cortex, and are not only incorporated into it passively at the primary bone-forming sites, periosteum, growth cartilage and endosteum, discussed above.

An early account of vascular neogenesis occurring in compact bone is that of Volkmann (1863). Regrettably the circumstances of his observations were forgotten and instead his paper gave rise to a concept, difficult to eradicate, that vessels lying in transverse canals still bearing his name are a hallmark of normal cortical vascular architecture. Actually, Volkmann recorded the finding of newly formed vessels which appeared to erode the cortex of a tuberculous metatarsal which he had excised from a peasant. (The operation appears to have been successful because the fortunate patient was able to walk 180 miles back to his own Land.) The observation is still valuable for pointing out that bone removal requires vascular participation, and that the arrangement of vessels in bone can alter in pathological circumstances.

Evidence for normally occurring vascular neogenesis is found in the writings of Zawisch-Ossenitz (1926, 1927), Pommer (1927), Weidenreich (1930), Schumacher (1935), Cohen & Harris (1958) and Schenk & Willenegger (1964). These investiga-

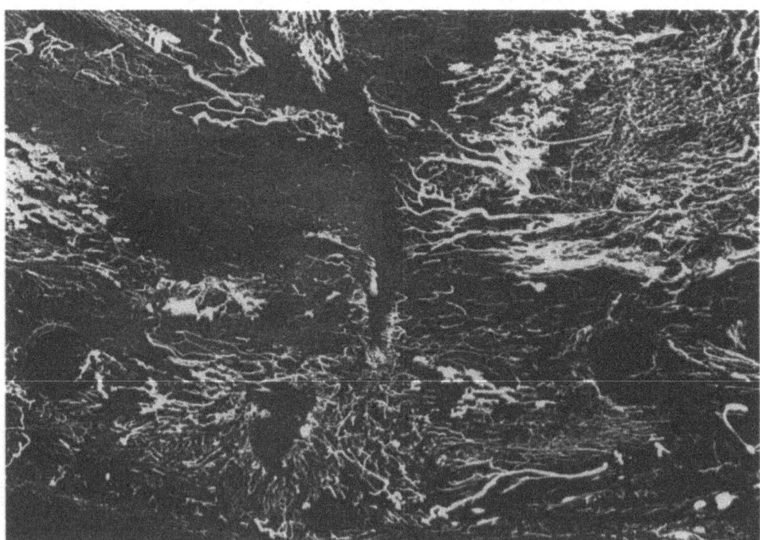

Fig. 9.29. Vascular neogenesis in the bone cortex of a rabbit humerus after fracture: longitudinal section. (Micropaque perfusion; Original magnification ×4)

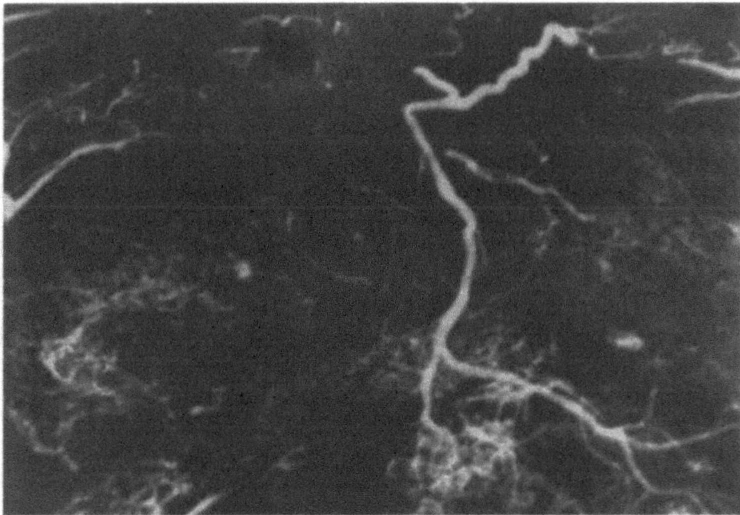

Fig. 9.30. New vessels growing from a periosteal artery and forming a stellate vascular figure (Gefässstern) in the marrow of an ischaemic tibia. (Microangiograph; Original magnification ×17)

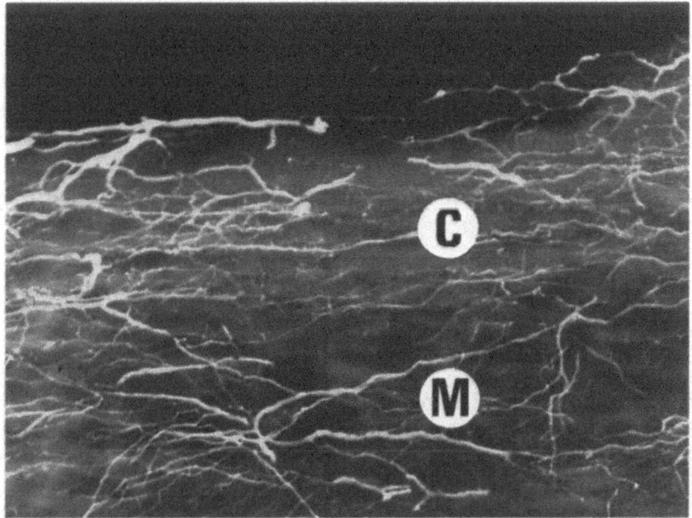

Fig. 9.31. New arterial channels growing in the cortex of an ischaemic human tibia. M, Marrow; C, cortex. (Original magnification ×4)

tors describe two main groups of vascular canals in compact bone. In one group, the canal on cross-section shows a smooth rounded outline and is surrounded by the concentric lamellae of an osteon, or appears interpolated between two circumferential lamellae of surface bone ("interlamellar canals" of Weidenreich). The other type of canal is much less common. It has a crenated or jagged border and shows no orderly relationship to lamellae. The latter type of canal, cutting across lamellar systems, suggests the early stage of formation of a new canal breaking through old bone deposits. From such a starting point, Zawisch-Ossenitz described the formation of a new canal, followed by its gradual filling up with lamellae and final obliteration of the contained vessel. She concluded that new bone canal formation required vascular neogenesis and that continual renewal of bone took place based on blood vessels. Later writers then developed the idea of vascular neogenesis and internal erosion of the cortex. In particular, canals with blind endings containing blood vessels were described in detail, supporting the fact of normal continual vascular renewal in bone cortex. In fracture repair, such new vascular canals are held to bring about primary union of the bone fragments, providing the fracture has been well reduced and maintained in fixation.

Given sufficient time, vascular neogenesis may modify the three vascular patterns found in tubular bone cortex of young individuals, resulting in the formation of the longitudinal pattern described in adult man by classical authors. Some evidence for this may be found in Heřt and Hladíková (1961), who described ingrowth of vessels from the medullary aspect of the cortex, with a subsequent superimposition of a longitudinal pattern on the primary vascular network.

In conclusion, it should be emphasized that there are no firm grounds for apportioning an osteolytic function to vascular endothelium. The process of osteonic renewal demands prior removal of bone, but the weight of histological evidence points to this as being carried out by mesenchyme cell derivatives and not by the vessels themselves in the Haversian canals. Nevertheless, the vascular lattice of compact bone is a labile structure and forms the basis of those events of internal reconstruction and ionic exchange which are essential to the metabolic function of bone. Hence, the possibility is not to be excluded that those factors which affect bone deposition and removal, and collagen and calcium turnover, do so not only by a direct action on bone cells and salts, but also by influencing the properties of vascular endothelium such as membrane permeability and its capacity for neogenesis.

Periosteum

Many authors (Barkow 1868; Langer 1876; Brookes & Harrison 1957; Morgan 1959; Novak 1959; Nelson *et al.* 1960) describe how large branches of the vessels which supply neighbouring muscles pass on to the fibrous layer of the periosteum and form at intervals several vascular circles round the shaft which are in series with the circulus articuli vasculosus. Longitudinal anastomotic chains are also found associated with the borders of bones, for instance the arteries of the linea aspera of the femur. From these vessels a network is built up in the fibrous periosteum comparable in density (about 10 to the square inch) with that associated with other fibrous membranes, e.g. the interosseous membranes of the appendicular skeleton, or the dura mater (Fig. 9.32). Offshoots from this plexus then form a capillary network in the osteogenic layer right against the bone surface.

At sites of fleshy muscle attachments, the situation is more complex. Here the fibrous periosteum is extremely tenuous, so that the intramuscular and periosteal circulations are continuous. Brookes (1958b) and Brookes *et al.* (1961) have shown that in areas of muscle attachment the periosteal capillaries are directly

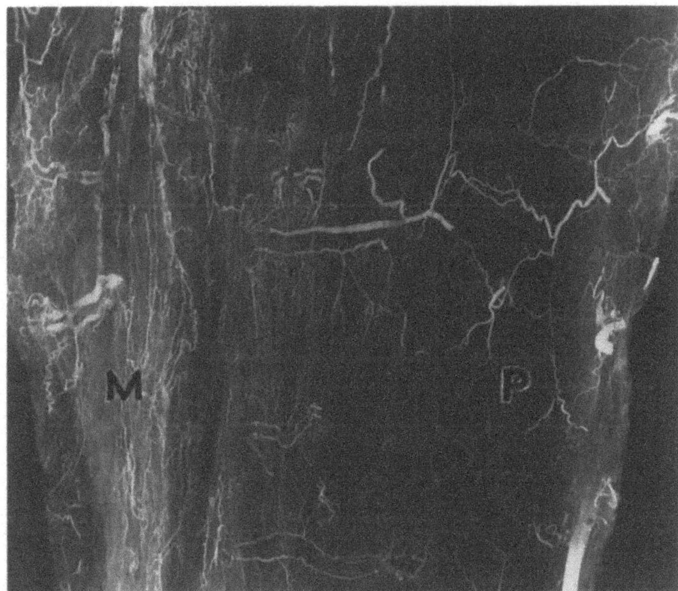

Fig. 9.32. A cuff of periosteum removed from a human tibia and laid out flat to show periosteal vascularity in subcutaneous area (P) and where muscles have a fleshy attachment (M). (Angiograph; Original: Natural size)

confluent with the perifibrillar capillaries and interfascicular venules of the attached muscle (Figs 8.14, 9.37). Where the shaft has no muscle attachments, periosteal capillaries are in connection with the vessels of the fibrous periosteum. The periosteal capillaries are also in direct continuity with those of the underlying bone cortex (Fig. 9.37).

Morgan (1959), however, described arteries passing from periosteum to cortex. Such perforating arteries have not been seen by many workers who have carefully looked for them (Caeiro & Mainetti 1932; Anseroff 1934; Brookes *et al.* 1961; Nelson *et al.* 1960; Brånemark 1958; Tilling 1958). Furthermore, the general type of vascular connection between periosteum and bone cortex is readily apparent from surface inspection of macerated bones. At low powers of the microscope these are seen to be marked by a profusion of gutters, the tertiary foramina of Testut (1880), which are uniform in calibre and orderly in orientation (Figs 9.33, 9.34), reflecting the radiate pattern of vessels in the underlying bone. These are the channels of vascular union between the periosteal capillaries and the cortical vascular mesh, and indicate that this union takes place exclusively at the capillary level.

Bone cells and endothelial cells

Syncytial character of osteocytes

Since Schwann (1839) propounded the cell doctrine, anatomists have been circumspect before granting a group of cells the status of syncytium. Nowadays this

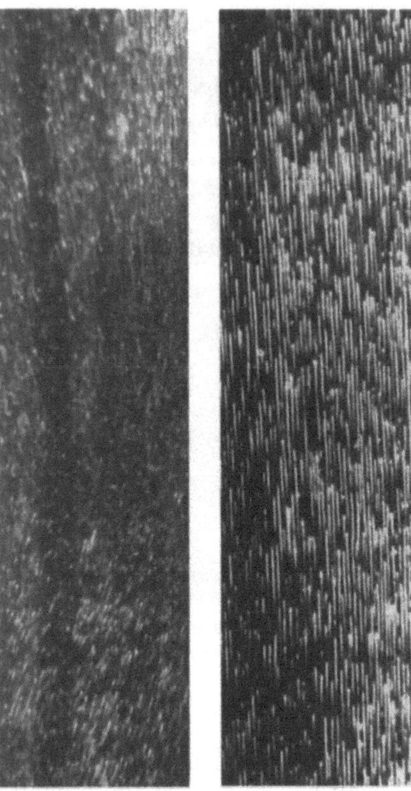

Fig. 9.33. (*left*) Surface view of the tibia of a kangaroo after blocking the openings of the tertiary foramina of Testut with chalk. The mouths of the foramina indicate the fan-shaped vascular pattern in periosteal bone cortex. (Original magnification ×4)

Fig. 9.34. (*right*) The tertiary foramina of Testut in the lower third of a kangaroo tibia. They all open outwards and downwards and are uniform in size. (Original magnification ×4)

term is being rendered increasingly out of date by electron microscopy, and "plasmodium" is to be preferred to indicate those cells formed by nuclear division without cytoplasmic division, for example muscle fibres, giant cells and the plasmodial trophoblast of the chorion. Leonhardt (1967) considers that "syncytium" should only be applied in its original meaning to a group of cells, in contact by means of cell processes, whose boundaries, if not obvious in the LM, are as likely as not demonstrable in the EM.

It is held by many that the osteocytes of bone comprise a syncytium wherein cell is continuous with cell through cytoplasmic processes. Suffice it to say that as regards the osteocytes, no EM photograph has ever been published which suggests that these cells form a plasmodium. For the osteocytes, buried alive in hard bone substance, the possibility exists that the cytoplasmic processes which these cells undoubtedly possess might make a syncytial contact with one another in the extremely fine canaliculi of bone. The claim that the syncytial character of osteocytes has been repeatedly observed requires further reinforcement.

Origin of bone cells

A more important conjecture that bone endothelium gives rise to a whole range of bone cells requires detailed examination.

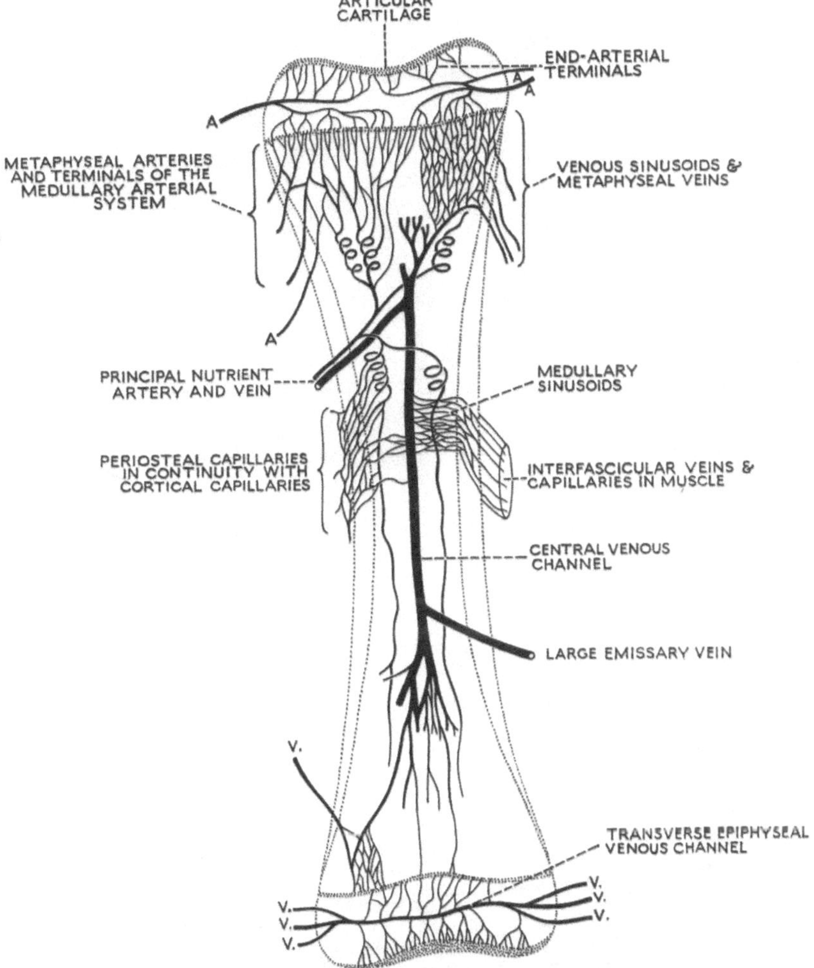

Fig. 9.35. Vascular organization of a long bone in longitudinal section.

Vascular change, the burgeoning and decline of cortical capillaries, at first received emphasis in studies on bone renewal and repair. Later writers have emphasized in this context the origin of osteoclasts from the monocyte-macrophage cell line. In addition, the view is now current that bone endothelial cells give rise to osteoblasts and, by engulfment of the latter by bone substance, osteocytes. Hence, the *diphyletic* proposition that osteoblasts and osteoclasts concerned in the laying down and remodelling of bone are not closely related.

Because osteoblasts have not been seen to divide in histological preparations even where active bone formation is occurring as in, for example, the growing cortex, an osteoprogenitor cell was postulated by Young (1962) as the source of osteoclasts, osteoblasts and osteocytes. The conjectured origin of osteoprogenitor cells from vascular endothelium was urged by Trueta, principally on the basis of the generally observable, and not to be denied, intimate relationship

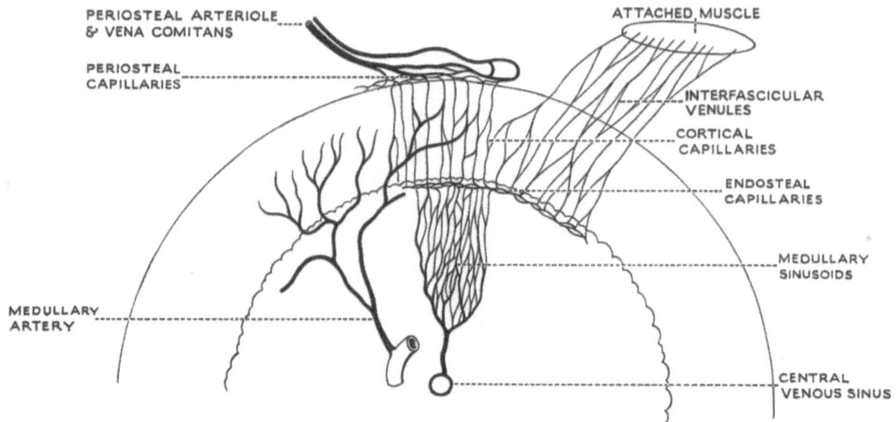

Fig. 9.36. Cross-sectional plan of blood supply of bone cortex in youth.

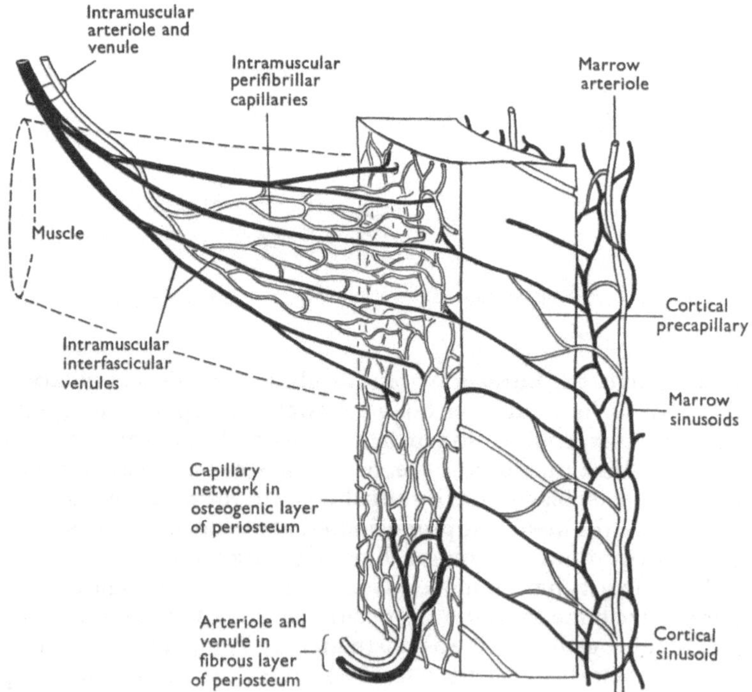

Fig. 9.37. Vascular connection between bone marrow, cortex, periosteum and attached muscle.

between blood vessels and bone (Fig. 8.35). The authority of older workers is attested by Keith (1927), whose review of the subject to the Royal Society of Medicine forms a valuable source-guide to the literature. Nevertheless, one cannot read more into the writings of von Haller (1763) or of Hunter (1772) than that blood vessels, "if not the actual bone builders, are an essential factor in its production".

It can also be fairly stated that Macewen (1912) never said nor offered evidence that osteoblasts were directly derived from capillary endothelial cells. On the contrary, he believed that capillaries and the blood circulation were an extremely important factor in osteogenesis, which is not the same thing. In describing his glass tube experiments he wrote: "Some of the capillary vessels became surrounded by bone formation, their lumen being gradually narrowed by the ingrowing osteoblasts so as to resemble Haversian canals, and occasionally the vessels in these spaces became obliterated by the prolific osteoblastic ingrowth". Or again, "It was obvious that the bone cells were deposited abundantly where the capillaries were numerous".

In 1920, Macklin had established from his studies of bone repair that bone-forming cells proliferate from subperiosteal connective tissue cells and in broken Haversian spaces. (Bone petalling (Jarry & Uhthoff 1960) is a technique to potentiate the Haversian source of osteoblasts in the treatment of delayed union of fractures.) The investigations of Leriche & Policard (1926) led them to the *monophyletic* conclusion that the same type of cell in almost any locality, either within or outside the skeleton, can participate in bone removal and formation depending on its microenvironment. That cell they believed to be a fibroblast. Moschcowitz (1916) and various other investigators of heterotopic bone formation rightly pointed out that osteocytes and fibroblasts have a common origin during embryogenesis.

Yet it still remains to be demonstrated that an endothelial cell in a bone capillary, even in fetal life, can in any circumstance spawn off an osteoprogenitor cell which then differentiates into osteoblastic pathways. Sir Arthur Keith (1927), in his speculative essay, was uncertain as to his own belief in this matter because he was only prepared to identify the local osteogenic cells of Leriche & Policard as budded off from "the capillary system". The cells were derived alternatively from "vascular endothelium" or "vascular sheath cells". In modern times, the discriminatory powers of the EM and molecular biological techniques have not resolved the problem.

Oni *et al.* (1993) have used the lectin *Ulex europaeus* I-peroxidase (UEP) which distinguishes tumours of vascular origin from other tumours (Holthofer *et al.* 1982; Walker 1985), and also monoclonal antibodies specifically raised against endothelial cell proteins (Pringle & De Bono 1988). UEP was used to study lectin binding in early adult human tibial fractures, and osteotomies of adult rabbit tibiae. Monoclonal antibodies were used on samples obtained from eight adults undergoing open reduction of tibial diaphyseal fractures. Bone trabeculae, osteoblasts and chondrocytes showed no evidence of lectin binding or antibody uptake, whereas the endothelium of adjacent blood vessels was clearly stained. Osteogenic cells adjacent to endothelial cells were not stained. The total lack of staining of the bone cells opposes the notion that endothelial cells give rise to bone cells, as proposed by Trueta (1963). On the other hand, in a review of the many proposed functions of endothelium, Hansen (1993) includes extravascular migration of endothelial cells and their transformation into osteoprogenitor cells.

Factors acting on blood flow in cortex

Vasoactive drugs

Dohler *et al.* (1995) have studied the effect of vasoactive drugs on cortical capillaries. They injected, in a well-controlled experiment, a single intravenous bolus of adrenaline, ATP or insulin in mice, and a piece of tibial diaphysis was removed and examined by transmission EM. Adrenaline increased the luminal width and endothelial thickness. ATP caused endothelial cells to flatten. Injected insulin was associated with a thick endothelium in the Haversian canals, possibly as a result of hypoglycaemia. The authors argue that luminal expansion and endothelial thickening reflect a decreased extravascular space in the canals, and oedema of cortical bone substance. Intracortical perfusion pressure might then decrease and the bone perfusion rate increase. ATP, on the other hand, increases the extravascular space and reduces transcapillary diffusion time. Importantly, their work suggests that there are specific insulin receptors in bone capillaries.

In an *ex vivo* canine tibia model (Dean *et al.* 1992), perfused with oxygenated Krebs–Ringer solution at constant flow, a noradrenaline dose–response curve was obtained. After 30 minutes perfusion a second curve was generated. Drug attenuation was determined by the total area under the curve. Adrenergic receptor antagonists 1 and 2 stopped the constrictor effect of noradrenaline. Calcium antagonism had a lesser effect in attenuating smooth muscle contractility. Beta adrenergic receptor blockade caused only a slight but consistent reduction in reactivity.

Prostaglandins

Kapitola *et al.* (1994) have examined bone blood flow in spayed rats. Flows were measured by microspheres in the tibia and distal femur. They found that spaying increased the cortical blood flow rate, as well as the uptake of ^{45}Ca radio-calcium. Aspirin in the rat feed cake was used to suppress prostaglandin production. They found aspirin abolished significantly the blood flow increase induced by spaying. There was also a decrease in tibial bone density and ash weight. The authors argued for a role for prostaglandins, probably PGE_2, to account for the increased bone blood flow in spayed rats.

Temperature

The effect on bone blood flow of cooling the knee joint in an ice wrap for 20 minutes was measured by triple phase technetium bone scans on 21 humans. The opposite knee acted as a control. Scans were obtained on completion of cooling. All iced knees demonstrated decreased arterial bone blood flow and decreased bone uptake of ^{99m}Tc, reflecting reduced blood flow and metabolism; *c.*40% for flow and 20% for uptake. The reduced flow and cell metabolism might well limit cell death in severe traumatic injury. See also Servelle (1948) for the effects of increased heat on bone growth.

Alcohol

Alcohol abuse is associated with osteopenia and bone fractures, especially in senescence. Bikle *et al.* (1993) studied 27 subjects, aged 26–68 years, with a record of 10 years of alcohol abuse. Seventeen of them were found to have spinal compression fractures by routine X-ray examination. Bone density fell sharply with age; spinal bone density fell two standard deviations in 15 subjects below normal-age matched controls. Osteomalacia was absent, but the total surface area of cancellous bone was increased. Although vitamin D metabolites were normal, parathyroid hormone levels in many cases were elevated as shown by urinary cAMP levels.

Smoking

Daftari *et al.* (1994) transplanted autologous cancellous bone into the anterior chamber of the eye in 24 rabbits. Half were given nicotine, the other half received placebos. Revascularization of the implant was followed by slit-lamp and fluorescein angiography. The authors pointed out that pseudarthrosis after spinal fusion is more frequent in smokers than non-smokers. Here, the results showed that nicotine caused delayed revascularization of the graft, and more grafts became necrotic, as compared with the placebos. Nicotine clearly inhibits revascularization of autologous bone grafts. (See also “Regulators and mediators”, in Chapter 8.)

Chapter 10

Cartilage canals

Certain minute tunnels containing blood vessels and known as cartilage canals (Figs 2.18–2.20, 10.1) are generally found in the cartilaginous epiphyses of the fetal appendicular skeleton, not only in mammals but also in birds and amphibia. They are also reputed to occur in the adult skeleton in persisting blocks of hyaline cartilage, e.g. the laryngeal and costal cartilages. The most frequently studied group is that which develops in the cartilaginous extremities of

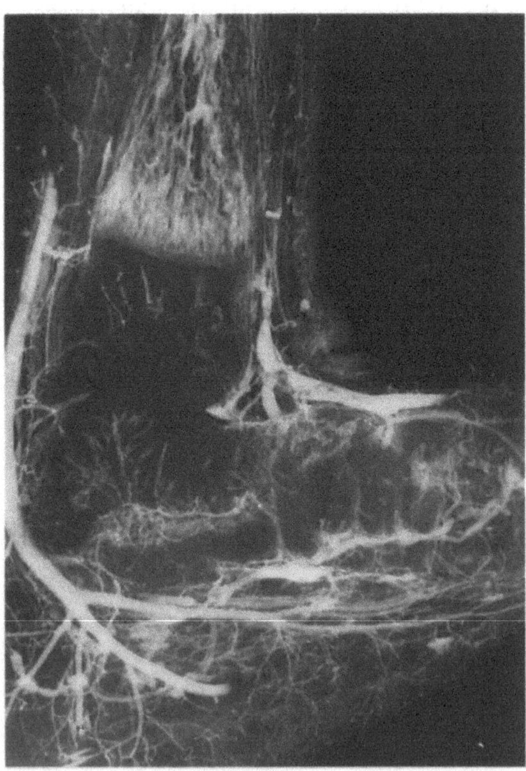

Fig. 10.1. Microangiograph of a human fetal ankle joint and tarsus, showing vascular cartilage canals. (Original magnification ×4)

the long bones. The vessels which they contain are the forerunners of the epiphyseal nutrient arteries and veins and their ramifications in bony epiphyses. Over the years a sizeable literature has grown up, especially on the Continent, about the vascular cartilage canals. Nevertheless the mechanism controlling their development is still largely unknown, and their significance in cartilage nutrition and in the initiation of centres of ossification has still to be accurately defined.

Relationship to ossification

That a relationship exists, however, between the establishment of centres of ossification and the presence of cartilage canals has been known since Prochaska (1810, quoted by Langer 1876) first drew attention to these structures. It would appear that no investigator for nearly 100 years, apart from Langer (1876), and he might well be the only one, has referred to Prochaska's original observation. The omission is here rectified:

> Es entstehen nämlich seiner Zeit in dem Knorpel einige Blutgefässe welche sich meistens aus dem angrenzenden Knochenteil dahin zu verlängern scheinen, und mit den Gefässen erscheinen auch schon die ersten Ossifikationspunkten, welche nach und nach einen knochigen Kern bilden.

The author (M.B.) has not been able to trace the "little known booklet" of Prochaska to which Langer refers, and makes use of his quotation:

> At the appropriate time several blood vessels can be found in the (epiphyseal) cartilage which in the main appear to grow in from the adjoining part of the bone. With the appearance of these vessels, points of ossification are discernible which gradually form a secondary centre.

The passage does not appear in Prochaska's Latin *Disquisitio* of 1812. For Prochaska then, the cartilage canals derive in the first place from the vessels coating the cartilaginous epiphyses.

Mechanisms of cartilage growth

Superficial apposition

A word is necessary on the mode of growth of the cartilaginous extremities of fetal bones, because the way in which these grow must influence the possible mechanisms of growth and enlargement at the disposal of the canals themselves. Bruch (1852) pointed out that the cells of the perichondrium merge with the epiphyseal cartilage cells in a spatial sequence of four or five cells, changing in morphology from flattened periosteal cells to plump chondrocytes embedded in hyaline matrix (Fig 11.3). Bruch therefore considered that the cartilage block grew, like bone, by apposition at the epiphyseal surface. Harris (1933), however, maintained that growth of human cartilaginous epiphyses took place interstitially to a major extent.

Interstitial growth

A zone of mitoses can be observed below the surface of the enlarging fetal epiphysis, which gives rise to chondrocytes which pack principally in a central direction and produce the bulk of the cartilaginous epiphysis. To a lesser extent, daughter cells may also pass towards the surface. The mitotic zone is found in postnatal life as the germinal layers of the growth and articular cartilages. The daughter cells of the latter cartilage exhibit, before maturity, both inward growth towards the epiphyseal centre, and outward growth towards the surface of the articular cartilage. The germinal zone of a growth cartilage, however, is polarized for outward growth only, towards the metaphysis.

Cartilage canal development

The age of the individual when cartilage canals first make their appearance is specific for each cartilage organ. In the human fetus it varies from about 4.5 cm CR length (11 weeks) for the distal epiphysis of the radius to about 12 cm CR length (16 weeks) for the epiphyses in the knee joint, or even later for the short bones of the hand (Langer 1876; Gray & O'Rahilly 1957; Watermann 1961).

The canals become more numerous and complex in arrangement as growth of the cartilage proceeds. Each canal, according to Langer (1876), contains a leash of small vessels. Brookes (1971) has demonstrated by intravascular barium sulphate perfusion that the canals branch considerably in second trimester human fetuses. In each branch a small arterial channel and accompanying venules open into an expanded portion at the blind end of the canal (Figs 10.2, 10.4). More recently, Skawina *et al.* (1994b) have studied the development of cartilage canals in the proximal femoral epiphysis of similar human fetuses, using corrosion casting and scanning EM. Vascular hairpin loops develop first from the perichondrial vessels. Capillary glomeruli form at the club-shaped leading ends now observed to be in cartilage. As the vascular unit lengthens it becomes embedded deep within the cartilage. Additional capillaries grow towards the surface, coating the original

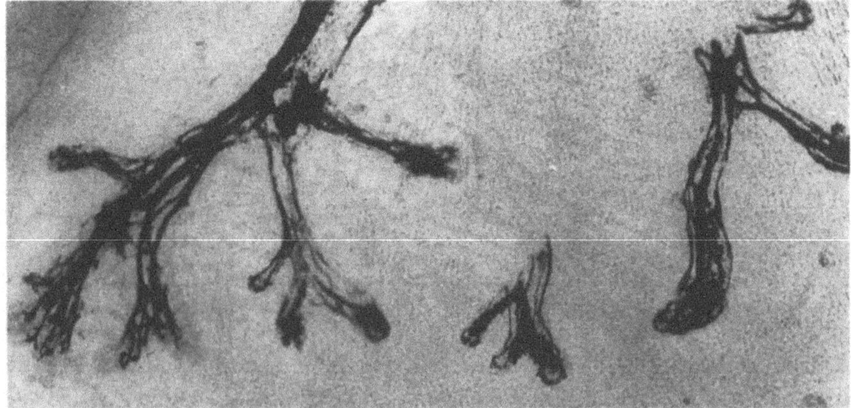

Fig. 10.2. India ink preparation of vascular leashes in human cartilage canals. (Original magnification ×22)

arteriole and venule; and the stem canals undergo repeated dichotomy forming tree-like structures. These are descriptive events which do not in themselves explain the mechanisms whereby the cartilage canals form, enlarge and bifurcate.

Mechanisms of cartilage canal development

Passive inclusion

The manner in which the canals and their contained vessels develop is still not known with certainty. Haines (1933) considered that the vascular canals arose by passive inclusion of perichondrial vessels into the epiphysis which grew by surface apposition. His opinion that the canals did not arise by vascular invasion, was reinforced by the observation that chondromucin was absent from subperiosteal cartilage as well as from the cartilage matrix immediately surrounding a canal. Furthermore, he pointed out that the hyaline cartilages in the tadpole's tail at metamorphosis are removed by leucocytes. For canals to be formed by erosion, he would have expected a leucocyte invasion of fetal epiphyses, a histological feature which is, however, absent.

Vascular invasion

On the other hand, the proponents of vascular invasion as the mechanism for cartilage canal formation are numerous. Some workers have described patches of *cartilage degeneration* which precede the inroad of the canals (Von Friedlander 1904; Bidder 1906; Hintzche 1931; Carlson *et al.* 1995). These may possibly serve as *chemotactic foci* attracting the growth of perichondrial capillaries inwards, or may be an expression of defective cartilage nutrition.

Eckert-Möbius (1924), Kajava (1919), Hintzche (1928) and Hurrell (1934) thought that the further growth and branching of the canal vessels might be aided possibly by a *chondrolytic vascular endothelium.* Watermann (1961), confirming Stump (1925), made histological observations on which he based the interesting opinion that canals are formed by *internal chondrolysis* by the epiphyseal chondrocytes; these lyse themselves free from their capsules in advance of an ingrowing blood vessel, which thereby finds its canal already prepared for it. Brookes (1971) studied cross-sections of canals, and pointed out that canal expansion must entail chondrolysis. In the chick, the vascular endothelium itself is not chondrolytic (Fig. 10.3, *overleaf*). On the contrary, light microscopy indicates that chondrolytic canal expansion may be ascribed to:

- The mesenchyme cells which surround the blood vessels in the canal, and
- The chondrocytes in the canal wall, lysing themselves free of their capsules and contributing to the mesenchymal content of the canals.

The question of the chondrolytic activity of cartilage cells will be examined in more detail in the case of growth cartilage and its invasion by vascular mesenchyme from the metaphysis.

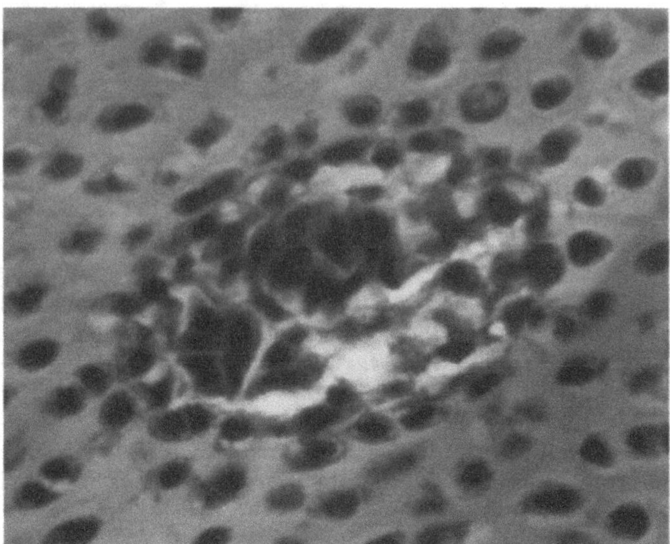

Fig. 10.3. A cartilage canal in a chick embryonic tibia; mesenchyme cells expanding the canal by eroding its wall. (Original magnification ×540)

With the advance of fetal life, the canals become more complex and develop an elaborate branching pattern. Anastomoses between terminal branches do not occur, which would argue for *vascular invasion with chondrolysis* being significant in the development of the full complement of cartilage canals. Lack of anastomoses also opposes the notion of canal origin by passive inclusion of the perichondrial capillary network during surface accretion. With the onset of ossification, the vascular mesenchyme as a unit undoubtedly becomes chondrolytic, removing calcified cartilage and making room in which osteogenesis can take place in the centre of the epiphysis. EM studies may help to resolve the question of chondrolytic activity in early canal development. In particular, closer examination may confirm that it is not the vascular endothelium itself which is chondrolytic, but rather the cells of the ever-present loose connective tissue closely associated with the capillaries. In the confined spaces in the depths of a canal these exiguous cells, notoriously difficult to stain, could easily be confused with a growing bud of endothelial cells.

Spatial organization

Haines, who studied the canals in serial section, did not remark on their having any precise spatial organization. If, however, recent studies on the main arterial patterns in adult human femoral epiphyses (Tucker 1949; Trueta & Harrison 1953; Rogers & Gladstone 1950) are compared with the patterns of the cartilage canals in the human fetus, it will be seen that the two are remarkably similar. The main vascular pattern of an adult bony epiphysis is outlined by the cartilage canal pattern in the corresponding fetal epiphysis (Brookes 1958a). The canal vessels are the precursors of the epiphyseal arteries and veins, and foreshadow the pattern of vascularization of the bony epiphysis.

Nutrient function

It is generally accepted that cartilage canals participate to some extent in the nutrition of epiphyseal cartilages, maintaining them alive and promoting their growth. The nutritional role has been related to the size of the cartilage mass involved. According to Haines, the main function of the canals is "the nutrition of cartilages too large to be supplied by diffusion of nutriment through their substance" He also states that "every large block of cartilage has its cartilage canals: no small block has them" More evidence is required before this opinion can be accepted without modification. In the human fetal carpus at any rate, although no canals develop in the os centrale or triangulare when present (Gray & O'Rahilly 1957), they are numerous in the rest of the cartilaginous carpal elements and even put in an early appearance in the cartilaginous sesamoids of the hand. Although, as Haines points out, cartilage canals may be absent in rat epiphyses prior to ossification, they are present even in the epiphyses of human phalanges, e.g. as early as 11 cm CR length (15 weeks) when the tiny blocks of cartilage are presumably sufficiently small to survive by diffusion of nutriment, without the aid of internally located vascular canals. Again it would appear that cartilage canals in a very small cartilage block serve as vascular precursors of the vessels of the future ossified cartilage, rather than obligate nutritive vessels.

Recently, Carlson *et al.* (1991) have studied the growth of cartilage canals and their vascular content in the femoral condyles of female pigs (3.6–71.0 kg). In the age range studied, the number of canal vessels decreased as the pigs increased in weight. Spontaneous foci of cartilage necrosis were also observed in this normal material, associated with necrotic blood vessels in the neighbouring canals. Experimentally, the blood supply to the canals was surgically interrupted on the medial condylar surface. This caused necrosis of the vascular content of canals as well as necrosis of the related epiphyseal cartilage itself. The authors concluded that a defect in the canal blood supply to the epiphyses was implicated in the pathogenesis of osteochondritis. The results also emphasize the dependency of long bone cartilage epiphyses on an adequate blood supply from cartilage canal vessels.

Carlson *et al.* (1995) have also examined cartilage canals in femoral condyles, distal tibia and proximal phalanx of horses less than 18 months old. In foals less than 3 weeks old, cartilage canals had patent blood vessels in all sites, but were absent from all sites by 7 months. The authors report, remarkably, the presence of lesions suggestive of osteochondrosis in a third of the sites, increasing to 50% in horses 2 months old and upwards. Principally the medial femoral condyle and distal tibia were involved. All lesions between 3 and 5 months were associated with necrosis of blood vessels in cartilage canals. The authors suggest that a defective vascular supply in cartilage canals is the cause of ischaemic cartilage necrosis. Some of the supposed osteochondrotic foci may be normal, attracting the growth and development of cartilage canals. (See "Vascular invasion" above.)

Epiphyseal ossification

The role of cartilage canals in the onset of secondary centres of ossification is problematical. They probably furnish the osteogenic blastema, i.e. the vascular mesenchyme which destroys the cartilage at the centre of ossification. The blastema then builds up bone trabeculae in the epiphyseal marrow and lays down a bone plate next to the growth cartilage. However, because of the early appearance of the canals and their extensive development prior to ossification, it is most unlikely that a direct causal relationship exists between the state of canal development and the time of onset of ossification in a secondary centre (Bidder 1906; Hintzche 1928). On the contrary, there is no relationship between the order of first appearance of the canals and the order of onset of ossification, or even chondrification, of the various skeletal elements in which the canals are found.

Initiation of ossification

When the idiosyncratic times of onset of secondary centres of ossification (Nesbitt 1736; Gray 1989) are further considered, it is understandable that one seizes, almost with relief, a *phylogenetic* or *genetic* explanation of these baffling phenomena. It is no doubt true that genetic mechanisms ultimately control canal development and ossification times, but in the epiphysis itself ossification will ensue when the environment, conditioned by the canal vessels, is appropriate. This, in its broadest sense, represents the *nutritional control* of secondary ossification, and was hinted at by Parsons (1905), Carey (1929) and Eckert-Möbius (1924). Future investigation of the circulation in cartilaginous epiphyses indicating the locally active mechanisms, neural and chemical, which control the haemodynamic conditions within the epiphysis, will probably elucidate the way in which the canal contents and the cartilage interact, and how the local physicochemical conditions necessary for ossification are brought about.

Ossification site

It has been said that the arrangement of cartilage canals determines the site of the secondary centre (Bidder 1906). Against this, however, is the fact that the distal ends of most human phalanges and the proximal ends of metacarpals, do not acquire secondary centres at all but undergo endochondral ossification from the marrow. Nevertheless they develop their complement of cartilage canals. The other epiphyses in these bones acquire both canals and centres of ossification.

Sources of the cartilage canals

In their layout, cartilage canals can be subdivided into two groups, the more considerable one passing from *non-articular surfaces* towards the centre of the cartilage mass, destined to become a long bone epiphysis or perhaps an irregular bone. The other, smaller, group is found in the epiphyses of fetal tubular bones originating in or close to the *ossification groove* of Ranvier and spreading out below the growth cartilage (Figs 10.4, 10.5). It is noted that the vessels in the latter canals are the forerunners of a subchondral circulatory network, with special features peculiar to itself, which is found close to the epiphyseal aspect of the growth cartilage.

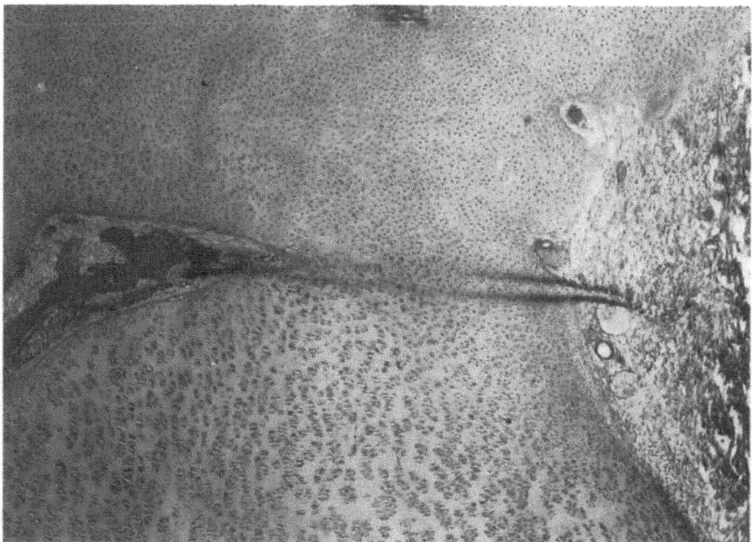

Fig. 10.4. A cartilage canal originating from Ranvier's groove. Such canals lie close to the growth cartilage. (Human humerus; Original magnification ×31)

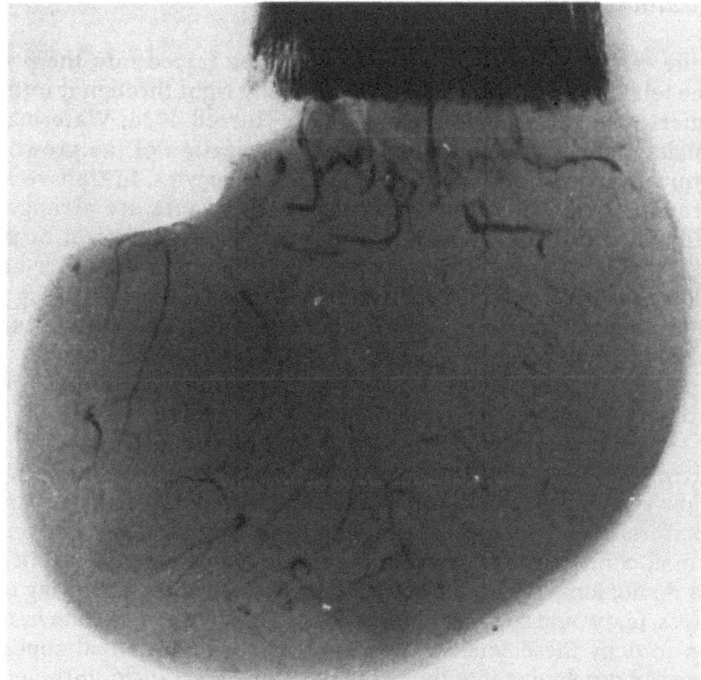

Fig. 10.5. Radiograph of cartilage canals in the condyle of a femur. Note communicating canals close to bony metaphysis. (Human fetus, 22 cm CR length; Original magnification ×8)

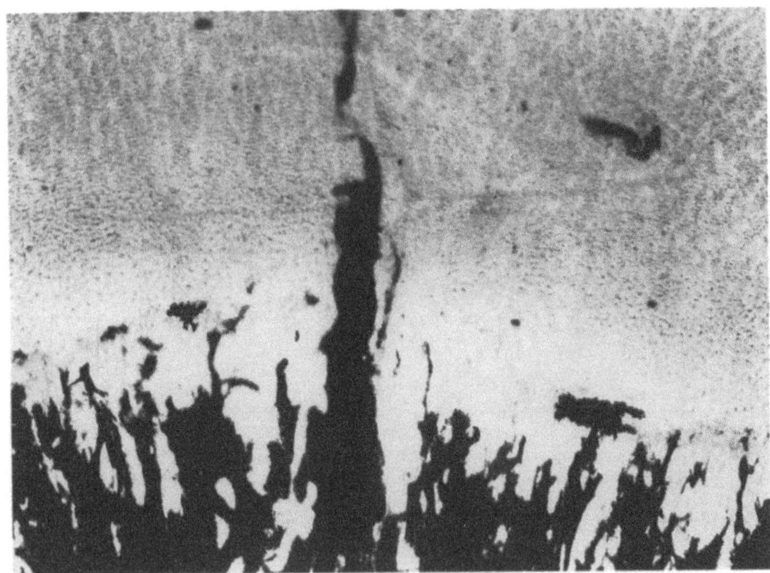

Fig. 10.6. India ink preparation of a communicating canal passing from marrow to epiphysis. (Human fetal tibia, 28 cm CR length; Original magnification ×72)

Communicating canals

Some of the canals from Ranvier's groove can be traced into the proliferative zone of the fetal growth cartilage and occasionally right through it into the metaphyseal marrow (Langer 1876; Haines 1933; Hurrell 1934; Watermann 1961). These canals might possibly influence the organization of the growth cartilage into its typical vertical columns of isogenic chondrocytes. In transverse sections taken through the proliferative zone, the chondrocytes are arranged radially around any such included vessel as if in response to chemical or nutritional influences emanating from it (Sharpey & Ellis 1856). On the other hand, some vessels pierce the growth cartilage from the metaphyseal marrow (Fig. 10.6), terminating blindly in the epiphyseal cartilage or joining up with the canal vessels (Prochaska 1810, quoted by Langer 1876; Langer 1876; Parsons 1905; von Eggeling 1935; Brookes 1958a). This second group of "communicating canals" contains blood vessels and an occasional bone trabecula.

Bidder (1906) strongly favoured the view that these canals conveyed osteogenic cells, derived from the metaphysis, which were then responsible for bone formation in the epiphyseal centre of ossification. He emphasized that cartilage canals, except for his "perforantes" (i.e. canals of the communicating type), contain only capillaries and small connective tissue cells, which are almost featureless. In particular, these cells do not look anything like the osteoblasts seen in the growing metaphysis. Nevertheless, few would support Bidder today in his contention. Rather, there seems no reason to deny these small featureless cells of mesenchymal appearance, the pluripotency of developing into the cell population necessary for forming a centre of secondary ossification; in much the same way as the exiguous mesenchyme cells of the primary vascular irruption give rise to the bone marrow in the shaft.

Centrifugal canals

After the formation of a secondary centre of ossification, new centrifugal canals are formed which radiate outwards through the cartilage, postnatally. These aid in the spread of vascular mesenchyme through the epiphysis, replacing cartilage with bone trabeculae and marrow. The vessels of the centrifugal canals at a later stage are found crossing the epiphyseal bone plate. They reinforce, then finally replace, the subchondral vessels in those canals which originated in Ranvier's groove. In this way a specialized subchondral circulation on the epiphyseal aspect of the growth cartilage is developed (Fig. 11.2). Finally, only the articular and growth cartilages remain of the original epiphyseal cartilages, and communicating vessels are no longer in evidence.

Chapter 11
Growth cartilages

As a tissue, growth cartilage, or the growth zone, forms a specialized layer in epiphyseal cartilages which constitute the extremities of fetal tubular bones (Fig. 11.1). In the event of a secondary centre of ossification developing in the epiphysis, the growth zone becomes sandwiched between the spongiosa of the epiphysis and the metaphysis, and is thereby converted into a cartilaginous *growth plate* (Fig. 11.2). A growth zone or plate is also often referred to as a growth cartilage, i.e. an organ, no special distinction being made between the fetal and postnatal structure. Because they are of paramount importance to the mechanism whereby bones increase in length, the blood supply of growth cartilages and the morphological interrelationships between cartilage, blood vessels and osteogenesis have engaged the attention of many investigators.

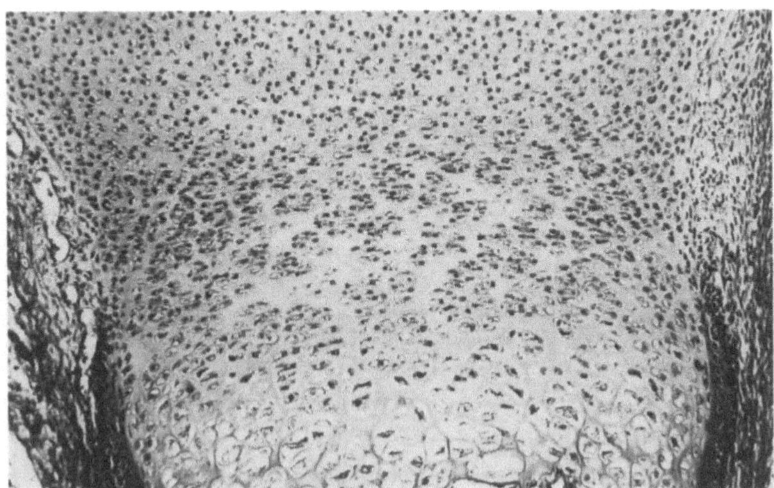

Fig. 11.1. The growth cartilage in a 28 cm CR length fetal phalanx. Note vertical orientation of clumps of hypertrophic cells. The smaller, proliferating cells are arciform, bounded by Ranvier's ring. (Original magnification ×67)

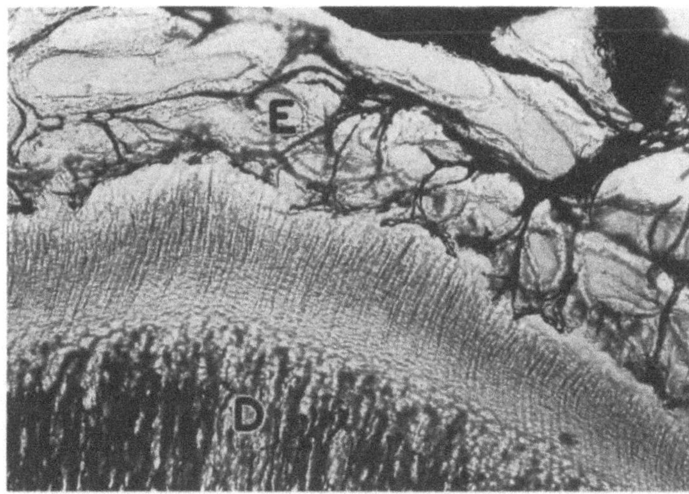

Fig. 11.2. Growth cartilage of a rabbit femur. E, Epiphyseal subchondral vessels below the bone plate; D, metaphyseal subchondral vessels. (Original magnification ×90)

Perichondral vessels

The early cartilaginous primordia of long bones in the 7th week of embryonic life depend for their nutrition on diffusion of substances from perichondrial vessels. With the development of a primary centre of ossification, a growth zone is formed flanked by Ranvier's ossification ring and groove which gives attachment to the periosteum-perichondrium of the growing bone (Figs 10.4, 11.1). In fetal life and until maturity, fibrocellular tissue fills in the groove (Fig. 11.3, *overleaf*); here also is a plexus of small perichondrial vessels derived from the circulus vasculosus. It seems reasonable to suppose that diffusion from capillaries in Ranvier's groove supplies nutrients to the rim of the growth cartilage, which forms a portion of the wall of the groove. Direct penetration of vessels into the growth cartilage from this site does not occur in postnatal life, although early in fetal life, vascular cartilage canals do arise in the floor of the groove. They penetrate into the undifferentiated cartilage epiphysis to ramify as a distinct canal group close to the epiphyseal aspect of the growth zone.

In growing postnatal bone, the vascular plexus on the rim of the growth plate is very obvious in perfused preparations. Brodin (1955) showed that fluorophors injected intravenously diffuse from the perichondrial plexus into the edge of the plate. In the experimental rabbit, Trueta & Amato (1960) have also observed that the rim of the plate survived after necrosis of most of the plate had occurred, following destruction of the epiphyseal tissue. It is clear that the perichondrial plexus of vessels is normally responsible for the nutrition of a thin annulus of chondrocytes at the periphery of a growth cartilage. This may, however, be very important for growth and expansion of the cartilage in its lateral diameter. Just how this takes place is not known with certainty. It could be a consequence of cell division in the edge of the germinal layer of the growth cartilage, occurring so that daughter cells move transversely and not in an axial sense as in the cartilage generally.

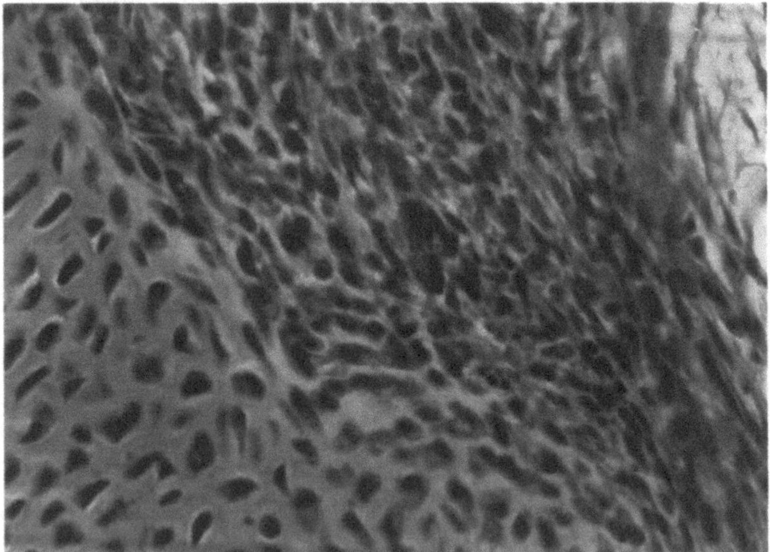

Fig. 11.3. Mesenchyme in Ranvier's groove, showing gradation from fibroblasts, through prochondrocytes, to chondrocytes. (Chick; Original magnification ×490)

On the other hand, the cytology of the ossification groove suggests that mitosis in vascular perichondrial mesenchyme contributes cells (prochondrocytes) which are incorporated into the edge of the expanding growth plate (Fig. 11.3).

Metaphyseal subchondral vessels

In growing animals, small arteries in the metaphysis pass towards the growth cartilage. Their arteriolar subdivisions, which neither branch nor anastomose, form the arterial feed-in of a subchondral vascular network, sometimes referred to as M-side juxta-epiphyseal vessels. Vascular loops are formed from which vertical collecting vessels arise. These, by retrograde confluence in the metaphyseal cancelli, give rise to the dense venous sinuses characteristic of the region.

The literature shows lack of unanimity of opinion with respect to several features of the metaphyseal subchondral circulation.

Arterial supply

According to Trueta & Amato (1960), two-fifths of the arterial blood supplying the metaphyseal subchondral circulation in the 3-month-old rabbit is derived from metaphyseal nutrient arteries. Lewis (1956), however, considers that in the early human fetus the arteries supplying this circulation are branches of the principal nutrient artery alone, and that later the metaphyseal nutrients become an additional source. It seems probable that the developmental stage reached by the skeleton, and whether one is dealing with a "growing" or "non-growing" growth plate, influences the proportion of arterial blood contributed by each nutrient group. (See also "Blood supply of metaphyses" in Chapter 2.)

The sinusoid network

According to Ranvier (1875), single vascular loops invade* the cartilage. The convexity of the loop occupies the space between two adjacent vertical matrix partitions and the most proximal cartilage capsule, i.e. there is one loop for each isogenic column of chondrocytes. Furthermore, in Ranvier's account, cartilage destruction "ne se fait pas dans une direction quelconque, mais seulement dans le sens de la croissance des vaisseaux", i.e. the direction of invasion is strictly in line with the direction of vascular growth. All vertical bars of matrix are thereby preserved. According to Langer (1876), each end-artery terminates in a tuft of capillary loops, each tuft being intimately associated with a small group of chondrocyte columns. The venous ends of the loops freely anastomose. The accounts of Ranvier and Langer, like those of several modern investigators, were based on vascular perfusion techniques and the study of thick cleared sections. Both these authorities justifiably command the respect of all who have followed in the pathways they pioneered. Because the point is relevant to the problem of the morphogenesis of cancellous bone, the evidence is worth examining further.

Isogenic columns or clumps

Ranvier's description of a discrete system of vascular loops, each related to a column of chondrocytes, is echoed by Testut & Latarjet (1948) and Bloom & Fawcett (1962). However, the photomicrograph exhibited by the latter authorities does not support the "one column–one loop" concept of vascular invasion implied in their text. Trueta and Morgan (1960) do, however, give it further substance by their work on the tibia of the 3-month-old rabbit. On the other hand, the work of Dodds (1930) on the human fetus and de Marneffe (1951) on the caudal vertebrae of the postnatal rat indicates that in some situations, and especially in fetal material, the sinusoid arrangement is more complex and diffuse.

Brookes (1963) and Brookes & Landon (1963) have investigated the juxta-epiphyseal region in fetal human and rodent material by a variety of methods. They find that sinusoid loops are dispersed over the surface of the calcified zone of cartilage in ill-defined clumps which freely anastomose (Fig. 11.4, *overleaf*). The vessels are varicose in appearance and show saccular and blind digital processes in agreement with the findings of Dahl (1934) and de Marneffe (1951), as indeed with those of both Ranvier and Langer in their original treatises (Fig. 11.5, *overleaf*). A clump of sinusoids is related not to a single chondrocyte column but to a group, so that in the wake of the invasion of cartilage by marrow, only stout vertical matrix bars survive the chondrolytic process; the many finer ones, and the transverse matrix

* The word "invade" is used here and elsewhere in a descriptive sense to record the appearance of growth into and replacement of cartilage by vascular mesenchyme. It is neutral with respect to any of the mechanisms of cartilage replacement that might be operative; e.g. vascular erosion of matrix from without, or chondrolysis by the cartilage cells from within.

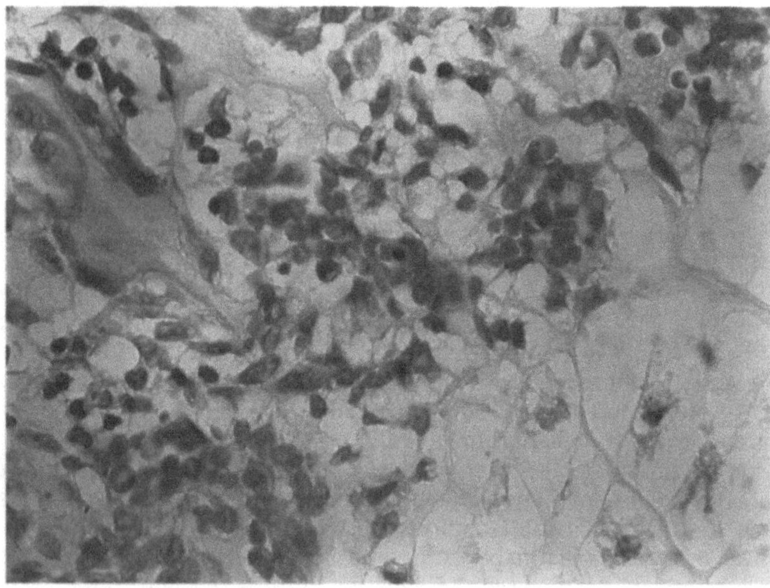

Fig. 11.4. An average paraffin section of the marrow–cartilage junction. The red cell masses do not appear to be extravasations. (Original magnification ×360)

bars, are destroyed. Both text and illustration in Ham & Leeson (1964) concur with this description, which in essence follows that of H. Müller (1858), the first investigator to give a detailed histological account of bone growth in length. Müller plainly states that invasion takes place not only vertically but transversely, so that columnar matrix is destroyed in addition to horizontal matrix partitions. The EM investigations of Anderson & Parker (1966) on postnatal rats also show that thin vertical matrix bars are removed by invading vascular mesenchyme.

If all vertical matrix bars survived, as implied by the "one column–one loop" school, then the pattern of young endochondral bone forming in the marrow would be congruent with that of the vertical bars in the calcified zone. This is not the case in fetal material, nor, according to de Marneffe (1951), does it happen in postnatal bones. Pratt's (1957) observation in the fetal rat that primary spongiosa (the layer between the calcified zone and the ordered bone deposits in the metaphysis) contains an irregular arrangement of matrix debris, also supports the view that matrix destruction is imprecise and does not leave behind a fine honeycomb of calcified matrix tubes in the metaphysis, as Trueta and Morgan (1960) described in the 3-month-old rabbit tibia. In transverse section, the metaphysis does indeed exhibit a trabecular honeycomb, but the spaces correspond to groups of chondrocyte columns and not to single columns.

The divergence in viewpoint as to whether cartilage matrix is invaded imprecisely or discretely may perhaps lie in differences between young and old growth cartilages. It is possible that as growth proceeds, the fetal condition represented by clumps of hypertrophic columns associated with juxtaposed sinusoid tufts, gives way to a more precise growth mechanism wherein the majority of cell columns, or matrix tubes, are associated each with its own varicose sinusoid loop. In this way calcified matrix would, with greater efficiency, be made available for endochondral bone formation in sites between the stem vessels of the subchondral circulation.

Open or closed subchondral sinusoids

Another problem that has been aired from time to time since Ranvier's day is whether the metaphyseal subchondral sinusoids are open or closed, i.e. whether microhaemorrhages from the sinusoid network occur or not. Van der Stricht (1892) was firmly of the opinion that the medullary sinusoids in general were closed in the avian material he studied. Nevertheless, he described how subchondral sinusoids arose by bifurcation of narrow rectilinear arteries and noted that red cells were present *outside* the sinusoid wall, lying free in the newly opened cartilage capsules. He also recorded his inability to see subchondral sinusoids by perfusion in mammals, and believed they were open in this situation.

Lewis (1956) studying perfused human fetal preparations, noted ampulla-like dilations of the subchondral sinusoids and concluded that they represented microhaemorrhages. Trueta & Morgan (1960), also working on perfused material, came to the same conclusion and speculated that the function of the microhaemorrhages might be to increase local phosphate concentration in the calcifying zone of cartilage, or to convey serum alkaline phosphatase to the calcification site.

It is noteworthy that Ranvier (1875), who examined this particular problem histologically, was sure that the endothelium is always closed. Other investigators, for example, Doan (1931), Dahl (1934), de Marneffe (1951) and Brookes (1963), utilizing perfusion techniques and LM, are also satisfied as to the closed nature of the sinusoids (Figs 11.5, 11.6, *overleaf*). Nevertheless, it must be admitted that results obtained by LM in this particular field of investigation must always be open to some doubt, which it can be hoped EM may go a long way to resolve.

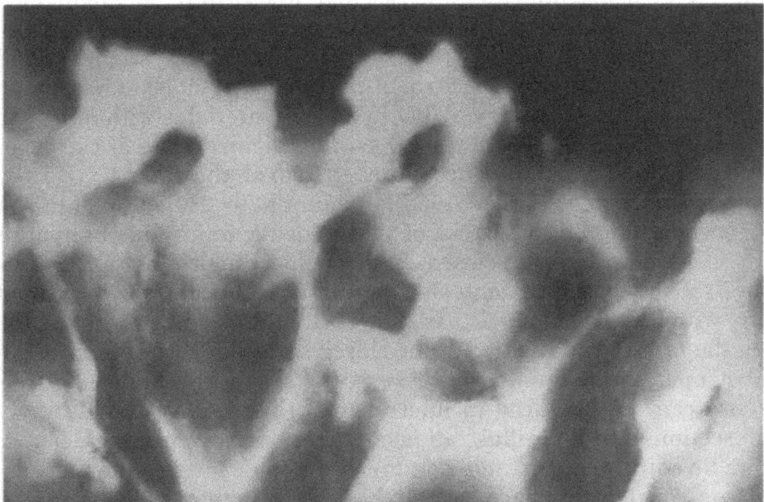

Fig. 11.5. Sinusoid loops in the metaphyseal subchondral circulation. (Human fetus; Original magnification ×600)

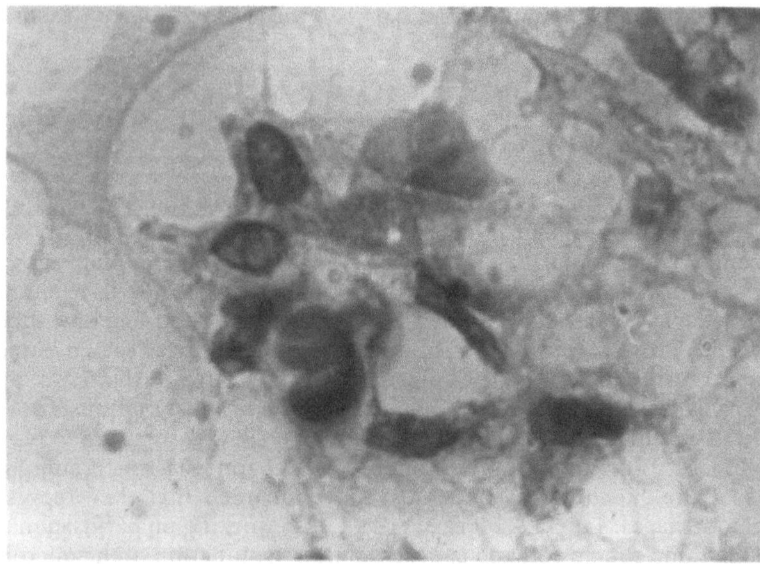

Fig. 11.6. High power examination of what may appear to be red cells lying free in chondrocyte lacunae often indicates the presence of vascular endothelium. (Original magnification ×880)

Brookes & Landon (1963) have examined with the EM the metaphyseal subchondral region of rat fetal femora perfused with osmium tetroxide fixative. The fetuses were perfused alive *in utero* through the umbilical artery a day before parturition, in order to avoid the real possibility of imperfect fixation and post-mortem retraction of the delicate subchondral vessels. This can occur only too easily when reliance is placed on post-mortem immersion fixation of what is the least accessible part of a limb, namely the skeleton.

In rapidly growing bone, where vascular microruptures might have been expected, they noted that when red cells were observed to be lying extremely close to the growth cartilage, they were separated from it by vascular endothelium (Fig. 11.7). Often the intervening strip of endothelial cytoplasm was about 40 nm (400 Å) thick or less. This presumably in no way interferes with ionic exchange, nor with the passage of enzymes, between the calcified zone of cartilage on the one hand and blood circulating in a closed system on the other.

However, Anderson & Parker (1966), in their EM investigation of this problem in rats, newborn and up to 3 weeks of age, made the following observations. The majority of the sinusoids are closed. In this respect their illustrations agree with those of Brookes & Landon, and show a thin endothelial layer in intimate relationship with cartilage matrix. In other situations, macrophages intervene between the matrix and the tips of the closed sinusoids. A minority of sinusoids are widely open in the opinion of these workers: endothelial defects are present whose size can be measured in micrometres (and hence should be visible in paraffin sections). In their illustrations of these open vessels, the defect is at the tip of the invading sinusoid and is at much the same level as the most advanced red cell, so that a haemorrhage beyond the vessels is not actually present. In addition, the most advanced red cells shown in "open" sinusoids are three to five red cell diameters from the nearest transverse bar. This situation, present in Anderson and

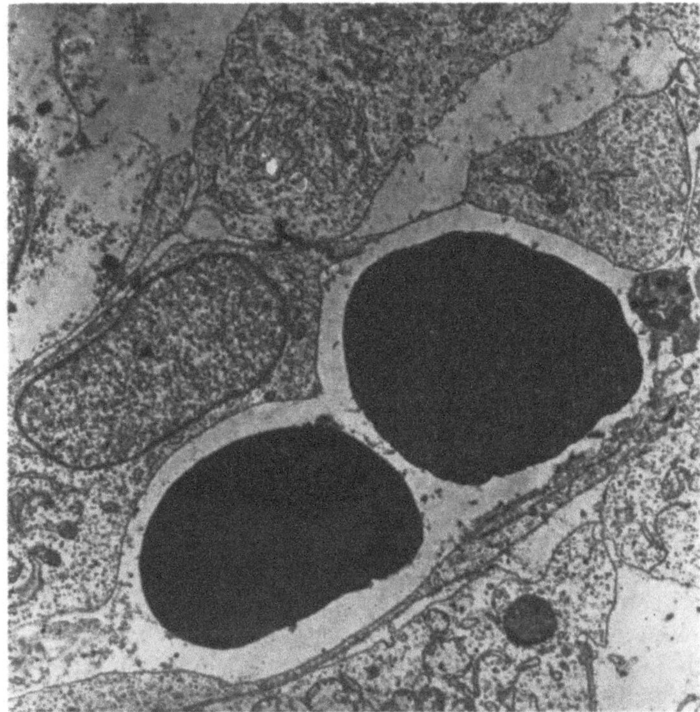

Fig. 11.7. EM of a longitudinal section of a closed juxta-epiphyseal sinusoid (fetal mouse femur). Note the extreme thinness of the wall in places, and the mesenchyme cells outside and not attached to it. (Original magnification ×5500)

Parker's principal visual evidence for open subchondral sinusoids, suggests a tearing of the endothelium during post mortem retraction away from an intimate contact with the cartilage. Furthermore, their illustrations derive entirely from work done on immersion fixed material: they write that abdominal aortic perfusion of their rats with fixative gave the same results.

Vascular endothelium and chondrolytic cells

The origin of the chondrolytic cell is debatable. The commonly held view is that it is a modified connective tissue cell, having only an ancestral connection with vascular endothelium in early embryogenesis. It is furthermore generally agreed that dissolution of the growth cartilage is brought about by circulating mononuclear cells and not by osteoclasts. The former cells in the metaphyseal subchondral region resemble in the LM either bone-forming cells (Bloom *et al.* 1941) or mesenchyme cells (Brookes & Landon 1963). Multinucleate osteoclasts are found only behind the forefront of the vascular invasion, not right against the cartilage (Park 1954; Brookes 1963). It is appropriate at this point to mention the suggestion which was put forward by Keith (1927) and others before him, and which has been renewed recently, that vascular endothelium may be the source of bone-forming cells, osteoclasts and chondrolytic cells.

Undoubtedly, bone substance is deposited and removed in the immediate neighbourhood of capillaries, an intimate relationship which has been remarked on by Wolff (1870), Gebhardt (1905) and Weidenreich (1923) as characterizing normal bone formation. It has also been observed and emphasized in the process of fracture repair by Bell (1823), Macewen (1912) and many others and in various ectopic ossification sites. In the latter group, Bürger and Oppenheimer (1908) described ossification in the walls of large arteries following the proliferation of the capillaries of the vasa vasorum; capillaries together with young connective tissue cells. This is the crux of the matter. A capillary is never present without the even more immediate and intimate association of connective tissue or mesenchyme cells, which derive from a mesodermal origin in earliest embryonic life. These extra-endothelial cells are always to be found in LM wherever there is a capillary in an osteogenic area, be it subchondral zone, Haversian canal, bone marrow, or fracture site (see "Origin of angioblasts" in Chapter 8).

It has long been recognized that the cells responsible for chondrolysis of cartilage are intimately related to the subchondral sinusoids. Ranvier, observing the closeness of the sinusoid loops to the calcified cartilage, emphasizes: "Il est impossible de ne pas reconnaître que les vaisseaux jouent un très grand rôle dans la resorption du cartilage d'ossification." On the other hand, in the term "bourgeons conjonctivo-vasculaires" Dubreuil (1929) reminds us that the subchondral vessels are not naked, but are packed in connective tissue. The aborted chondrolytic power of the subchondral metaphyseal circulation is suggested by the unusually thick cartilage found in clinical *rickets*, where only irregular inroads of mushroom-like processes of vascular mesenchyme occur (Park 1939).

Park's account has been confirmed in experimental rickets using vitamin D_3, by Hunter *et al.* (1991) who emphasized the integrity of the subchondral arterioles, sinusoids and venules, complete with basal membrane and pericyte coat. No organized growth front developed in contact with the hypertrophic zone of the growth plate. Vitamin D_3 repletion restored vascular invasion of the cartilage, in particular by attenuated endothelial cells lacking a basal membrane or pericyte coat. Hunter & Arsenault (1990) find that the invading vascular buds consist of squamous fenestrated endothelial cells, which even in daughter cells are held together by tight junctions. Normal vascular subchondral morphology, however, was restored in 4 days (Hunter *et al.* 1991).

The persistence of the avascular cartilage growth plate in harmony with the subchondral vascular invasion, depends on its chondrocytes releasing messenger molecules which inhibit angiogenesis and vascular invasion. Hansen (1993) has reviewed this area and points out that one factor stops endothelial cell proliferation and migration and inhibits endothelial collagenase released during invasion of the growth plate (Moses *et al.* 1990). Other factors produced by chondrocytes are basic fibroblast growth factor (bFGF), its acidic variety (aFGF) and endothelial cell growth factor (ECGF). All these stimulate proliferation and migration of endothelial cells, in a cell culture medium (Folkman 1985). It is held that vascular invasion of the growth plate results from angiogenesis stimulating factors overriding inhibitory factors. Initiation of invasion requires a trigger mechanism. This may be the release of bFGF from chondrocytes in the hypertrophic zone of the plate. Protease inhibition is maximal during chondrogenesis, but decreases as protease activity increases in the zone of calcification (Reddi & Kuettner 1981).

Plasmin, a potent peptidase released from circulating plasminogen by plasminogen activator (PA), peaks where the vessels invade. PA is presumably involved in destruction of cartilage matrix bars as the sinusoids advance (Desimone & Reddi 1992).

On the other hand, the EM evidence of Brookes & Landon (1963) shows that, apart from the ultrathin endothelial cytoplasmic barrier between cartilage and erythrocytes (see "The sinusoid network", above), clumps of endothelial-like cells are frequent. They differ in EM detail from typical endothelial cells, but resemble them far more than they do either a chondrocyte or a bone-forming cell, and can be equated with the mesenchyme cells of LM. Anderson & Parker (1966) refer to them as macrophages. These chondrolytic cells might, on the face of it, be budded off from subchondral endothelial cells actively growing into the cartilage. This possibility is strengthened by Cameron's (1961) EM investigation, in which he found collagen and bone crystals in endothelioid cells immediately flanking the calcified zone of cartilage. Furthermore, there is evidence of the phagocytic property of vascular endothelium in the marrow generally (see "Phagocytosis" in Chapter 8) and in other situations (Macklin & Macklin 1920; Cunningham 1922). Nevertheless, until more decisive evidence is available regarding the supposed direct descent of a chondrolytic cell from a sinus endothelial cell, the conservative view of chondrolysis as a function of a distinct and separate line of mesenchyme cells closely associated with, but not the daughter cells of, sinus endothelium, will probably find general acceptance.

Growth plate chondrocytes themselves are involved in the breakdown of the matrix bars and transverse partitions which surround them. As the cells of the hypertrophic zone approach the marrow, their lacunae become larger and the matrix bars become thinner. Under the EM a clear zone of matrix, free of collagen fibrillae, immediately surrounds these large chondrocytes. With thinning of a matrix partition, the part containing collagen is reduced to a minimum and finally vanishes when the clear zones associated with two chondrocytes fuse (Figs 11.8–11.12, *overleaf*). Hence, hypertrophy of the chondrocytes in a growth plate necessitates a chondrolytic activity on their part.

In support of this view it may be noted that in the cytoplasm of enlarging chondrocytes there is an abundant granular endoplasmic reticulum (Fig. 11.10), indicating a high level of protein, including enzyme, synthesis. Furthermore, lysosomes and "myelin" figures increase in frequency the nearer the cells are to the marrow (Fig. 11.12). Collagenase has been identified at least in liver lysosomes (Schoefl 1963). Histochemical investigation of rat growth cartilages shows that the cells of the hypertrophic zone contain hydrolytic enzymes, cathepsin, and acid and alkaline phophatases.

It is apparent that large chondrocytes are equipped for the chondrolytic function indicated by microscopy. In particular, they themselves participate in the dissolution of mucopolysaccharides and collagen in the matrix of growth cartilages. A similar phenomenon occurs in fetal epiphyses during the growth and development of cartilage canals. According to Watermann (1961), the epiphyseal chondrocytes lyse themselves free and thus contribute to the elongation of the canals.

As for the metaphyseal aspect of growth cartilages, it seems that the "invasive" description applied to the subchondral vascular tissue has misled many investigators in favour of granting it a destructive "storm-troop" character which it may not in fact possess. On the contrary, what we discuss as a subchondral

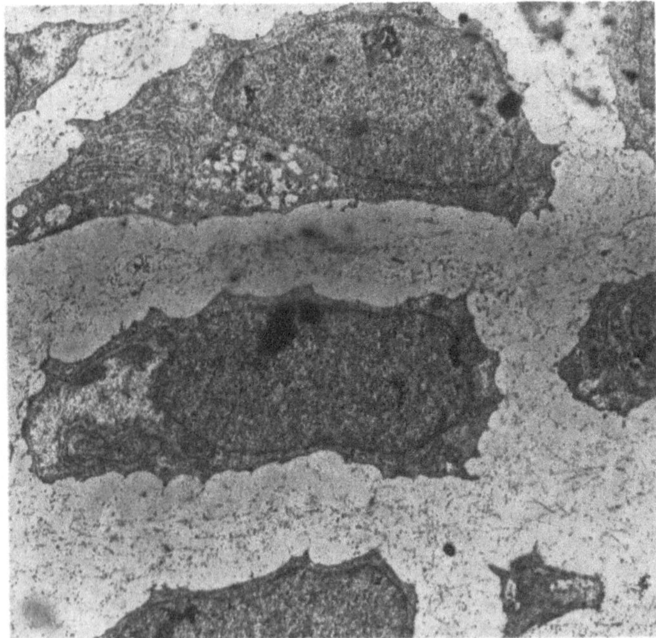

Fig. 11.8. EM of germinal cells in the growth zone. The cartilage matrix contains fine fibrillary collagen. (Fetal rat femur, Original magnification ×5500)

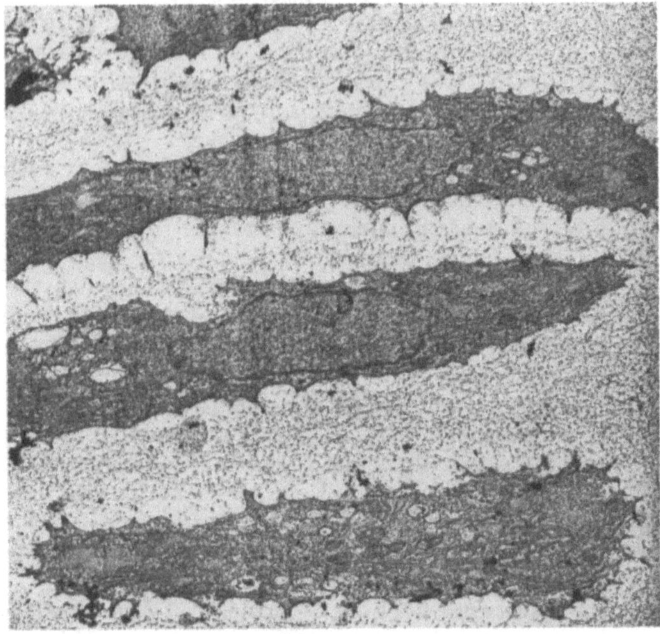

Fig. 11.9. EM of flat cells in the proliferative layer in the growth zone. The cytoplasm is electron dense, and is packed with granular endoplasmic reticulum and granular material. (Original magnification ×5500)

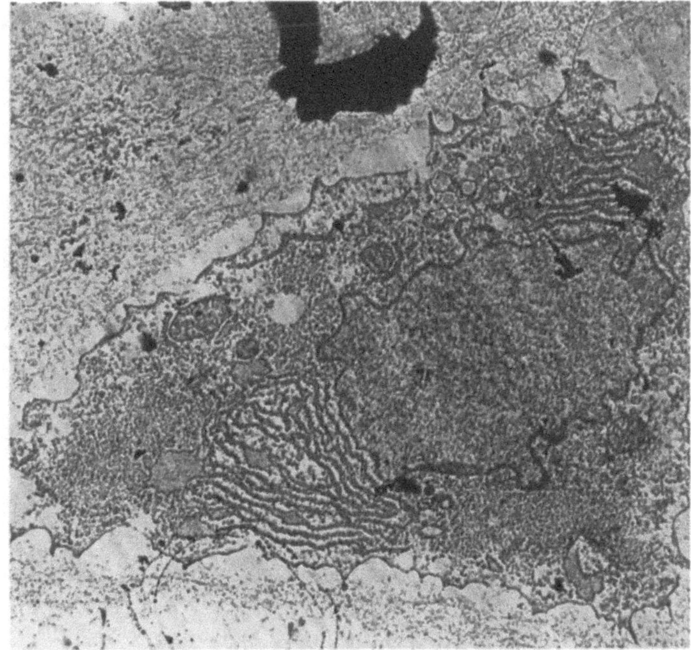

Fig. 11.10. EM of a hypertrophic cell in the growth cartilage. An abundant granular endoplasmic reticulum and clouds of glycogen granules are in the cytoplasm. (Original magnification ×8000)

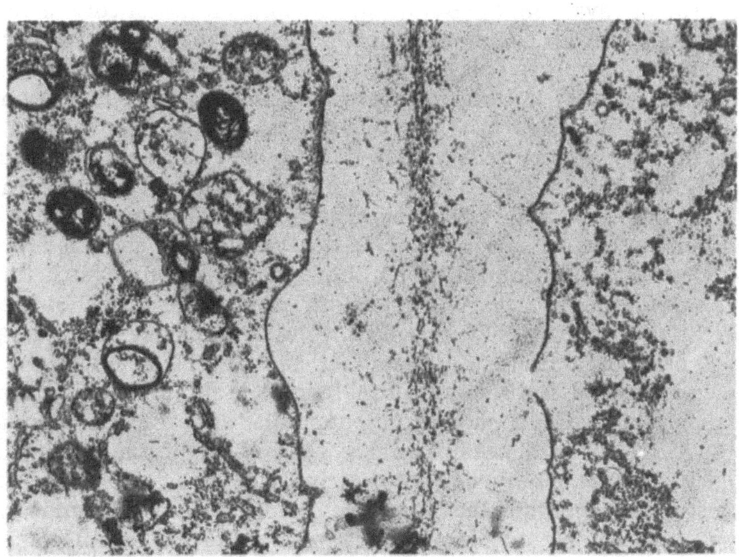

Fig. 11.11. EM of two hypertrophic chondrocytes in the growth cartilage near to the marrow. Note the loss of collagen in the narrowing matrix partition between them and the presence of cytoplasmic lysosomal bodies. (Original magnification ×10 000)

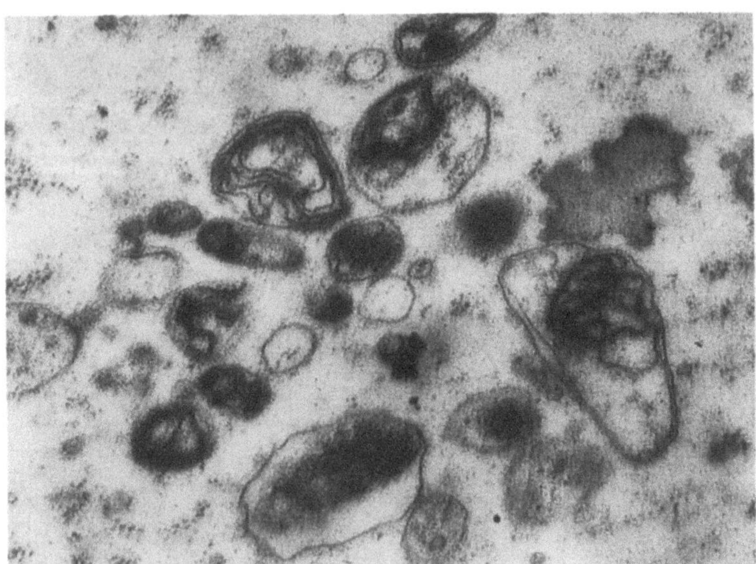

Fig. 11.12. Lysosomal figures in the cytoplasm of hypertrophic chondrocytes. (Original magnification ×60 000)

chondrolytic cell may possibly be concerned only with mopping up the debris of lysed calcified cartilage which was primarily disorganized and broken down by the large chondrocytes in the cartilage itself.

Stump (1925) was of the opinion that the buds of vascular mesenchyme which he observed invading the growth cartilage were made up of syncytial masses. These, as growth advanced, differentiated into an endothelial core in continuity with a growing sinusoid. The more peripheral cells of the bud moved proximally and differentiated into osteoblasts, which remained behind the invasion front, flanking the blood vessels, to participate in endochondral bone formation.

Trueta (1963) gave osteoclasts, osteoblasts and chondrolytic cells a common origin from the endothelial cells of the general bone vasculature, the pathway of differentiation being influenced by environmental differences within the bone. Against this, however, is the well-documented fact that osteoclasts derive from the mononuclear-macrophage cell line. In the EM the cell population of the vascular buds in the subchondral zone shows a gradation of structure from undoubted endothelial cells, through intermediate endothelioid cells, to undoubted bone-forming cells, the most significant change being the gradual acquisition of an organized endoplasmic reticulum. Yet it is to be expected that vascular endothelium and the cuff of mesenchyme immediately in front of it, both mesodermal in origin, should present similar appearances, although these are not identical. The evidence of Oni *et al.* (1993) using lectin binding and antibodies raised against endothelial cell proteins, clearly suggests that osteoblasts do not derive from endothelium. Hence, until direct descent of chondrolytic cells (the third claimant of an endothelial ancestry) from subchondral vascular endothelium is demonstrated beyond doubt, it seems safer to regard chondrolysis at the growth plate as a function of perivascular mesenchyme, proliferating and differentiating in pure race separately from endothelial development.

Vascular and trabecular pattern

From a study of typical growth plates with well-marked column formation, the conclusion may be attractive that the vertical matrix partitions which survive erosion account for and impose a similar order on endochondral bone trabeculae. Certain facts throw doubt on this general proposition, which would make metaphyseal structure secondary to the guiding trabeculae, "travées directrices" (Ranvier 1875; Dubreuil 1929) derived from the vertical spans of the growth cartilage. It has been shown (Pinard 1952; Brookes 1963) that in early human fetal growth cartilages, chondrocytes are not necessarily vertically arranged, but can be disposed on the arc of a circle delimiting the primary marrow, i.e. they are arciform in layout (Figs 4.8, 11.1). Metaphyseal vessels and bone trabeculae lie, however, side by side in postnatal bones and both are disposed vertically in the bony long axis. Again, in normal postnatal material, chondrocytes are by no means always found in unbroken columns extending from the amorphous to the calcified zone, without any directional change. For example, in the periphery of the growth plate of a rib, the chondrocyte columns are oblique until the hypertrophic zone is reached (Fig. 11.13). Similar appearances can be found even in such a typical growth plate as that at the lower end of the femur (Fig. 11.14, *overleaf*). Hence, it is only the hypertrophic cells which are generally aligned with the metaphyseal vessels (Fig. 11.14). Other examples can be found in an experimental growth plate and metaphysis raised ultrasonically at the lower end of the femur, *outside* its shaft (Figs 11.15–11.18, *overleaf*). Column formation in the neocartilage is at best poorly indicated, although the arrangement of the bone trabeculae and vessels is typically metaphyseal. In both normal and abnormal material, the constancy of metaphyseal vascular and trabecular pattern is remarkable, and is not dependent on the form of the matrix bars in the growth cartilage. On the contrary, the growth of sinusoids in the subchondral region is in advance of

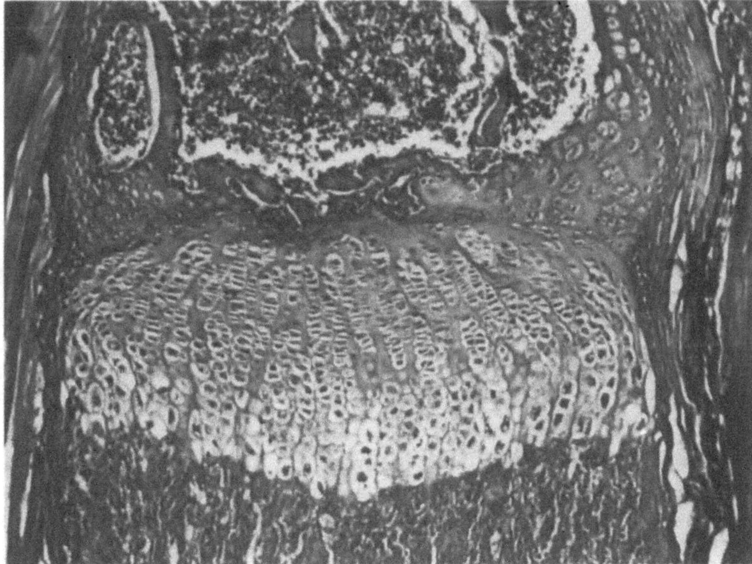

Fig. 11.13. Growth cartilage in the head of a rib. The proliferative cells radiate outwards, but the hypertrophic cells are in line with metaphyseal blood vessels and trabeculae. (Original magnification ×90)

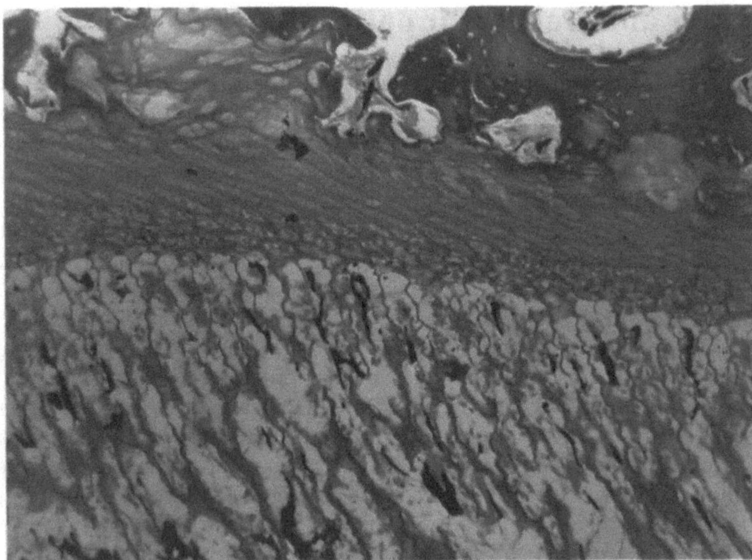

Fig. 11.14. Oblique columns of proliferating cells in the periphery of rabbit femoral cartilage. Only the hypertrophic cells are in line with metaphyseal vessels and trabeculae. (Original magnification ×90)

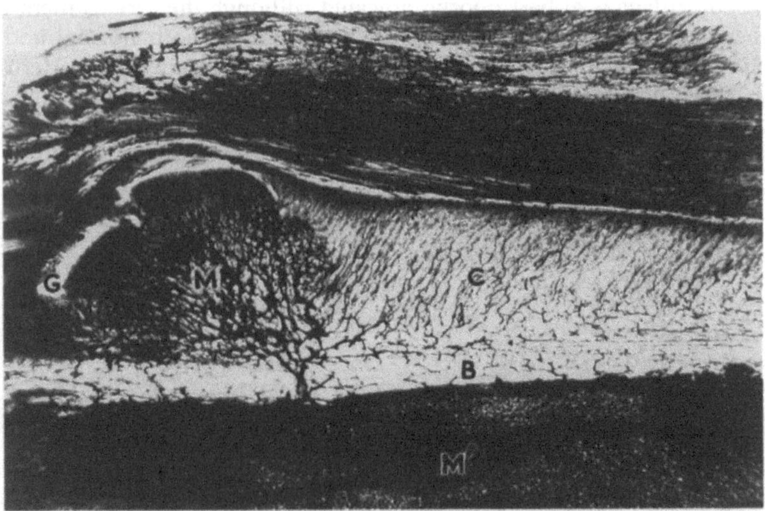

Fig. 11.15. After ultrasonic irradiation of the femoral metaphysis in a rabbit, a new cortex (C), metaphysis (M) and growth cartilage (G) have formed outside the old cortex (B) and marrow (M'). The new metaphyseal vascular pattern is indistinguishable from normal. (India ink; Original magnification ×24)

the differentiation of osteoblast cells from the mesenchyme of the vascular buds. As growth in length proceeds, the subchondral mesenchyme cells are left behind, to lie between sinusoid endothelium and surviving bits of cartilage matrix on which bone deposition occurs. That is to say, bone trabeculae are built up in the metaphysis parallel to *already ordered vessels*. It is therefore contended here that the pattern of endochondral bone trabeculae is secondary to that of the vessels about

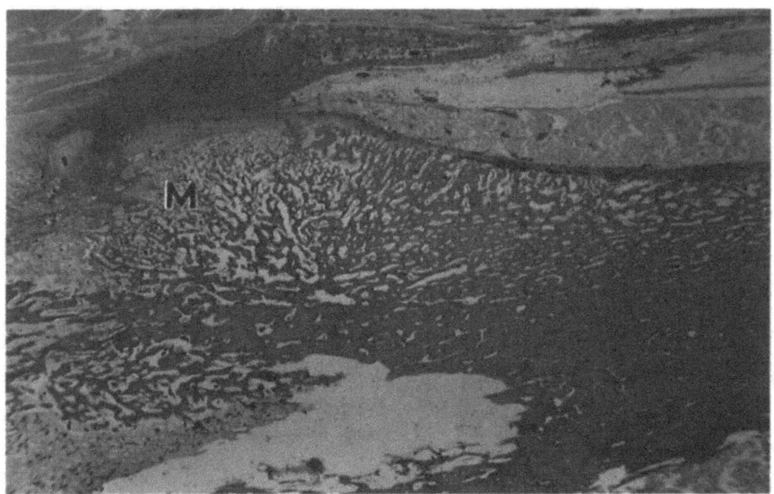

Fig. 11.16. The pattern of the new metaphyseal trabeculae (M) is the same as the vascular pattern in Fig. 11.15. (Original magnification ×24)

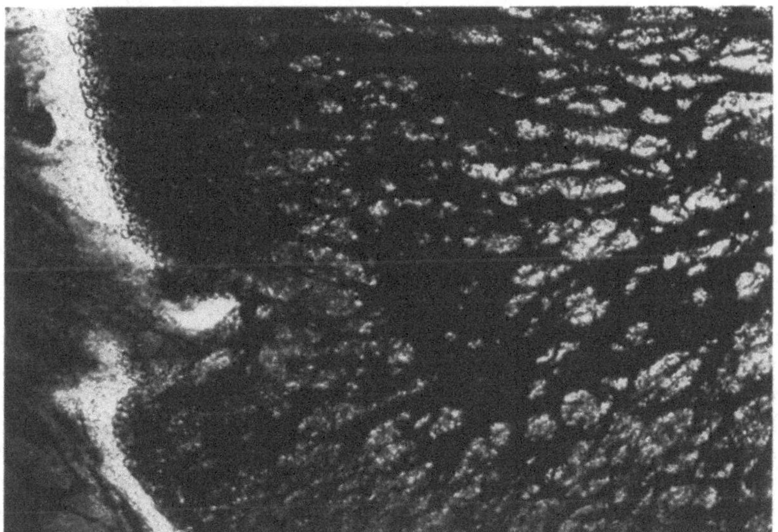

Fig. 11.17. New metaphyseal vessels associated with an abnormal growth cartilage after ultrasonic irradiation. (Original magnification ×225)

which they form. It is the metaphyseal vessels which order the disposition of the bone trabeculae.

Mechanism of bone elongation

The essential mechanism controlling the growth of vessels in the metaphysis and the emergence of their distinctive pattern is as yet poorly understood. It is

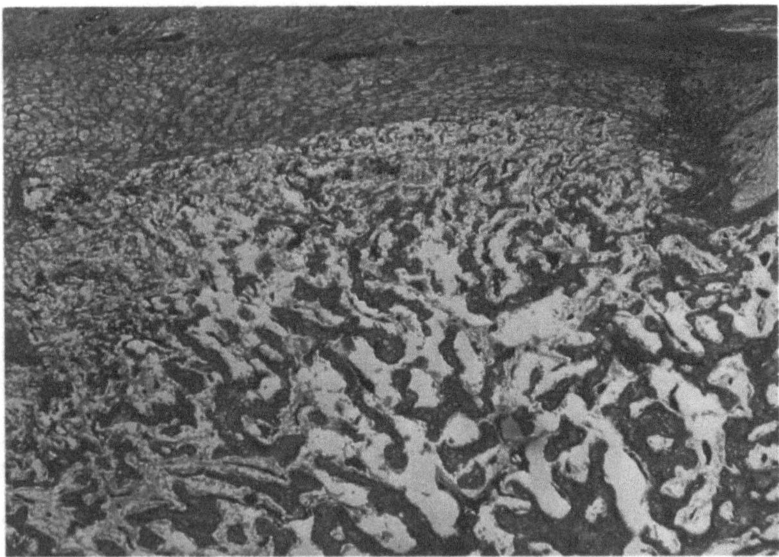

Fig. 11.18. Abnormal growth cartilage corresponding to Fig. 11.17, and spongy bone associated with it. (Original magnification ×340)

apparent that the growth front of the vessels is in the subchondral region and that they grow *into* the cartilage plate.

Molecular factors, stimulatory and inhibitory, are now known to interact between the the growth plate cartilage and subchondral vascular plexus (see "Vascular endothelium and chondrolytic cells", above).

Vitamin D_3 is well known to be a specific metabolite of hypertrophic chondrocytes (E. Kodiček, 1962, personal comunication). Its absence in rickets is the cause of the thick uncalcified growth cartilages found in this condition and of the failure of the chondrocytes to break down the matrix partitions near the marrow cavity. In the absence of matrix dissolution, the vascular mesenchyme of the marrow no longer advances and bone elongation ceases. In addition to the large number of molecular factors affecting longitudinal growth in this region, can be added the fact that growth cartilage chondrocytes respire anaerobically, utilizing the Emden–Meyerhof pathway of glycolysis (P. Kunin, 1966, personal communication). In the course, however, of normal cartilage development and dissolution, it might be expected that physiological gradients in the concentration of acid metabolites, lactate, CO_2 tension and pH of local tissue fluid, would radiate out into the subchondral zone from each cartilage lacuna, and thus impose a vertical order of growth on the adjacent vascular mesenchyme; providing, of course, that vascular endothelium is responsive to such stimuli.

That this may be so is suggested by similar phenomena in wound healing and acute inflammation, wherein the breakdown products of connective tissue protein, local acid pH and changed blood gas tensions probably form a background against which new capillaries are attracted into the damaged region. In the course of experimental fracture repair, perfusion technique shows that new blood vessels grow towards, as if attracted to, the anaerobically respiring cartilage masses necessary for soft callus formation, as well as towards damaged bone

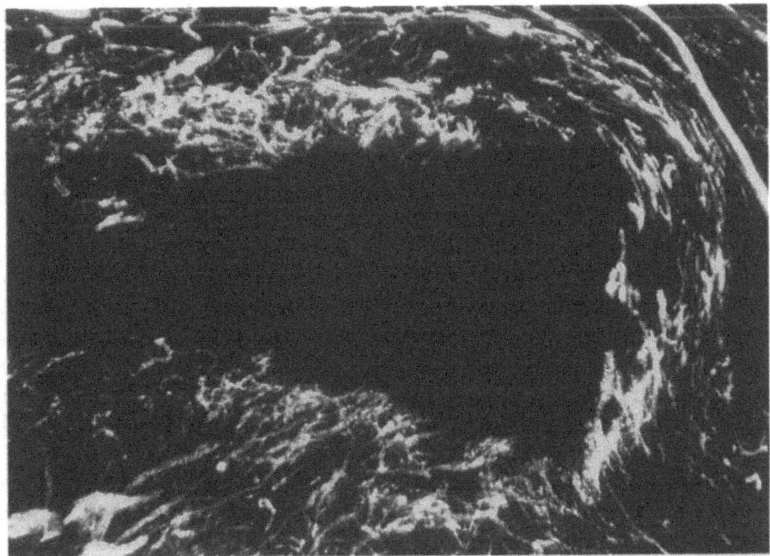

Fig. 11.19. Blood vessels growing towards osteotomized bone cortex 2 weeks postoperatively. (Microarteriogram; Original magnification ×24)

debris in the fracture site (Fig. 11.19). The crushed tissue contiguous with surgical screws, driven in for internal fixation of a fracture, seems to provide a particularly powerful stimulus directing the growth of new vessels, which in perfused preparations appear to focus on to the Vitallium screw itself (Fig. 11.20).

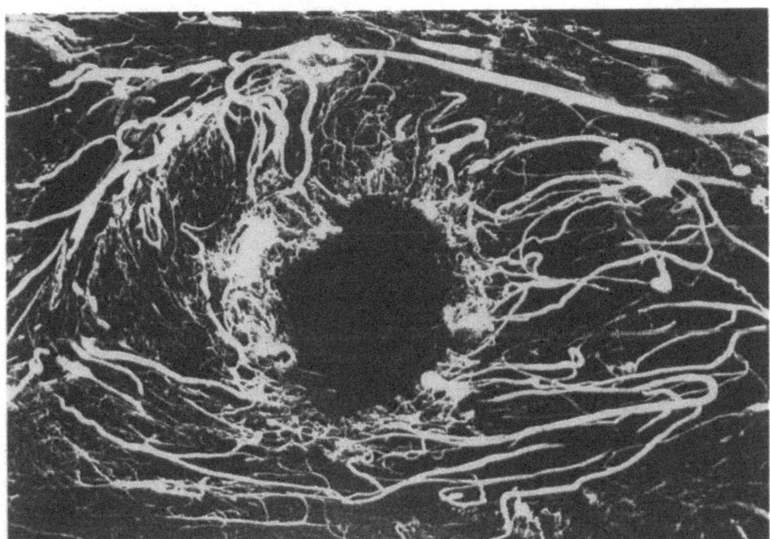

Fig. 11.20. Medullary blood vessels growing towards the site of a fixation screw, applied after humeral osteotomy. (Rabbit microarteriogram; Original magnification ×26)

Further examples may be quoted suggesting that an acidic region exercises a stimulating action on the growth of new capillaries in bone. Volkmann (1863), for example, described the growth of new vessels into a chronic tuberculous metatarsal. Jaffe & Pomeranz (1934), in another classical paper, described capillary erosion of ischaemic bone in arteriosclerotic disease.

The vessels attracted into the growth plate carry with them their mesenchymal cuff, which participates together with the chondrocytes in the breaking down of matrix, thus releasing into the primary marrow the proximal row of chondrocytes. Whether these cells survive or die in their new medullary environment is not known with certainty. At one time it was commonly held that the chondrocytes survived the vascular invasion from the metaphysis and gave rise to red blood cells and other marrow elements (Kassowitz 1881). The release of the last chondrocyte shown in EM (Figs 11.21–11.24) suggests that it dies. However, Holtrop (1965) carried out experiments on transplated growth plates utilizing ^{3}H-tritiated thymidine labelling and radioautography. She suggested that chondrocytes live on in the marrow and give rise to osteoblasts. There is no reason to doubt that chondrocytes, while they are in the cartilage plate, are very much alive and dependent on nutritional resourses emanating from blood vessels lying nearby. Even in the hypertrophic zone the chondrocytes, if not released into the marrow by vascular irruption, can live on in a considerably thickened cartilage, e.g. in rickets, or when a marrow infarct is produced (see "Blood supply of growth cartilages, below).

It seems, therefore, that in the mechanism of bone elongation, a reciprocal relationship exists between the growth cartilage and the blood vessels of the

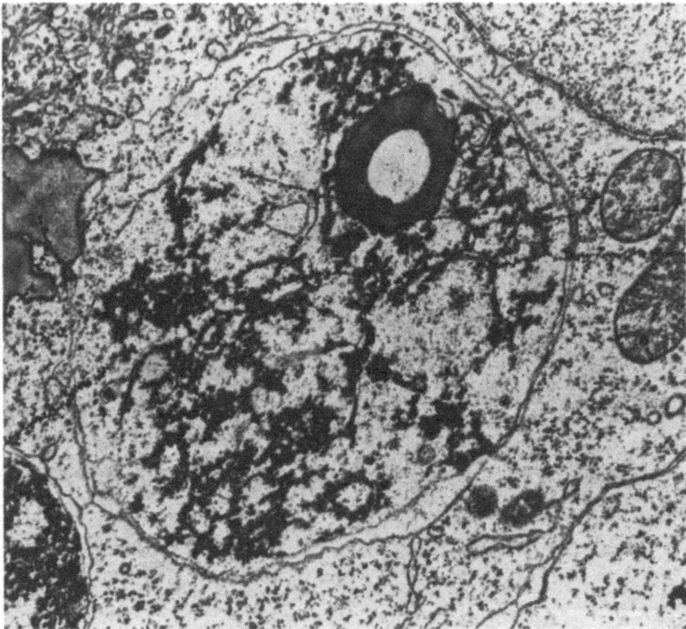

Fig. 11.21. EM of nuclear debris engulfed by a macrophage lying immediately against the calcified zone of growth cartilage. (Original magnification ×47 000)

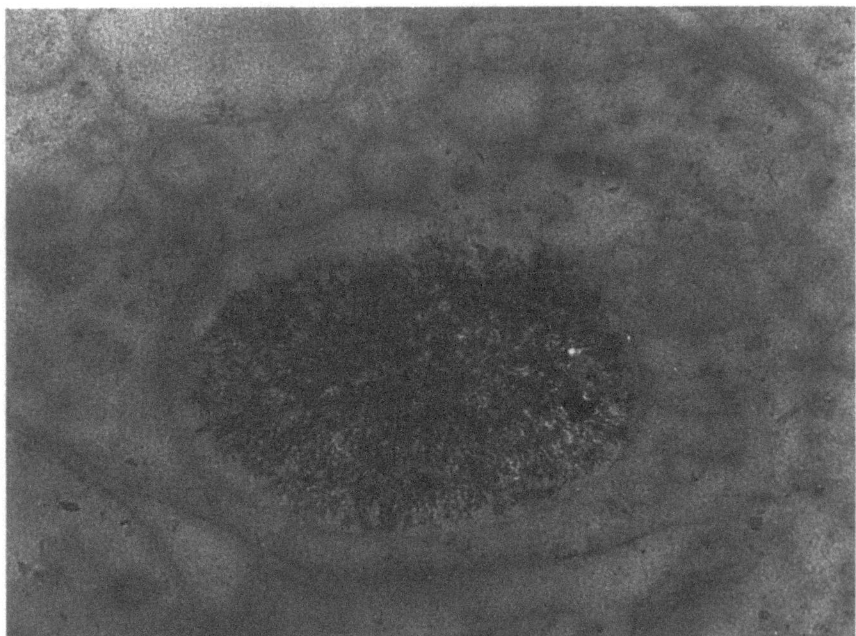

Fig. 11.22. EM of bone crystals engulfed by a juxta-epiphyseal mesenchyme cell. (Original magnification ×57 000)

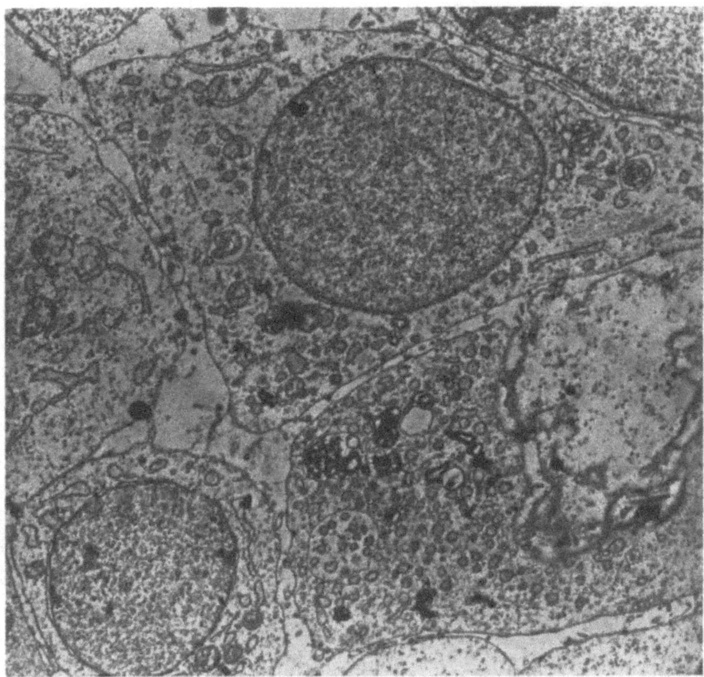

Fig. 11.23. Lysosomal figures frequently occur in the cytoplasm of juxta-epiphyseal mesenchyme. (EM; Original magnification ×5000)

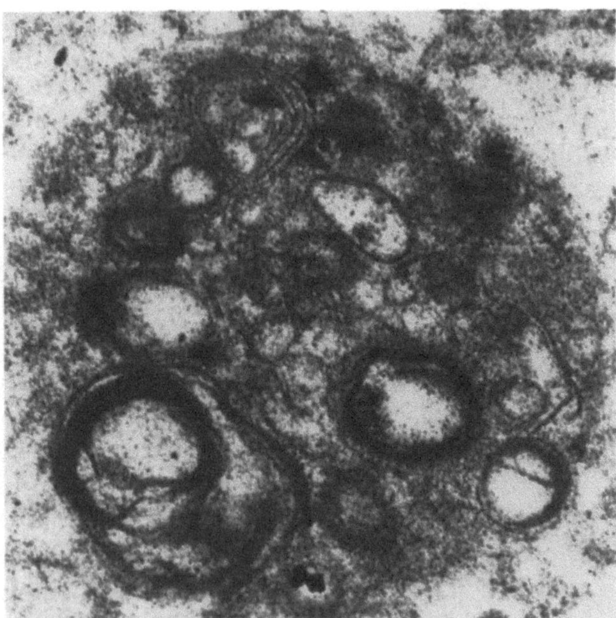

Fig. 11.24. High power view of a typical large lysosome found in juxta-epiphyseal mesenchyme. (EM; Original magnification ×50 000)

subchondral zone. The cartilage is essential for promoting the growth of vascular mesenchyme in an ordered fashion that results in the emergence of a characteristic metaphyseal bone structure. On the other hand, the blood vessels of the subchondral zone contribute to cartilage nutrition, possibly in the normal animal only to the extent of the chondrocytes of the calcified and hypertrophic zones. Nevertheless, the pathway of diffusion of nutritive elements from sinusoids to cartilage may well be an important factor in the acquisition by growth cartilages of their typical columns in the course of development.

In the bone-forming system envisaged here, chondrolytic activity by large chondrocytes in the fetal growth cartilage attracts in, i.e. provides the growth stimulus for, the vessels and associated mesenchyme in the subchondral zone. The mesenchyme erodes the calcified hypertrophic cartilage. The vessels are the source of nutritive and molecular diffusion gradients passing into the cartilage, which with increasing age, direct chondrocyte development into vertical parallel columns. In the long-established growth cartilage this subtle interrelationship of vessels and chondrocytes probably accounts for the precision and efficiency with which vertical matrix bars, the "travées directrices", are delivered to the metaphyseal ossification site, aptly placed for bone building in relation to the vessels already there. It will come as no surprise that this delicately balanced endochondral growth system, in which the vascular component is the primary and essential constituent, is easily disturbed by a wide variety of agents such as bacterial toxicity (Acheson 1960); vitamin, hormone and ionic derangements (Hartles & Leaver 1961; Simpson *et al.* 1950; Asling & Evans 1956); and mechanical factors (Arkin & Katz 1956; Siffert 1956).

Vessels crossing the cartilage

Blood vessels do not usually cross the growth cartilage (Harris 1929) to irrigate the epiphysis, although this may happen in the upper femoral epiphysis in young individuals. Tilling (1958) has observed vessels crossing the growth plate in calves, and Spira *et al.* (1963) in young rabbits when secondary centres of ossification were taking over the cartilaginous epiphyses. In the human fetus likewise, vessels normally cross growth cartilages as "communicating canals" (Fig. 10.6, Brookes 1958a), but they are scarce. Vessels also cross the cartilage when it is dying at the approach of epiphyseal synostosis and when it is subjected to abnormal mechanical influences (Gelbke 1950) entraining high compression forces across it.

Epiphyseal subchondral vessels

It is generally conceded that the metaphyseal subchondral circulation participates in the nutrition of growth cartilages at least to the extent of supplying the raw materials for calcification in the hypertrophic zone. Whether it does more than this, i.e. whether and to what extent it maintains alive the cells of a definite part of the growth plate, is another matter. It is known that when the metaphyseal circulation is obstructed, both cartilage erosion and increase in bone length cease. The cartilage, however, does not die and may become considerably thicker than normal (Kistler 1934; Foster *et al.* 1951; Trueta & Amato 1960).

These facts have suggested to some that normally the metaphyseal subchondral vessels may have an almost exclusively erosive function, while the full thickness of the cartilage is maintained alive from an anatomically distinct circulation found on the epiphyseal aspect of the growth plate (Fig. 11.25). Trueta & Morgan

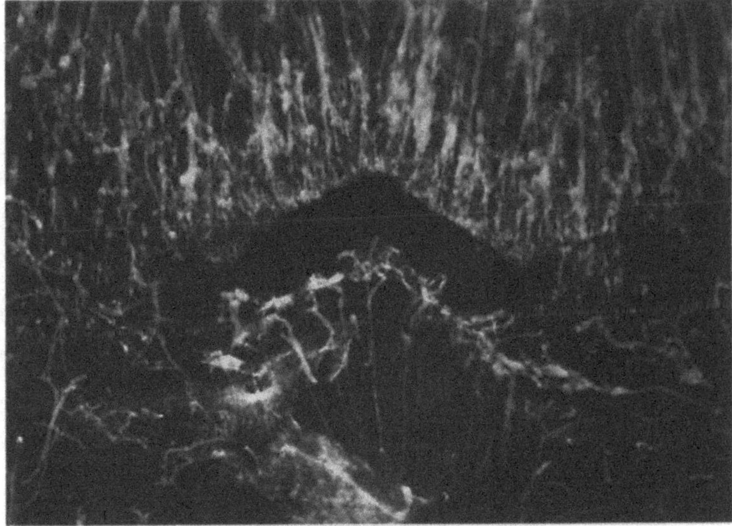

Fig. 11.25. Microangiograph showing the two different circulations associated with a growth plate. (Rat; Original magnification ×27)

(1960) drew attention to the vascular characteristics of this circulation in the rabbit. They pointed out that arterioles pierce the epiphyseal bone plate lying against the germinal zone of the cartilage (Fig. 11.2). The arterioles then give rise to sinusoids, in a duck's foot layout, in closest proximity to the stem cells of the cartilage columns. The collecting sinuses then re-cross the bone plate in separate foramina and pass into epiphyseal collecting sinuses. Trueta & Amato (1960) observed that destruction of this circulation leads to death of the cartilage. In their experiments, chondrocyte proliferation ceased but erosion and bone substitution from the metaphyseal aspect went on, resulting in the formation of a bone bridge uniting epiphysis and metaphysis across the surviving part of the cartilage plate. In Holdsworth's experiments (1966), the bridge was fibrous.

Although a prime nutritive value has been accredited to the epiphyseal subchondral circulation, it is to be borne in mind that in the fetal period, growth cartilages are formed and eroded before such a circulation exists. Moreover, cartilage canals which might nourish the growth cartilage do not form in man until about the 4.5 cm stage, when the growth cartilage is already well established. Ionic [$^{32}PO_4$] transfer has been shown to take place in dogs across the cartilage from metaphysis to epiphysis after destruction of epiphyseal nutrient vessels (Prives *et al.* 1959). It may also be noted that certain growth cartilages normally occur which consist of a central germinal-proliferative layer sandwiched between two hypertrophic zones (Fig. 11.26): for instance, between the secondary centre for the tuberosity of the tibia and the proximal metaphysis of that bone; also between the basi-occiput and the basi-sphenoid. Such cartilages have a bimetaphyseal vascular supply and the germinal cells are wholly dependent on it. Furthermore, the growth plate in the condyle of the mandible is continuous with the articular cartilage of the temporomandibular joint. In this instance no blood

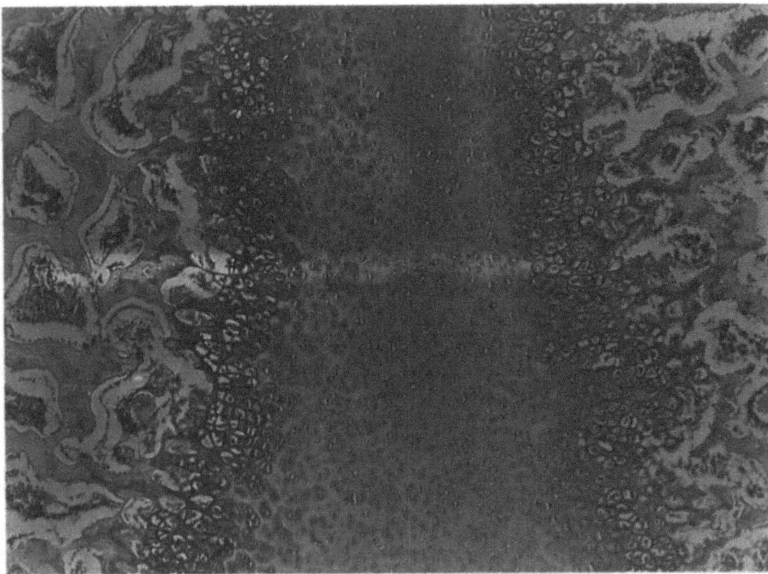

Fig. 11.26. Paraffin section through the growth cartilage separating the rabbit tibial tuberosity from the superior epiphysis. See also Fig. 4.11. (Original magnification ×45)

supply exists except through the metaphyseal subchondral circulation to nurture the main bulk of the growth cartilage.

In the interesting experiments of Selye (1934) and Hellstadius (1947), part of a limb of a rat was amputated and regenerative processes were studied. A new growth cartilage was formed at the distal end of the femur or ulna, and some bone elongation took place. Presumably the metaphyseal subchondral circulation regenerated and, in the absence of an epiphyseal counterpart, was competent to further bone growth. Nevertheless, it is probable that some blood supply to the new growth plate was also derived from the surrounding soft tissue.

In the face of this evidence from normal and experimental material, the case for predominance of the epiphyseal subchondral circulation in cartilage plate nutrition diminishes. When Trueta & Amato's experiments are more closely considered, it is noteworthy that a bone bridge did not form in all cases. Furthermore, destruction of the epiphyseal vessels was carried out within the epiphysis; the nutrient extra-osseous vessels were not severed as in the experiments of Prives and her co-workers quoted above. Holdsworth (1966) also carried out extra-osseous severance of epiphyseal vessels in some of his experiments. Neither the articular nor the growth cartilages died as a result of the ensuing ischaemia. Cellular proliferation was reduced, or even ceased for a short interval, but normality was soon restored because the possibility of there being an intra-osseous circulation at all had not been abolished by experimental interference. Essentially, bone bridges form when germinal cells of the growth plate are destroyed, by whatever method, e.g. during intracancellous vascular destruction, radiation or ultrasonically.

The investigations of Dale & Harris (1958) and of Briant *et al.* (1961) are also illuminating. They found that in epiphyseolysis in children, the line of separation runs through the hypertrophic cells of the growth plate. If the separated epiphysis maintains its nutrient supply, then the attached cartilage continues to proliferate. If the epiphyseal nutrient vessels are torn, the whole epiphysis, bone and cartilage die. The above authors concluded that the epiphyseal circulation normally maintains the germinal and proliferative zones of the cartilage.

Finally, as will be shown later (Chapter 17), there is now reason to believe that the rate of blood flow in the metaphysis is considerably greater than that in the adjacent epiphysis, so that any notion of predominance of the epiphyseal circulation for cartilage plate nutrition seems to be tenable only in the sense that normally this circulation maintains alive the germinal cells. Further investigation may well show that provided the basis for a circulation exists in the epiphysis, i.e. the vessels themselves are still intact, epiphyseal ischaemia can still be compensated by the metaphyseal vessels with survival of cartilage.

Blood supply of growth cartilages

In conclusion, the available evidence strongly suggests the following:

- A growth plate, whatever its anatomical situation, derives its nutrition from the nearest available sources, and a functional reserve exists which to a certain extent allows circulatory deficiencies to be compensated.
- The perichondrial circulation normally supports the outermost rim of the cartilage at all ages.

- In the fetal period, metaphyseal nutrition supports the full thickness of the growth cartilage, aided by a few cartilage canals.
- Postnatally the epiphyseal subchondral circulation normally supplies the germinal and proliferative layers. In abnormal circumstances it can also support the full thickness of the growth plate.
- Postnatally the metaphyseal subchondral circulation is normally responsible for maintaining alive the cells of the hypertrophic and calcified zones: the cartilage matrix nearest to the marrow cavity is continually removed by the subchondral venous plexus and associated mesenchyme, in participation with the hypertrophic chondrocytes of the bone plate, spongy bone being substituted in its stead.

Chapter 12

Synovial joints – 1

Terms of reference

Throughout this chapter and Chapters 13 and 14, reference will be made to *articular* or *joint cartilages*. These rest on the *articular lamella of bone* or *articular bone plate*, covering over the *articular vascular plexus* conveying the blood of the *articular circulation*. In long bones, the epiphyseal bone mass intervenes between the *articular cartilage* and the *growth cartilage*. The growth cartilage is in contact with two specialized *subchondral circulations*, on the epiphyseal and metaphyseal aspects of the cartilage. Growth cartilages are discussed in Chapter 11.

Vascular anatomy

William Hunter, in his extraordinarily perceptive paper of 1743 on articular cartilages, wrote:

> Where-ever the Motion of one Bone upon another is requisite, there we find an excellent Apparatus for rendering that Motion safe and free: We see, for Instance, the Extremity of one Bone moulded into an orbicular Cavity, to receive the Head of another, in order to afford it an extensive Play. Both are covered with a smooth elastic Crust, to prevent mutual Abrasion; connected with strong Ligaments to prevent mutual Dislocation; and inclosed in a Bag that contains a proper Fluid deposited there, for lubricating the Two contiguous Surfaces. So much in general.

Epiphyseal vessels

Many nutrient arteries arise from the circulus articuli vasculosus and ramify within the epiphyses of long bones, supplying the spongy bone and bone marrow included in the structure of a synovial joint. Some small intra-osseous branches pass directly towards the specialized subchondral circulation on the epiphyseal aspect of the growth cartilage discussed in Chapter 11. But in the main, the arterial branches pass through the intertrabecular spaces towards the articular cartilage and the remaining non-articular surface of the epiphysis. Intra-osseous arcades are found between these radiating vessels, about three or four tiers in the condyles of the human femur (Nussbaum 1923). On the other hand, the sinuses and sinusoids of epiphyseal cancellous bone are highly irregular in calibre and arrangement, and in no sense accompany the arteries. A similar radiate layout is present, but the occasional arterial anastomoses are matched and dwarfed by innumerable and voluminous venous connections. The largest of these form prominent sinuses orientated transversely to the axis of the central venous sinus in the shaft of the bone (Figs 8.7, 8.30, 8.34, 8.40).

The pattern of the intra-osseous arteries, converging on the centre of the epiphysis and then radiating outwards, is reminiscent of the pattern of the vascular canals in the cartilaginous epiphyseal precursor. In the case of epiphyses in the human hip and knee joints, the gross arterial pattern is the same as the cartilage canal pattern present in the fetal condition, and remains largely unchanged throughout life. The same applies to the patella and the small bones of the tarsus, whose pattern of arterialization is on a par with that of the cartilage canal pattern present in the human fetus, the larger nutrient vessels converging on to the site of ossification, and radiating towards the articular cartilages and non-articular surfaces. (See Fig. 10.1, showing the lower tibial cartilaginous epiphysis and the cartilage canals of the talus.)

Judet *et al.* (1955), studying the vessels in the head and neck of the femur, considered that the pattern of the large epiphyseal vessels was not related to the trabecular architecture. Since the latter is of a labile character responsive to changes in the mechanical stresses applied to the epiphysis, it seems that bone mechanics do not play an important role in the development of the epiphyseal vascular pattern. Rather, the large vessel pattern is the result of particular growth mechanisms controlling the emergence and development of vascular cartilage canals.

Articular vessels

Perfusion preparations of long bone epiphyses show many fine arterial terminals, possibly end-arteries, passing towards the articular bone plate which supports the articular cartilage. Sinusoid loops of unusual length are then formed (Fig. 8.32) which do not show the blind endings, saccular expansions and varicosities so typical of metaphyseal vessels where these abut against the growth cartilage (Fig. 11.5). On the contrary, the articular sinusoids show only mild and gradually occurring irregularities in calibre.

Histological preparations show that the articular loops reach, here and there, into the calcified zone of cartilage, but not beyond it into the superficial uncalcified layers. Barnett *et al.* (1960) believed that a few vessels do reach out beyond the calcified zone. In the average section, articular vessels are usually separated from the joint cartilage by a few osteonic lamellae or fine bone trabeculae (Fig. 12.1). The articular bone plate, however, is incomplete in the sense of being like a sieve, so that some fine blood vessels often lie against and touch the calcified zone of the joint cartilage. The vascular loops anastomose at their venous ends. The sinusoid network so formed lies parallel to the cartilage, and in small mammals drains over a short distance into the venules of the epiphysis and thence into the larger collecting sinuses. In human subjects, well-defined articular venous sinuses develop, which although maintaining a connection with the general collecting sinuses of the epiphysis, keep to the articular zone

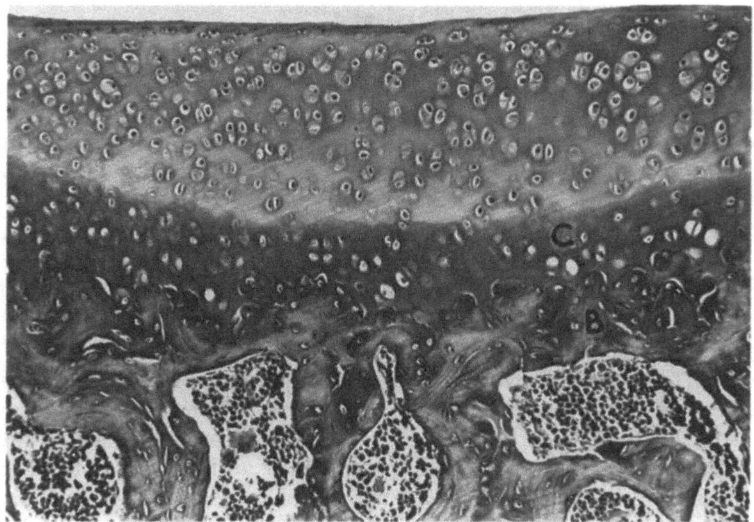

Fig. 12.1. Section through normal rat articular cartilage. **B**, Articular bone plate; **C**, calcified zone of cartilage. (Original magnification ×150)

and empty into Hunter's vascular circle close to the articular margin (Crock 1967).

The existence of a specialized articular circulation in synovial joints would appear to be beyond doubt on morphological grounds. It exists as a zone of fine vessels, still largely radiate in layout, bordering the dense vasculature of the epiphysis. The latter is distinguished by its greatly dilated and irregular venous vessels, whereas the subarticular region is characterized by a fall-off in vascular density when contrasted with the epiphysis as a whole; and also by the long and tortuous sinusoid loops which are quite different from those found in relation to growth cartilages (Fig. 8.7).

It may be assumed that where structural specialization of a vascular bed is present, special functional demands are subserved by the circulation in question. It is possible, but very doubtful, that the articular vessels are solely concerned with the formation and maintenance of the articular bone plate. The near presence, however, of the joint cartilage, perforations in the bone plate and vascular projections reaching to the calcified zone, demand a close examination of the extent to which the articular circulation participates in the nutrition of the articular cartilage.

Early investigators were never in any doubt that the articular vessels revealed by perfusion preparations were nutritive. For example, Hunter (1743) pointed out that:

> The larger Vessels, which compose the vascular Circle, plunge in by a great Number of small Holes. From these again, there arises a Crop of small short Twigs, that shoot towards the outer Surface; and whether they serve for nourishing only, or if they pour out a dewy Fluid, I shall not pretend to determine.

Of necessity, the fields of vascular anatomy and joint development, the structure and physiology of synovial membrane and articular cartilage, and the mechanisms of joint lubrication must all be gleaned for evidence which might help to formulate an answer.

Development of synovial joints

Toynbee (1841) enquired into the nutritive sources for the growth of avascular organs such as joint cartilages, the lens, vitreous, nails, horn, feathers and teeth. He was impressed by the constant near presence of vascular plexuses in intimate relation to these structures, which for him indicated that they were dependent on the plexuses for their nutrition.

With special reference to joint cartilages, Toynbee described, in bovine and human material, how in the late embryonic period the whole epiphyseal cartilage is avascular and is nourished by the vessels in the surrounding mesenchyme. With further growth and development, the articular cartilage becomes sandwiched between vascular mesenchyme in the joint space and the main bulk of the epiphyseal cartilage vascularized through cartilage canals. The vessels superficial to the joint cartilages, however, subsequently retreat and a synovial cavity is formed between the two articulating epiphyses at the beginning of the fetal period. After the formation of an ossification centre and the spread of cancellous bone in the epiphysis, the articular vascular plexus takes over the nutrition of the joint cartilage, and an articular bone plate is formed.

> Articular cartilage in the adult state is principally nourished by fluid derived from the vessels of the cancelli of the bone to which it is attached, which exudes through the coats of those vessels and makes its way into the substance of the cartilage through an intermediate lamella of bone.

The articular bone lamella, according to Toynbee, was not pierced through by the vessels of the articular circulation, which nevertheless:

> have the function of supplying the articular cartilage with a nutrient fluid and they do so without entering into its substance.

The above account by a great classical investigator, taken together with the laconic statements of William Hunter, emphasizes the function of the articular circulation as nourishing the joint cartilage and supplying "a dewy Fluid", the synovia, to the joint space. Of course, their conclusions were deficient in experimental support and entirely neglected the nutritive role of synovial fluid, but with more excuse than belongs to some modern investigators who make no reference at all to the presence of the articular vessels, known to science for more than 250 years.

Toynbee's account of joint development has been amply confirmed by many workers, particularly by Haines (1947), Streeter (1949) and Gardner & Gray (1950), who supply further details. The joint is first defined by two *mesenchymal condensations*, the forerunners of the articulating epiphyses participating in the formation of the joint. With *chondrification* at the height of the embryonic period (7th week), a mesenchymal interzone remains between the two cartilaginous epiphyses. Another, *orbicular condensation* then defines the vascular primitive capsule, enclosing a mass of mesenchyme between the cartilaginous primordia. The central part of this mass, the *intermediate layer* of Haines, is avascular (Fig. 12.2). Taking the knee joint as an example, the peripheral annulus of mesenchyme enclosed by the primitive capsule, gives rise to enarthrodial structures such as discs, menisci and fat pads (MacConaill 1932). The articular cartilages develop from those chondroblasts which lie in *chondrogenous zones* of condensed mesenchyme, sandwiching Haines' *intermediate avascular layer* (Gray & Gardner

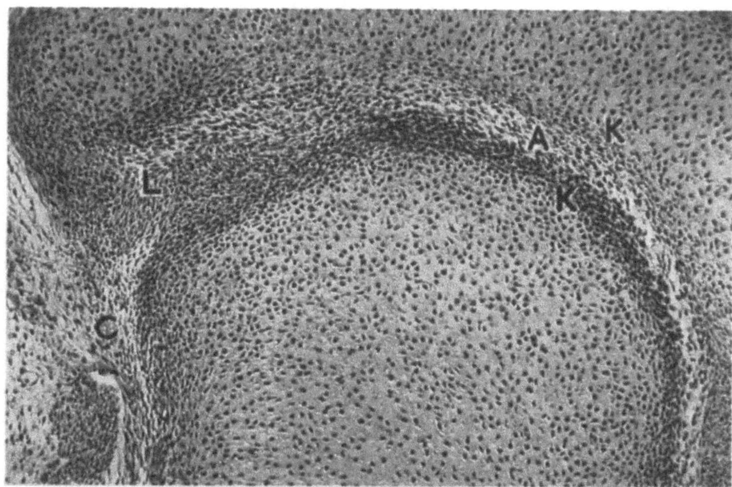

Fig. 12.2. Section through the hip joint of a 7-week-old human embryo. K,K, Chondrogenous zones; A, avascular zone; L, ligamentum teres; C, capsule. (Original magnification ×75)

1950). In the early fetal period the principal features of individual synovial joints can already be recognized; only the synovial cavity is lacking.

Formation of the joint cavity

At 9 weeks, according to Streeter (1949), cavitation appears in the interzonal mesenchyme, at first peripherally but spreading rapidly towards the centre, with the consequent emergence of a *synovial cavity* and its contained *synovial fluid.* Interzonal cavitation may be the result of *mechanical forces,* when the joint cartilages rub against each other with the acquisition of muscular contractility in early fetal life (Barcroft 1946). At that time, histogenesis of muscle is far from complete (Nicholas 1950). Tensions within the joint produced by early fetal movements would make the existence of blood vessels in the interzonal mesenchyme untenable. This might explain the persistence of a membrane and subsynovial vessels derived from Hunter's circle, which even in the adult can be found superficial to the joint cartilage at its rim. Here the vessels are not subjected to mechanical forces during joint movement or in weight-bearing. On the other hand, Gardner (1950) suggested that *mucolytic enzymes* released by the primitive synovium may be the basis of interzonal liquefaction and the formation of a joint space. Davies (1950) suggested a third mechanism, that of *cell retraction.* The cytoplasmic processes of the interzonal primitive mesenchyme cells are withdrawn, thus allowing viscous extracellular fluid to coalesce into a mass and push the differentiating synovial cells to the periphery of the joint.

Chapter 13
Synovial joints – 2

Nutrition of articular cartilage

Aseptic necrosis of bone

The concept of a synovial nutrition of joint cartilage arose from a consideration of the pathology of small loose cartilaginous bodies in joints, or "joint mice". These were described by J. Hunter (1790), who believed that they arose from a *sanguineous effusion* into the joint which, becoming vascularized and organized, was transformed into a cartilaginous loose body. For Hunter, joint mice were of synovial origin. Klein (1864) described an allied condition of massive *spontaneous demarcation* in the knee joint, wherein a large piece of femoral condyle with associated articular cartilage was dehisced from the epiphysis. König (1887) reviewed the subject, coined the name osteochondritis dissecans for the condition, and emphasized that a demarcation or dissecting process in spongy bone was basic to the development of loose bodies, large or small, in joints.

Surgeons still debate the extent to which arterial (Axhausen 1926) or venous thrombosis (Burrows 1941) of articular vessels may contribute to the genesis of this condition, as also the role of trauma in its aetiology. It is conjectured that trauma, if violent, depresses the joint surface, fractures underlying trabeculae and damages epiphyseal blood vessels. Nevertheless, loose bodies in joints not only occur but continue to thrive for long periods, kept alive as suggested by Hildebrand (1896) and many others by the synovial fluid.

Synovial nutrition of joint cartilage

Strangeways (1920) related the significance of this phenomenon to the normal nutrition of articular cartilage, objecting that it seemed unreasonable for fluid to pass from articular vessels, through the articular bone plate and the calcified zone of cartilage, in order to reach what he considered were the more active cells in the superficial layers of the cartilage. His histological studies of four joint mice showed a continuing but slow growth of cartilage and bone within the loose body, as well as the presence of osteoclasts and internal remodelling. Because pathological loose bodies in synovial joints could thus demonstrably grow, Strangeways concluded that "the articular cartilage of joints may derive some, if

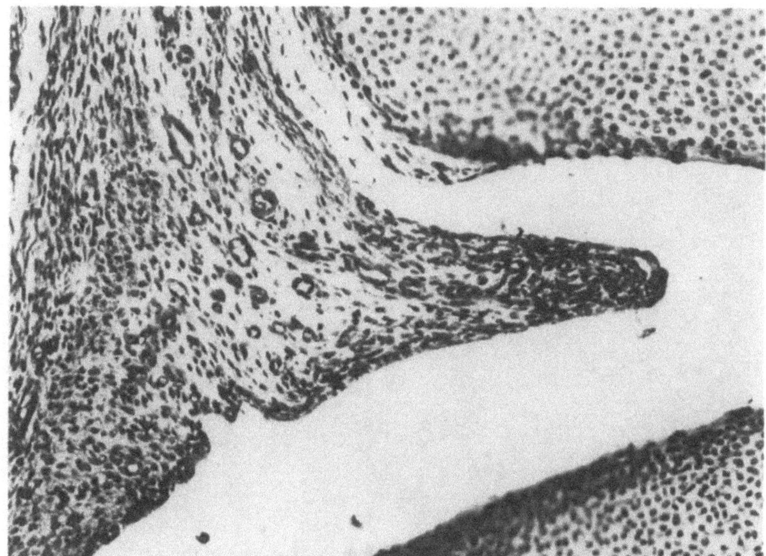

Fig. 13.1. A fold of vascular synovial membrane in a fetal interphalangeal joint. (Original magnification ×60)

not the greater part of its nourishment from the synovial fluid". He also made explicit the origin of synovial fluid from the vessels of the synovial membrane, a view which today finds ready acceptance.

Synovial membrane

The synovial membrane is a layer of cells resting on a highly vascular connective tissue and lining the fibrous capsule of the joint (Figs 13.1, 13.2). It sometimes exhibits fatty or fibrous features as well as the areolar form which predominates. The synovial cells do not form a uniform unbroken monolayer, but show at least two cell types differing in ultrastructural detail, which may be found stacked in several layers (Barland *et al.* 1962). They are irregular in shape and do not exhibit desmosomes or intercellular cytoplasmic bridges. They do not fit together accurately as in the pleural or peritoneal membranes, so that cellular discontinuities that are sometimes extensive may exist, bringing synovial fluid and subsynovial vascular tissue into direct contact (Hueter 1866; Lever & Ford 1959).

Synovial vessels

The capsule of a synovial joint is related to several arteries and veins which derive from Hunter's vascular circle and form extracapsular periarticular anastomoses (Fig. 2.22). The irregular plexus so formed is observable by naked eye in dissecting-room specimens. Davies & Edwards (1948) point out that branches from this superficial plexus then pass longitudinally between fibre bundles and establish cross-connections to build up a ladder-like vascular pattern in the substance of

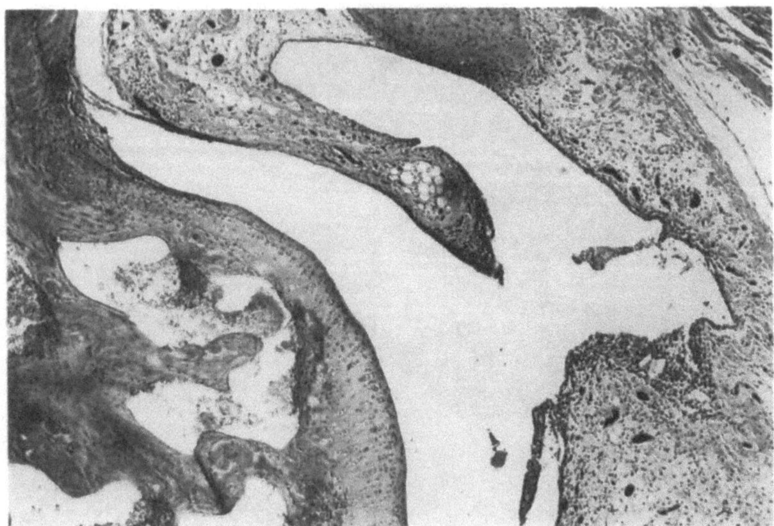

Fig. 13.2. The variable thickness of synovial mesothelium is shown in this section through the rat knee joint. (Original magnification ×53)

the fibrous capsule and ligaments alike. Very few of these "second order" vessels are continuous with the intra-osseous vasculature. Anastomoses are established, however, at bone–ligament or bone–capsular junctions with periosteal vessels. The latter lie on the non-articular surfaces of the bony epiphyses in a subsynovial position.

Numerous twigs from Hunter's circle help to establish synovial vascular plexuses, especially in those parts of the synovial membrane which are reflected from the fibrous capsule on to intracapsular bone. Many more "third order" branches from the periarticular vessels pierce the fibrous capsule and ramify in the areolar subsynovial tissue. This supports a surface layer of synovial cells (synovial intima, or mesothelial layer) which faces the joint cavity. In the subsynovial tissue, two or three superimposed and intercommunicating vascular plexuses are formed, the deepest forming a dense capillary network in immediate contact with the mesothelial layer. The subintimal plexus is far denser than the other subsynovial plexuses. "It is always separated from the joint cavity either by synovial cells, collagenous or reticular fibres, or a layer of amorphous tissue" (Barnett *et al.* 1960); an observation which bears witness to the variable morphology of the synovial membrane. It is also reported by the above authors that veins are remarkably abundant in subsynovial tissue forming dense plexuses. Valves are unusually numerous and occur frequently even in subintimal venules. The venous structure of the synovial circulation suggests a powerful absorptive function, as well as productive.

Turnover of synovial fluid

In recent times, it has become possible to study Starling's forces in joint cavities and in the synovial microcirculation, because of the discontinuous synovial cell layer and easy access to the extracapillary matrix between synovial capillaries and synovial cavity. Hydrostatic pressure, plus the difference between colloid osmotic pressure in blood plasma and joint fluid, yields the capillary pressure in the synovial capillaries; 24 mmHg according to Ahlqvist *et al.* (1994). The hydrostatic pressure and colloid osmotic pressure difference both oppose filtration of fluid from plasma into joints. An unexpected outcome of these studies has been the finding that a substantial part of the hydraulic resistance to fluid transport between blood plasma and joint cavity, resides in the serous membrane rather than in the capillary endothelium. It has also been shown that under appropriate boundary conditions, synovial fluid can simultaneously be filtered into the joint cavity in some regions where the intimal cells directly overly the capillaries, but in a reverse direction into the subsynovium, in other regions where serous cells are lacking, thus producing a rate of turnover of synovial fluid (Levick 1995).

Composition of synovial fluid

The analysis by Bauer *et al.* (1940) of bovine synovia has been adduced as a considerable support to the *membrane theory* of origin of synovia. These workers found that in chemical composition, synovia resembled a dialysate of blood plasma with the addition of hyaluronic acid, a characteristic constituent of synovial fluid and resposible for its viscous properties. Hyaluronic acid is a polymer of roughly equal amounts of glucuronic acid and *N*-acetyl glucosamine. It is non-sulphated, but on the other hand contains abundant COO– groupings which give the molecule a markedly polyanionic character. One would expect that glucose would be a principal raw material for its cellular synthesis.

The non-electrolytes in synovia are identical with those of plasma and in much the same concentration except that, according to the above workers, synovial glucose is much reduced in strength at 66 mg per 100 ml compared with plasma glucose values of 100 mg per 100 ml at least. The ionic constituents of synovia are found in concentrations in general accord with the Donnan theory of membrane equilibrium. Synovial chloride and bicarbonate have the same concentration as in the plasma, but sodium and potassium are decreased (Bauer *et al.* 1940).

The protein content of synovia, although lower than that of blood plasma (about 2 g and 7 g per 100 ml respectively) shows a markedly raised albumin/globulin ratio of about 4 : 1 as against 1 : 5 in plasma (Platt *et al.* 1956; Schmid & MacNair 1956; Decker *et al.* 1959). Indeed, the synovial proteins are of small molecular weight, none being larger than γ-globulin (mol. wt. 160 000). Fibrinogen, lipoprotein, clotting factors, and other giant macromolecules found in blood plasma are not normally present (Bauer *et al.* 1940; Cho & Neuhaus 1960). The proteins present in synovia are, however, identical in general with plasma proteins, with one certain and important exception, i.e. a specific protein which is bound covalently to hyaluronic acid to form a hyalurono-protein complex (hyaluronan). This protein was detected by Preston *et al.* (1965) by repeated ultrafiltration of bovine synovia. It was not possible to dissociate it from hyaluronic acid without depolymerizing the latter. It was isolated by Hamerman *et al.* (1966), whose immunological investigations showed that it is not a plasma protein.

In fine, the synovial fluid shows chemical features suggesting it is formed in part as a dialysate of plasma, to which a hyalurono–protein complex has been added. The plasma in question lies in the subsynovial vascular plexus, which is undoubtedly rich, the subintimal capillaries being especially densely packed. The venous morphology of the subsynovial plexus clearly indicates that fluid absorption is a major function of the synovial membrane, as well as on the arterial side a producer of synovia. It is therefore necessary to examine further two other features of the synovial apparatus which have been adduced in support of a synovial origin of synovial fluid. On the one hand it is said that synovial cells secrete a protein–hyaluronate complex, or hyaluronan. It is also contended by many that the low glucose content of synovial fluid is the result of its cellular utilization in the synthesis of this macromolecule which confers on synovia its viscid character and "Spinnbarkeit" (Gunter 1949).

Synovial cells and hyaluronate

Considerable effort has been expended to substantiate the synovial origin of hyaluronic acid. With the LM, Castor (1960) described the synovial cells as possessing prominent cytoplasmic processes and exhibiting numerous vacuoles. The vacuoles might represent polysaccharide globules before extrusion into the intercellular matrix of the synovial mesothelium.

Many polysaccharides are chromotropic, i.e. instead of staining orthochromatically (blue) with basic dyes such as Methylene Blue, Toluidine Blue, Cresyl Violet and others, they exhibit metachromasia, i.e. reddish-purple staining. Metachromasia with Toluidine Blue is shown in mast cell granules, found scattered in the subsynovial connective tissue. These granules, however, are resistant to histochemical incubation with hyaluronidase and therefore do not represent hyaluronate inclusions; they represent heparin (Davies 1942; Asbø-Hansen 1950; Meyer 1957; Horváth 1959). A weak metachromatic staining with Toluidine Blue was shown by Hamerman & Ruskin (1959) to be restricted to the intercellular matrix of the superficial layers of synovial cells. The reaction was presumed to indicate hyaluronate because it was abolished by streptococcal hyaluronidase. Nevertheless, Hamerman & Schubert (1962) were of the opinion that hyaluronate is probably not chromotropic at all, and hence cannot be demonstrated with certainty by metachromatic procedures.

A direct proof of the production of hyaluronic acid by synovial cells has been repeatedly attempted by many workers (Grossfield *et al.* 1955; Kling *et al.* 1955; Castor 1957; Castor & Fries 1961) relying on tissue culture techniques. In successful cases of *in vitro* propagation of cells derived from synovial membrane, the presence of hyaluronic acid in the culture medium has been demonstrated by a variety of methods including microelectrophoresis (Curtain 1960). Nevertheless, several objections have been raised to the interpretation of the results as unequivocal demonstrations of hyaluronic acid production by synovial mesothelial cells *in vivo*. These include the uncertainty that tissue explants from inside joints might not include subsynovial cells. Fibroblasts are known to produce hyaluronic acid, which has also been demonstrated in cultures of skin, bone and subsynovial tissue (Hamerman & Schubert 1962). Because hyaluronate occurs as the sole mucopolysaccharide only in synovial fluid and the vitreous of the eye, it does not follow from its demonstration in a culture medium that the formative cells are synovial.

Cells *in vitro* can lose much of their *in vivo* morphology, metabolic characteristics and genetic expression (Ross *et al.* 1962), in exchange for the selective advantage of rapid multiplication in the new environment offered by the culture medium. As Frazer & McCall (1965) pointed out, it is common experience that epithelial cultures are difficult to propagate, whereas fibroblastic hyaluronate-producing cultures are comparatively easy to maintain. Only the most rapidly established pure synovial cell line, preferably obtained without repeated subculture, is capable of supplying an unequivocal answer to the question of hyaluronate production by synovial cells. On the other hand, EM might, if sufficiently refined, help to determine the place of the synovial cell in the schema of joint function.

Barland *et al.* (1962), in their EM studies of human synovial membrane, described two types of mesothelial cell. Most of the synovial cells belonged to a group exhibiting a prominent Golgi apparatus, numerous vacuoles, intracellular filaments, mitochondria and pinocytotic vesicles. A small number of cells showed large amounts of granular endoplasmic reticulum, which are clearly closely related to the abundant, characteristic cells of the synovial mesothelium. That they represent the synovial progenitor cell is indicated by the occurrence of cells with a mixed ultrastructural morphology in synovial cell cultures (Castor & Muirden 1964). Their complement of granular endoplasmic reticulum does, however, suggest that a minority of synovial cells are actively engaged in protein synthesis for export. These cells may possibly be the source of some of the enzymes found in synovial fluid (Davies 1967), as well as the specific protein which enters into combination with hyaluronic acid to form hyaluronan. Collagen fibres are not found in the intercellular spaces of the intimal cells. Nevertheless, the preponderant cell type occurring in the intimal layer of the human synovial membrane possesses ultrastructural features, numerous vacuoles and pinocytotic vesicles which indicate an absorptive, phagocytic function.

Synovial absorptive function

The absorption of water by the synovial membrane was shown by Edlund (1949) in his perfusion experiments on joints, to be slow and continuous as long as the hydrostatic pressure of the perfusate was below 9.5 cmAq. At this critical pressure, the synovial tissues suddenly appeared to give way. There was an abrupt increase in the rate of flow of the perfusate into the joint which was increased by further elevations in the perfusion pressure, very much as if the perfusion were taking place in loose connective tissue (McMaster 1941).

Simple solutes and small molecules injected into the synovia of the living joint have been detected within 30 seconds in the systemic circulation (Rhinelander *et al.* 1939; Adkins & Davies 1940). Colloids, on the other hand, may leave the joint through subsynovial lymphatics. Bauer *et al.* (1933) found that egg albumen and horse serum albumin injected into the joints of dogs did not reach the systemic circulation when the lymphatic connections had been blocked. India ink particles have been found in the regional lymph nodes within minutes of injection into the joint cavity. It has also been known for many years that the synovial membrane rapidly takes up Neutral Red, Trypan Blue and other dyes introduced into the synovial fluid, as well as carbon particles and blood. The transport of this wide range of materials from synovia to subsynovial tissue, blood vessels and lymphatics, presumably requires the activity of either the intimal cells, subsynovial macrophages or both.

That the intimal cells have an absorptive function and participate in clearing the synovia of detritus has long been established. For example, Clarke (1928) injected Trypan Blue into the knee joints of rabbits. The intimal cells at first took up the dye in small quantities and in time became heavily stained with Trypan Blue-containing vacuoles. At the same time, the subsynovial macrophages became loaded with stored dye. Vaubel (1933) recorded that the vacuoles in his synovial cell cultures took up Neutral Red. To this may be added that most of the intimal cells had a profuse content of pinocytotic vesicles, giving a sure indication of a considerable absorptive capacity. Subsynovial macrophages certainly store dyes and particulate matter, once these have crossed the synovial intima. Adkins & Davies (1940) also observed that large particles introduced into the joint space were taken up by macrophages which remained in the subsynovial layer for an indefinite time. Blood extravasated into the joint space in the event of fracture is absorbed and gives rise to considerable haemosiderin deposits in the subsynovial tissue. Clarke (1928) also described the migration of subsynovial macrophages and synovial intimal cells into the synovial fluid, where they took up Trypan Blue and then returned to the synovial membrane. Beyond the synovial macrophages, absorption is carried out by either the subsynovial blood vascular plexuses or the lymphatics.

From the evidence quoted above, it would appear that during synovial absorption the blood vascular route is largely utilized by water, solutes and substances of small molecular size. Large particles, colloids and proteins find their way into the lymphatics draining the synovial membrane.

Fluid production by capsular synovium

In order to sustain the theory of synovial fluid production by the synovial membrane, more direct evidence is required than is yet available of the passage of fluid, solutes and large molecules from subsynovial blood vessels *into* the joint space. It is known that bacteria and carbon particles injected into the blood stream can be found in the subsynovial macrophages, and it is believed that acute inflammation of a joint can occur when this barrier to bacteraemic invasion breaks down (Kuhns & Weatherford 1936). These workers also traced intravascularly injected Trypan Blue as far as the subsynovial tissues. Fluorescent immune complexes and fluorescent aggregates of γ-globulin injected intravenously have been successful in labelling "rheumatoid factor" in the synovial membrane of patients with rheumatoid arthritis.

These experiments do not, however, serve as a demonstration of the normal passage of substances from the blood stream into the synovial fluid. More persuasive evidence has been offered by many workers both for proteins and for electrolytes. For example, Bennett & Shaffer (1939) have shown that intravenously injected egg albumin appears in the synovial fluid of rabbits in as short a time as 10 minutes. Others have noted the rapid appearance in the synovia of electrolytes injected into the blood stream (Cajori *et al.* 1926; Fisher 1929; Zeller *et al.* 1940, quoted by Bauer *et al.* 1940; Brodin 1955; Salter & Field 1960). Nevertheless, it still cannot be stated on this evidence alone, that proteins and large molecules, or even water and electrolytes, normally pass from the subsynovial vascular plexuses into the joint spaces through the whole area of the synovial membrane, in particular that part of it, the major part, which is related to the fibrous capsule. If this were so, one might expect mucopolysaccharides such as the metachromatic chondroitin sulphates B and C and mucoitin sulphuric acid, which are normally found in vascular connective tissue matrix, to be washed into the joint space as well as hyaluronic acid. As far as is known, hyaluronic acid is the only polysaccharide found in synovial fluid.

Fluid production by transitional synovium

Water, electrolytes and small molecules could for example enter the synovia from a restricted region of membrane, the portion that is reflected on to intracapsular bone and covers the rim of the joint cartilages. Here, indeed, numerous capillary loops form a delicate lacework border (Figs 2.21, 2.22) for the periosteal vessels springing from Hunter's vascular circle, and are separated from the joint space by a single layer of flattened synovial cells. The established facts that small ions introduced into the circulation rapidly gain entrance to the synovial fluid (Cajori *et al.* 1926), and that the constituents of the synovia resemble a dialysate of plasma (Bauer *et al.* 1940), do not indicate which "membrane" is utilized. The general, capsular synovial membrane has an intima of variable morphology, being thick, thin or even absent, but possesses only a proven *absorptive* capacity.

Further evidence is required before it can be stated with certaintly that water, electrolytes or proteins normally dialyse from the capsular blood plasma across vascular endothelium, a substantial subsynovial matrix, and the intimal cells. On the other hand, the narrow band of synovium attached to the articular margins has a different vascular morphology, Hunter's vascular mesentery, with a capillary density which is markedly greater than that in the general capsular network; the synovial intima is exceedingly thin, and the tissue on which the membrane lies is also peculiar to this region, namely fibrocartilage.

Transitional fibrocartilage, as it is termed, is a junctional region between the hyaline articular cartilage on the one hand, and the periosteum covering the non-articular surface of the epiphysis, on the other. At the rim of a joint cartilage the otherwise preponderant hyaline material becomes packed with collagen bundles, easily visible in the light microscope (Fig. 13.3, *overleaf*). Deep to the transitional zone is the thin articular lamella of bone. Superficial to it is a membrane of areolar connective tissue, coated with a single flattened layer of synovial intimal cells and containing the terminal loops of Hunter's vascular circle. (Some authors seem to understand that this *linear* terminal vascular border is the whole of Hunter's circle. According to his original description, Hunter was referring to a *zonal* vascular border of the joint, about half an inch wide, in which the vessels were arranged "as in the mesentery".) The fibroblasts associated with the vascular loops are said to be intermediate in form between the rounded cells found in the fibrocartilage of the transitional zone, and those found in the capsular subsynovial tissue, which are spindle shaped and exhibit long cytoplasmic processes. The fibrocartilage becomes continuous over a short distance with the fibrous layer of the periosteum to which the fibrous capsule of the joint is attached.

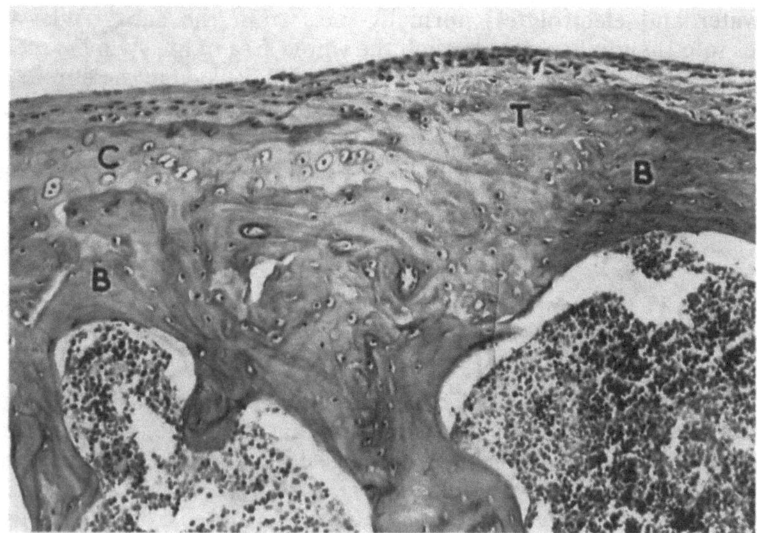

Fig. 13.3. Section through the transitional zone (T) of cartilage in a rat femur. **B,B**, Bone: **C**, calcified cartilage. (Original magnification ×150)

The transitional zone, in contrast to the rest of the joint cartilage, shows considerable powers of cell proliferation and repair, and is the site of pathological productive processes resulting in osteophyte or chondroma formation. The anatomical peculiarities of this region, especially its rich subintimal vascularity and the proliferative capacity of its subintimal cells, have been noted by many, although no investigational reports are available on synovial fluid formation with particular reference to this special portion of the synovial membrane.

The supposed origin of hyaluronate, at least, from the general synovial intima is still in doubt. Renewed inquiries may show that this substance is produced in the transitional zone, where the characteristic flattened intimal cells, the rounded subintimal fibroblasts, and even the abundant vascular endothelium itself all represent possible sources of hyaluronate.

It is common surgical knowledge that the operation of synovectomy, if radical and taking in the region of the transitional zone, can sometimes result in a "dry joint" prone to the development of intra-articular adhesions. Possibly in these instances where the synovium overlying the transitional zone is removed, the production of a dialysate is severely hampered. The transitional zone is particularly rich in capillaries; the mesothelial barrier to diffusion is peculiarly thin; conditions for dialysis would seem to be perfect.

The thinness of a membrane, however, is not proportional to its permeability. Glucose, when injected intravenously into calves, is known to appear rather slowly in the synovial fluid (20 minutes) as compared with 10 minutes for thiocyanate (Zeller *et al.* 1940, quoted in Bauer *et al.* 1940) or 10 minutes for egg albumen (Bennett & Schaffer 1939) in the case of the rabbit. Other proteins appear more slowly in the joint cavity after intravenous injection. These results indicate that the "synovial barrier", i.e. those structures comprising the membrane across which plasma dialysis takes place, may not be inert with respect to the transport of materials through it. On the contrary, complex enzymatic processes may be involved as well as physicochemical factors affecting diffusion rates. If Hunter's mesentery and the synovium of the transitional zone are in part the site of synovial fluid production, then trans-synovial transport may show some analogies with trans-placental transport, which selectively influences the rate and direction of passage of a wide range of substances including both ions and macromolecules (Needham 1931; Harrison 1961).

Chapter 14
Synovial joints – 3

Joint lubrication and cartilage nutrition

It is seen that the theory of synovial nutrition of joint cartilages is defective, in that the manner and site of production of the synovial fluid are both uncertain. Nevertheless, it may still be asked how the fluid actually gets into the cartilage. Because of the importance of hyaluronate in the composition of synovia, and the central position accorded it as the substance which endows synovia with special mechanical properties, it might be expected that the mechanism of joint lubrication might give some indication of the relationship of joint mechanics to cartilage nutrition. Unfortunately joint lubrication is an unsolved problem, there being almost as many theories as there are investigators, and "all ably defended by impenetrable thickets of applied mathematics" (McCutchen 1967). Nevertheless, it is appropriate to consult the various hypotheses that have been put forward, bearing in mind that for present purposes the reference is to joint nutrition.

Theories of lubrication

MacConaill (1932, 1967) propounded the theory of hydrodynamic lubrication – that during movement, a thin film of synovia lies between the cartilages in the load support zone of a synovial joint. The film persists in this position because of relative motion during rolling and sliding between the two surfaces and the viscous character of the fluid (hydrodynamic entrainment). Charnley (1959) showed, however, that in human joints, articular cartilages could move freely on one another at low friction values without benefit of synovial fluid. He introduced the theory of *boundary lubrication*, in which essentially it is envisaged that a monolayer of hyaluronic acid molecules is adsorbed on to the surface of the joint cartilage, like the pile of a carpet. This physical arrangement separates the two articular cartilages. Under load, squeeze films of fluid are pressed out of the cartilages and lubricate the joint. Movements can then take place with low friction at high shear rates. Both the hydrodynamic and the boundary theory of lubrication in their undeveloped form offer nothing by way of clarifying the problem of cartilage nutrition, i.e. whether it derives from the synovial fluid or the subarticular vascular plexuses in the bony epiphyses.

Dintenfass (1963) made allowance in his analysis for the fact that cartilage is deformable and non-Hookeian in its elastic properties; also for the non-Newtonian thixotropy of synovia, i.e. its increased viscosity at low shear rates. He claimed to have removed many of the theoretical objections to thin film lubrication in his *elastohydrodynamic theory.*

Fein (1967) investigated the friction and forces attendant on the movement of a deformable sphere on a flat surface. He considered not only that synovial joints are lubricated by squeeze films replenished by hydrodynamic entrainment but, quite remarkably, that all biological factors, such as the non-Newtonian character of synovia, the non-Hookeian properties of cartilage and boundary lubrication, are at best secondary factors hardly affecting the purely mechanical properties of synovial joints. If his view based on engineering principles is correct, the role of synovial fluid is purely mechanical and the function of the synovial membrane is reduced to the renewal of broken-down molecules, especially hyaluronate, which account for the fluid's viscosity.

Nevertheless, from the biological point of view it would seem almost certain that the nutrition of cartilage is intimately bound up with joint mechanics and the conservation of joint structure. For example, when joints are immobilized for a lengthy period (Evans *et al.* 1960) or compressed by apparatus designed to resist growth in length (Gelbke 1950; Salter & Field 1960; Trias 1961), the articular cartilages succumb to necrosis. It is also general experience that in the case of a variety of arthritic conditions, joint movement helps to overcome stiffness and pain. Experimentally, changes have been noted in the thickness of joint cartilage, indicating that at least the degree of hydration of the cartilage is related to the extent to which the joint has been mobile or otherwise. Ingelmark and Ekholm (1948) and Ekholm (1951) demonstrated an increasing thickness of the articular cartilage during joint movement, followed by a gradual thinning during rest after exercise. It is therefore unlikely that a theory of joint lubrication which has no linkage with the mechanism of joint nutrition will be sustained by future investigation.

Lewis & McCutchen (1959) and McCutchen (1967) have introduced a theory of what is termed *weeping lubrication* which recognizes the deformability of articular cartilage. It is based on the old observation that when compressed, joint cartilage oozes fluid on its surface, and that it quickly returns to its normal shape on release of the compressing force provided that this has not been excessive or prolonged. It might be thought that the fluid expressed from the cartilages when subjected to load would be sufficiently viscous to lubricate their relative motion hydrodynamically. Hyaluronate, however, has not yet been identified in joint cartilage. McCutchen (1967) in a recent review emphasizes that in weeping lubrication the expression of a viscous fluid is not envisaged, but a thin aqueous film is wrung out of the joint cartilage. This may help to maintain a thin film of hyalurate-containing fluid between the joint cartilages under load, which lubricates the joint surfaces and prevents their mutual contact and abrasion. Fluid may also be forced laterally through the substance of the cartilage and then out into the joint space around the load-bearing area. This is then returned to the cartilage, possibly by osmotic forces, when the compressed cartilages are released from load in a succeeding phase of movement. Weeping lubrication therefore indicates that joint movement and cartilage nutrition are linked, in the sense that the passage of water and solutes through the cartilage matrix is promoted by mechanical use of the joint. The precise nature of the lubrication mechanism, boundary or hydrodynamic, is however still unsettled.

Load and nutrition

The forces acting on articular cartilages are of the order of tons per square inch. This has led many to suppose that synovial nutrients such as glucose and electrolytes are forced into the depths of the avascular cartilage during the load phase (Ekholm 1953; Harrison *et al.* 1953). Marnell (1967) measured the "bottoming time" of synovial fluid (0. 55 second) acting as a squeeze film between two flat surfaces. His results give an indication of the time taken, under physiological loading, for the two cartilages in a joint to come together. Because most of the load phase in the hip joint during walking occurs for only 0. 6 second, Marnell suggests that increased synovial fluid pressure in the load support zone could give rise to fluid flow *into* the cartilage, dependent on its permeability Permeability experiments (McCutchen 1967) suggest a pore size of 6 nm (60 Å) for joint cartilage, but this quantity almost certainly varies with age, with the particular joint in question, and with many other factors.

Maroudas (1967) lends support to the view that nutrients are forced into the cartilage from the synovial fluid during loading, although for her, hydrodynamic squeeze films are apparently of no account in joint lubrication. On the contrary, from her experiments she deduces the possibility that a fine hyaluronate layer, 4 nm (40 Å) thick, will still persist at high loads of the order of 2×10^6 dynes cm^{-2}. Commenting on McCutchen's opinion that water *leaves* the cartilage under load, she adduces data which suggests that the resistance to tangential flow through a 250 nm (2500 Å) gap between cartilages and out into the synovial cavity is eight times the resistance to the flow of water *into* the cartilages. For Maroudas therefore, as for Marnell and others, synovial water passes into joint cartilages under load. McCutchen (1967), on the other hand, is of the opinion that fluid is expressed from the cartilage in these conditions. He also believes that a hyaluronate film would not be stable under high load, and that other considerations such as osmotic pressure and surface tension are involved in boundary lubrication in addition to the simple adsorption of hyaluronate to the surface of articular cartilage, if indeed this occurs at all.

It seems that biomechanical investigations into the lubrication of synovial joints have yielded little by way of firm evidence to help in elucidating either the mechanism of joint lubrication or the manner of cartilage nutrition. Joint movement, however, does appear to promote the transfer of fluid between synovia and cartilage. The extent and direction in which this occurs, and its relation to different phases of a cycle of movement, are all at present conjectural. It has been suggested that joint lubrication is not described by any single theory; rather, in a cycle of movement in a synovial joint successive theories, hydrodynamic, elastohydrodynamic, squeeze films, boundary and weeping lubrication, may all apply in different phases of the movement.

Articular nutrition of joint cartilage

Permeability of articular bone plate

For many years, the articular bone plate has generally been taken to be a major barrier to diffusion of nutrient substances from the articular vessels into the joint cartilage. It has been likened by biomechanists to an impermeable backstop applied to a disc of porous material, such as they use in their investigations of the viscosity of fluids and the engineering properties of cartilage. Histological preparations show that, in the main, the vessels are separated from cartilage by only a few lamellae or trabeculae of bone, depending on the age of the subject. The articular plate of bone is incomplete and some contact occurs between sinusoid loops and the calcified zone of cartilage. According to the valuable treatise of Barnett *et al.* (1960), vascular contacts may occur even with the more superficial, uncalcified zone. The porosity of the bone plate was noted by Fischer (1929) and ably demonstrated by Holmdahl & Ingelmark (1950), who estimated the amount of vascular contact present on the deep aspect of several different articular cartilages in rabbits. The values they gave range from 1.5% in the elbow to 7% in the knee, i.e. about 5% in general of the deep aspect of an articular cartilage may be in direct contact with the articular vascular plexus. The latter might therefore supply that much of the cartilage's nutrient requirement, provided that its metabolic rate is the same as in other tissues. This has been investigated by Rosenthal *et al.* (1941), who found that articular cartilage showed a marked glycolytic activity. The oxygen consumption, however, was low. According to Bywaters (1937), the metabolic rate of articular cartilage calculated with respect to weight is only 1/80 to 1/100 that of other tissues, yet when calculated as the rate per chondrocyte, Bywaters' results indicate that the metabolic level of cartilage cells is comparable to that of many other cells. However, the cellularity of cartilage is about a tenth of that of compact tissues. It is therefore likely that cartilage as a tissue requires only 10% of the nutrient supply usually accorded to other tissues. As we have seen, cartilage contact with the articular circulation may occupy 5% or more of its deep surface.

Berry *et al.* (1986) described the presence of defects extending through the bone plate into the basal cartilage layer of the adult human talus, made visible by the perfusion of fluorescent dyes. The authors offer the possibility that these are active pathways serving for the transport of nutrients to the cartilage. The fluorescent areas were noted, particularly in areas of intermittent cartilage loading. Lane *et al.* (1977) have studied the vascularity and remodelling of the articular lamella and calcified cartilage in human femoral and humeral heads. They found that in the femoral articular region the number of vessels per unit area fell by 20% from adolescence until the seventh decade, and by 15% until the sixth decade for the humerus. At all ages more vessels were present in the load-bearing areas of the articular cartilages; 25% more for the femur; 15% more for the humerus. More remodelling of the bone plate was noted in loaded areas at all ages. Levick (1995) in his review of microvascular architecture and exchange in synovial joints, points out that nutrient exchange in articular cartilage is "facilitated by a high density of fenestrated capillaries situated very close to the synovial surface". The fenestrations are preferentially orientated towards the joint cavity and not the articular lamella. Hadhazy & Varga (1976) studied regeneration of the articular cartilage in dogs. They found that in the early stage of regeneration the oxygen supply was predominantly from capillaries in the granulation tissue. Later, as the capillaries regressed from the regenerate cartilage, the oxygen was reduced (it is less cellular) but was sustained by diffusion from the synovial fluid and the articular vascular plexus. Recently, more information has become available bearing witness to the permeability of the articular plate. Clarke (1990) has produced clear images of bone and blood vessels in the articular region in humans, dogs and rabbits. He finds that there are cavities larger than 40 μm in the bone plate containing typical marrow elements. Capillaries run through the bone plate in cylindrical channels, surrounded by concentric bone lamellae. A majority of the channels are separated from the cartilage by bone. "A minority of these channels open into calcified articular cartilage", and are preceded by cell clumps cutting into the cartilage substance.

Nakano *et al.* (1986) have measured blood flow rate in pigs using radioactive microspheres (see Chapter 19). Blood flow rate in the femoral condyle was greater in 10-week-old pigs than in the proximal femur, patella, central tarsus and metatarsus. A significant ($P < 0.05$) age-associated decrease in flow rate was observed in femoral patellar and metatarsal cartilages. Most importantly, in epiphyseal cancellous bone, blood flow rate in the surface 2 mm layer was three to ten times greater ($P < 0.01$) than in the remaining deep cancellous bone in their femoral and tibial samples. It may be assumed that this peripheral epiphyseal zone coincides with the articular vascular plexus.

It follows from all the visual evidence referred to above, that the articular bone plate does not provide an analogy for an impermeable backstop, and that the articular circulation makes sufficient contact with the articular cartilage and has an abundant blood perfusion rate, comfortably accounting for at least 50%, if not more, of its glucose and oxygen requirements and also of water contributing to the synovia.

Sulphate and oxygen diffusion

That oxygen diffuses outwards from the epiphysis to the joint cavity appears not unlikely, in that sulphur takes this pathway through the cartilage. A single dose of ^{35}S administered as sodium radiosulphate is rapidly incorporated into the chondrocytes and reaches a maximal intracellular concentration in 2 hours. Thereafter, radioactivity passes from the cells into the matrix, the movement of the isotope being complete in about 6 days (Hall 1965). It is generally agreed that radiosulphate is ultimately incorporated into chondroitin sulphate, the characteristic polyanionic polysaccharide of joint cartilage. The initial concentration of the isotope in the chondrocytes, however, indicates that its uptake is not a purely passive substitution into existing sulphate groups in matrix mucosubstances, but that cellular activity is required for the production of radioactive ^{35}S-labelled polysaccharide molecules.

The earliest phases of radiosulphate incorporation into joint cartilage require careful examination. It would appear that after the first day, the superficial and intermediate zones of articular cartilage are more intensely labelled (Barnett *et al.* 1960). It has been suggested that these zones are sites of heightened polysaccharide production, in particular, of increased chondrocyte activity in the intermediate growing area (Carlson 1957). However, the monograph of Barnett *et al.* also shows an autoradiograph of ^{35}S incorporation 4 hours after injection of radiosulphate into a 2-day-old rat. The articular bone trabeculae are heavily labelled and the articular cartilage shows a fall-off in intensity of the label towards the joint surface. Further autoradiographic studies of radiosulphate uptake by joint cartilage within 1 hour of injection are clearly needed in order to define the direction of diffusion of the electrolyte in the matrix before it reaches the chondrocytes for processing into polysaccharide.

It is also to be borne in mind that the concentration of chondroitin sulphate as indicated by metachromatic staining (Hirsch 1944) is maximal in the basal region of the cartilage, a result which in itself supports the view that sulphate, like oxygen, may pass from the articular vessels into the overlying cartilage.

Centrifugal diffusion from articular plexus

A few other substances are known to be capable of passing through joint cartilage centrifugally, i.e. in a direction outwards from cancellous epiphysis to synovia. Ishido (1923) showed that a solution of *silver nitrate* injected into the marrow of a joint epiphysis could subsequently be detected in the basal portion of the overlying cartilage. If the silver nitrate solution was injected into the synovial fluid, on the other hand, the superficial portion of the cartilage was marked by silver deposits. This heavy metal, it would seem, can penetrate the cartilage with equal facility from both the articular plexus and synovial fluid.

Large *starch particles*, about 1 μm in diameter, were reported by Ingelmark & Sääf (1948) to enter the joint cartilage of a rabbit from its epiphyseal aspect, when the starch had been injected into the epiphyseal marrow. When injected into the synovial fluid, starch granules could not be detected in the cartilage matrix, except possibly in the transitional zone. When starch suspensions were injected intravascularly and the joints studied, granules of starch were found only in the basal zones of the joint cartilage. If Ingelmark & Sääf's work is taken to have significance beyond the particular case of starch granules, it would seem that macromolecules may gain access to joint cartilage from the articular circulation.

Ekholm (1951, 1953, 1956) investigated the occurrence in rabbit knee joints of *radiogold* ^{198}Au after the intravenous injection of radiogold chloride. This is believed to form a complex with serum protein. Penetration of the articular cartilages in the knee joint was evident an hour after injection. Autoradiographic procedures showed that the heavy metal gained access to the cartilage through both its superficial and deep aspects, but the basal zones exhibited a greater concentration of the isotope. Similar results were obtained using *radiophosphorus* ^{32}P injected intravenously as disodium hydrogen phosphate.

Cartilage permeability, vascular contact and blood flow

Ekholm further observed that radiogold uptake in the femoral knee joint cartilage was greater than in the case of its companion in the tibia. This effect may be due to differences in the structure of the cartilages, resulting in different permeabilities; to different degrees of articular vascular contact in the case of the two articular cartilages in question (Holmdahl & Ingelmark 1950); or to different haemodynamic conditions in the two epiphyses. It is known that in the case of the rat, the red cell volumes and rates of blood flow in diverse parts of the femur differ markedly (Brookes 1965, 1967b). Furthermore, the circulating red cell volume of the lower femoral epiphysis, as measured by the ^{51}Cr-labelling technique, is significantly greater ($P < 0.01$) than that found in the upper tibial epiphysis in the knee joint of young rapidly growing rats. It may well be that Ekholm's observation is an indication of a more rapid circulation in the femoral portion of the knee joint than in its tibial part.

Exercise, which causes cartilage to swell, also increased the uptake of radiogold in Ekholm's experiment, presumably because of an increased passage of nutrients from the articular circulation related to the load support zone. The increased radioactivity in the autoradiographs was confined to the central basal region of the joint cartilage and was not observed at its periphery. Hence, Ekholm was of the opinion that Hunter's mesentery was not a source of nutrients to the central area of an articular cartilage. His work, however, clearly supports the view that the articular circulation figures prominently in the nutrition of the central load-bearing area of joint cartilage, especially in exercise.

Brodin (1955) made use of the fluorochrome, sodium-3-oxypyrene-5,8, 10-trisulphonate, which gives a yellow-green fluorescence in ultraviolet light. He reported that this molecule rapidly gained access (in 30 seconds) to the joint cartilage, both from the synovia and from the articular circulation. Some 4 minutes after a single intravenous dose, the fluorochrome was largely confined to the deep portions of the cartilage. Brodin's observations also show that in as short a time as 15 seconds, the articular trabeculae (in rabbits) exhibit an intense fluorescence, an observation which calls in question the supposed impermeability of the articular bone plate. The intense labelling of the plate in the autoradiographic studies of many workers (Leblond *et al.* 1950; Amprino 1953) concurs with Brodin's illustrations. All this throws considerable doubt on the misleading proposition of Strangeways (1920), that access of nutrient materials to the articular cartilage from the intra-osseous articular circulation is ruled out by the intervention of the articular bone plate. On the contrary, autoradiographic and other visual evidence suggests that nutrient materials in tissue fluid can pass through the thin articular bone lamella and may be sufficient to sustain, at least in part, the metabolism of the articular cartilage. Nor is this to gainsay the importance of vascular contacts between cartilage and articular vessels which, as shown above, appear to be adequate for 50% of articular cartilage metabolism.

Changes in cartilage thickness

Several workers have demonstrated that exercise results in thickening of the articular cartilage (Hirsch 1944; Ingelmark & Ekholm 1948; Ekholm 1956) and that immobilization of a joint results in its thinning in the non-weight-bearing area. Presumably the work of the chondrocytes is related to strains undergone by the cartilage during joint movement, and exercise increases metabolism of the chondrocytes. It may be expected, therefore, that a cartilage made thick by a bout of exercise will show an acid trend in the pH of the microenvironment of the cells. An old investigation by Harpunder (1926) indicates that cartilage swells in an acid pH, but shrinks when placed in an alkaline medium. Eichelberger (1960), working on denervated knee joints in puppies, found that in these circumstances the articular cartilages were swollen because of an increased water content and an absolute decrease in the content of matrix solids. Her experiments may indicate that a disordered bone circulation depresses the synthetic powers of the chondrocytes, possibly because of an acid trend in their microenvironment. The source of the increased water content in these circumstances is obscure. As shown above, direct experimental evidence suggests that normally the articular circulation is a major source of nutrients to the articular cartilage. The absorptive aspects, however, of the circulation in relation to fluid movements and the removal of metabolites of chondrogenic origin, have as yet hardly been considered. Eichelberger's experiments could mean that water is absorbed from articular cartilage by the articular vessels, but collects in the joint matrix in the absence of movement or in the presence of circulatory derangement.

Venous congestion of the articular circulation and its effects on joint structure were examined by Bernstein (1933) in dogs, and by Brookes (1966a,b) in rats. Essentially, in the presence of a sustained circulatory impediment resulting from experimental venous ligation, thickening of the articular bone plate occurs together with epiphyseal sclerosis. An increase in the thickness of the calcified zone of the congested cartilage also occurs in rats after only 8 weeks of mild venous obstruction (Figs 14.1–14.4, *overleaf*). It would appear that articular venous obstruction produces an acid trend in the chondrocytes, and that a fall in the pH or a change in the Po_2 and Pco_2 may cause cartilage to swell as occurs normally in exercise, or to calcify excessively as occurs pathologically. The work of Eichelberger, Brookes and others, demonstrating cartilage change consequent on venous congestion, confirms that the articular circulation has a nutritive role with respect to joint cartilage, and suggests also that this role is absorptive.

Conclusions

If the results of the many investigational approaches that have been made in the field of joint vascularization are brought together at this point, the following tentative conclusions can be reached.

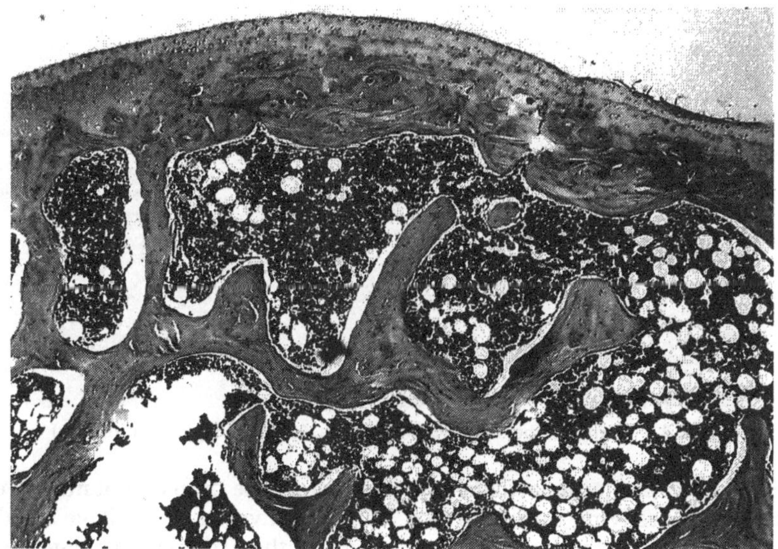

Fig. 14.1. Normal rat femoral articular cartilage and bone plate. (Original magnification ×75)

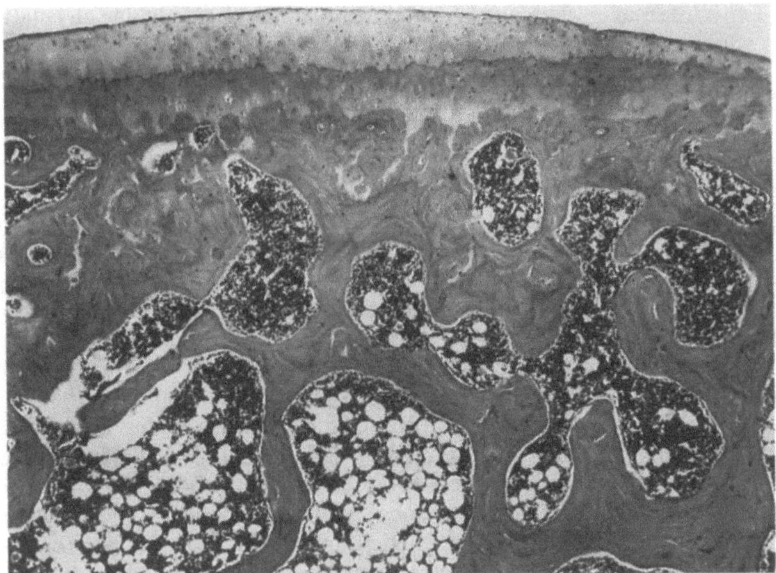

Fig. 14.2. Contralateral joint to Fig. 14.1, 8 weeks after femoral ligation. Bone trabeculae are thicker. (Original magnification ×75)

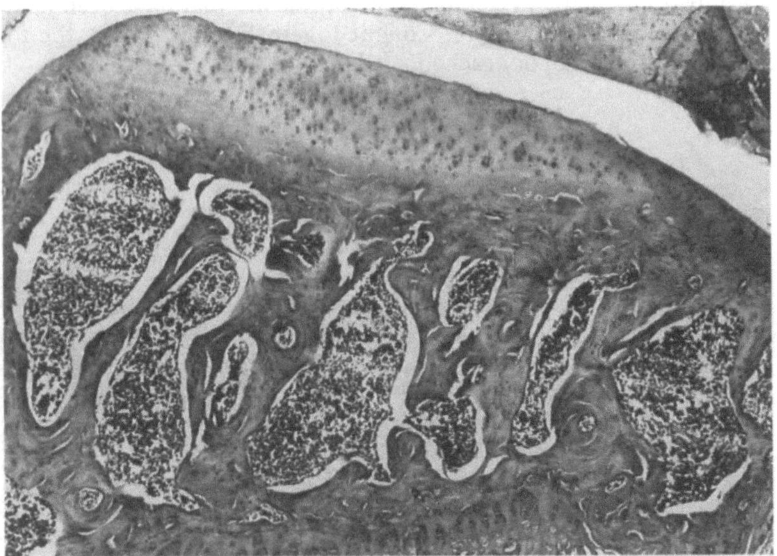

Fig. 14.3. Normal upper epiphysis of rat tibia. (Original magnification ×75)

- In embryonic life, joint cartilage is dependent on the diffusion of nutritive fluid from capillaries lying on its surface. Thereafter, vascular cartilage canals and synovial fluid together support the growth of the articular cartilage. In post-natal life, with the advent of epiphyseal ossification, the systemic skeletal

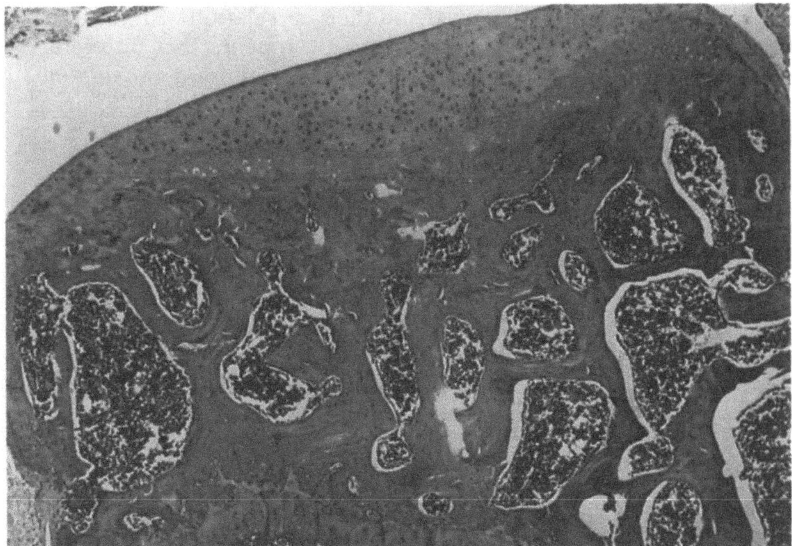

Fig. 14.4. The contralateral bone to Fig. 14.3 shows trabecular thickening after femoral vein ligation. (Original magnification ×75)

circulation ensures a rich blood supply to the bony epiphyses, as well as a sufficient supply to the fibrous capsule and ligaments of the joint and to any enarthrodial structures that may be present.

- An articular circulation is found in close relation to the joint cartilage, and a subsynovial circulation external to the general synovial intima. The subsynovial circulation is derived from periarticular vessels and lies between the intima and the fibrous capsule. At the rim of the articular cartilage, the subsynovial vasculature is formed by the border of Hunter's mesentery and lies between the intima and transitional fibrocartilage.
- The absorptive function of the capsular part of the subsynovial circulation is well established, but whether it is also the normal source of synovial fluid is uncertain. It is probable that the portion of the subsynovial circulation derived from Hunter's mesentery, and related to folds and recesses close to the articular margins of the joint, contributes to the production of synovial fluid, but to what extent is not decided. Even the source of the hyaluronic acid–protein complex in the synovia has still to be elucidated.
- Evidence is available that nutrient fluids, water and a variety of solutes can pass from the articular circulation into the articular cartilage and back again. The absorptive capacity of the articular circulation would also account to some extent for the removal of metabolic waste products of articular cartilage origin.
- Both the synovial fluid during joint movement and the articular circulation in capillary contact with the calcified zone share in the nutrition of the articular cartilage, probably to an equal extent. It also seems that alternating productive and absorptive phases in articular vascular function occur, depending on the phases of the joint cycle.

- The mechanisms of joint lubrication and their correlation with the dynamics of cartilage nutrition are unsolved problems. It appears that different mechanisms of lubrication apply in different phases of joint movement, which interlock with phasic nutritional inputs and absorption in living articular cartilage.

Chapter 15
Introduction to bone haemodynamics

Haemodynamics may be defined as the study of the physical characteristics of blood in circulation. It is only since the late 1960s that statements of more than qualitative value have become possible regarding the osseous circulation, and a plethora of techniques and studies since then have confirmed a sustained interest in this important subject. The principal relationships between such factors as driving and transmural pressures, flow rate, viscosity and tube dimensions which apply to any circulation, blood vascular or otherwise, have been seen to be relevant to the circulation in bone tissue. The evidence bearing directly on haemodynamics in bone, therefore, is considerably amplified in scope and meaning if, in assessing it, reliability is placed on fundamental generalities found to obtain in the circulation of other tissues.

Low or high pressure system?

Blood pressures inside the osseous circulation have not been measured, but are generally believed to be low. Such a view implies that the osseous circulation can be treated on the whole as a low pressure system.

In support of this hypothesis one could point to the extremely tenuous walls of the medullary sinusoids, which seem so fragile in the optical microscope and yet form a closed circulation. Furthermore, the tortuosities, undulations and fineness of calibre of the branches of the nutrient artery and other afferent vessels suggest that they are mechanisms for the reduction of the pressure of blood entering the capillary or sinusoidal vascular lattice. That the latter may function at low pressures is indicated by the manner in which many precapillaries arise from parent stems, coursing in the subcortical or endosteal zone of bone marrow. They come off nearly at right angles. According to Reynolds (1948), this type of arterial branching is a mechanism for the swift reduction of arterial pressure when the distance from artery to capillaries at the delivery site is small. There is also the well-known observation that when a bone is transected, blood oozes from the cut surface and does not burst out in jets, a fact which has been taken to be indicative of low medullary arterial pressure (Lamas *et al.* 1946). In addition, it may be pointed out that the vessels of bone marrow are intimately associated with nerve filaments (Zamboni & Pease 1961). Presumably the calibre of the vessels, venules as well as arterioles, can be altered by neural mechanisms, thereby modifying still further the blood pressure in the sinusoids and capillaries of bone.

Nevertheless, all the above evidence, while valuable in itself, can be accommodated by the view that the osseous circulation may function at different pressures in its diverse parts, and that the medullary circulation in particular represents a high pressure system. This hypothesis is grounded on the following observations.

Chemical exchange between blood and tissue fluid in any tissue takes place across the semipermeable endothelium of the vascular lattice. Two important factors affecting this exchange are capillary hydrostatic pressure and plasma osmotic pressure. The pressure within a capillary over that of the tissue fluid (transmural pressure) tends to drive plasma water and ionic solutes into the extravascular space, that is, it promotes filtration. The osmotic tension of plasma, on the other hand, promotes absorption into the vessel.

Although tissue fluid pressure is usually taken as atmospheric or subatmospheric in other microcirculations (Guyton & Hall 1996), this does not in general appear to apply in bone marrow. Stein *et al.* (1957) have shown in dogs by the use of electromanometers that the tissue pressures inside diaphyseal and epiphyseal marrows are different (50 : 12 mmHg), the diaphyseal pressure being particularly high; this trend was also found by Polster (1970) in the rabbit femur. In these experiments it should be noted that true *intravascular* blood pressures are not recorded. Pressure measurement is made via a hollow needle or trochar which is introduced through a cortical borehole into the marrow and, crucially, ensures a tight seal so that no leakage can occur. The tip of the needle rests in a mixture of bone tissue and blood, the composition of which depends upon the particular vessels damaged during insertion. It is usually accepted that the recorded pressure is primarily related to the intramedullary venous pressure (Michelson 1967; Wilkes & Visscher 1975). High tissue pressures in bone marrow are probably correlated with the absence of lymphatics in bone marrow and cortex (Anderson 1960), and with the peculiar situation of the vessels of the osseous circulation, encased as they are in unyielding bone cortex. Any increase in tissue fluid volume due to an excess filtration over absorption would result in a precipitate rise in tissue pressure and closure of the sinusoids, bringing the circulation to a stop. In any case the vessels can be kept open only if the transmural pressure is positive, that is, if the hydrostatic pressure in the capillaries does not fall below that in the extravascular space.

High tissue pressures of the order of 50 mmHg have also been recorded in the diaphyseal marrow of cats, dogs and rabbits by Bloomenthal *et al.* (1952), Herzig & Root (1959), Kalser *et al.* (1951) and Polster (1970). On the other hand, human diaphyseal marrow pressures are low according to Petrakis (1952) and Tocantins & O'Neill (1941), although human epiphyseal cancellous pressures are in the same range as those measured in animals (Arlet *et al.* 1968; Arnoldi *et al.* 1972, 1975). This may of course simply reflect a species difference in diaphyseal marrow pressures between man and other mammals investigated; or the different results may stem from the presence of an erythroid marrow in the case of the dogs, cats and rabbits referred to above, and to a fatty marrow in human investigations; or again, technical inadequacies may be the reason. Nevertheless, the results as a whole tend to support the view that the circulation in the red marrow of the diaphysis of many mammals is a high pressure system.

It is known that in most soft tissues the arteriolar mechanism reduces blood pressure from 90 mmHg or more in the arteries to about 35 mmHg at the arterial end of capillaries. In diaphyseal marrow it seems that the abrupt break up of arteries into arterioles, which is so characteristic of this region, results in delivery of blood to the vascular lattice at a pressure head much higher than is usually the case, possibly as much as 60 mmHg. The lower tissue pressure in the epiphysis would permit lower input pressures. The arcade systems in Hunter's mesentery already noted may well provide the means whereby the arterial pressure of blood is reduced to low levels prior to entering the epiphyses, distinguishing this component of the osseous circulation from the diaphyseal region. In both cases, transmural pressure must initially exceed osmotic pressure if filtration is to occur. Absorption of tissue fluid depends upon the transmural pressure being less than the osmotic pressure of the blood at the venous end of the sinusoid. Osmotic pressure is generally held to be about 20 mmHg. It follows that pressure in the collecting sinuses of diaphyseal marrow may be of the order of 55 mmHg, but will be very much lower in the epiphysis, possibly 20 mmHg.

If these figures for bone venous pressure are only approximately correct, the freedom of egress of blood from cancellous bone becomes readily explicable. Many authors have shown the extreme rapidity with which solutions, blood or even barium sulphate suspensions leave cancellous bone and enter the systemic venous system (Tocantins & O'Neill 1941; Leger & Frileux 1950; Harrison & Gossman 1955). Intra-osseous blood transfusion, when practised, would owe its success not only to the capacious venous vessels to be found in the spongy bone but also to intra-osseous venous pressures, which are higher than those found in the veins of the surrounding soft tissues.

Cancellous bone, when cut into, bleeds profusely. In the days when bleeding was still vigorously practised as a therapeutic measure, "la saignée osseuse" (Laugier 1852) had its adherents, and this suggests that bone venous pressures are not to be measured in mmH_2O but rather in mmHg. The high pressure hypothesis is supported by the following consideration of Bernoulli's equation:

$$E = P \,.\, A + mgh + 0.5(mv^2)$$

where E is the energy of a circulating fluid, $P \,.\, A$ represents the product of the lateral pressure and the surface area over which it acts, mgh expresses the potential energy, and $0.5(mv^2)$ the kinetic energy of the fluid. In accordance with the laws of conservation of energy, the Bernoulli equation describes the constancy of energy in a microcirculation. In particular, with blood velocities of high kinetic energy the lateral intravascular pressure is low, with a tendency toward collapse of the vessel wall. But where blood velocities are low, as they probably are in the profuse sinusoid vessels of the osseous circulation, the low kinetic energy of the system will be correlated with high intravascular pressures. This, as we have seen, is indicated by the available experimental evidence, thus strengthening the hypothesis that the circulation in the marrow is a high pressure system.

An interesting correlation between high marrow tissue pressure and the tenuous character of medullary sinusoids can be made by applying the Laplace equation:

$$T = rt$$

where T is the tension in the vessel wall, r its radius and t the transmural pressure. If t is small owing to the high tissue pressure of bone marrow, it follows that the tension in the wall of the vessels is also small. Hence in a high pressure system the endothelium of medullary sinusoids may well be as fragile as their appearance suggests, but nevertheless is not necessarily under a raised tension which might result in microhaemorrhages (see p. 157).

Regulation of intravascular pressure

From the foregoing, it is apparent that the physical regulation of chemical exchange across vascular endothelium, centres on the maintenance of capillary pressure at a level adequate for normal filtration and absorption.

It is known by dissection that numerous nerve fibres accompany the afferent vessels into a bone, and that many of the nerve fibres in bone marrow are sensible to painful stimuli including vascular distension (Bazett & McGlone 1928; Sugiura 1958; Helal 1965; Arnoldi *et al.* 1975). Bone cortex is insensible to pain according to Bichat (1801), Testut (1880) and others who have had the opportunity to enquire into the matter. The presence in the marrow of nerve fibres in association with sinusoids has been shown in electron micrographs (Zamboni & Pease 1961; Thurston 1982). There is sound evidence that some of these fibres are vasomotor in function, although the termination of a nerve fibre on a blood vessel has not been unequivocally demonstrated. Because of the abundance of sinusoids and collecting sinuses and the relative sparseness of arterial channels, it may well be that capillary pressure is influenced by the nervous control not only of arteriolar diameter, but more particularly of the calibre of the venous end of the medullary circulation.

Stein *et al.* (1957) have shown in dogs that the pulse pressure inside diaphyseal marrow was normally much higher than in the epiphysis (8 mmHg : 1 mmHg). Stein *et al.* (1958) were of the opinion that the differences observed by them in pulse and tissue pressures between diaphysis and epiphysis were independent of the systemic arterial pressure, and other authors have confirmed a general lack of correlation between mean arterial pressure and intramedullary pressure. Whilst Herzig & Root (1959) found a marked fall in femoral intramedullary pressure following occlusion of the femoral artery in dogs, Tøndevold (1983) showed an arterial pressure threshold (around 80 mmHg); below this threshold the intra-osseous pressure fell sharply. Both above and below this threshold level, however, intra-osseous pressure showed no correlation with changes in arterial pressure; in fact intra-osseous pressures remained largely constant, confirming the presence of autoregulative factors in bone (see below). Stein *et al.* (1958) found that adrenaline, noradrenaline and pituitrin may act locally on the intramedullary arteries, producing a fall in marrow pressures without a corresponding fall in the systematic pressure. Indeed, the latter could be simultaneously elevated. Whilst this is evidence for placing control of sinusoid pressure on the arterial side, the work of Stein *et al.* (1959) on tissue pressures in the presence of experimental arteriovenous fistulae point to a powerful venous control. In their experiments, pressure in diaphyseal marrow was unchanged in spite of high systemic venous pressure resulting from the fistulae. Presumably, neural control of sinuses is a factor to be reckoned with, the extent of which will become clearer as more evidence becomes available.

As mentioned earlier, control of the osseous circulation may also depend to a certain extent on autoregulatory mechanisms, acting independently of neural and chemical factors affecting the circulation from outside the bone. Autoregulation implies the maintenance of a constant tissue fluid volume despite variations in input pressure or rates of flow in the system. Local reflexes and the accumulation of vasoactive metabolites (Johnson 1974) may possibly regulate sinusoid pressure by affecting the arteriolar or venous resistance. But in the special circumstances of the medullary circulation, functioning as it does in an enclosed space, it seems more likely that variations in tissue pressure are more particularly important for the maintenance of adequate filtration and absorption, and hence of a tissue fluid volume compatible with normal nutrition. For example, a rise in input pressure would result in an increased transmural pressure, promoting filtration and thereby elevating the tissue pressure. The latter, however, automatically reduces transmural pressure and thereby promotes reabsorption at the capillary end. The rate of flow through the system in this instance may have increased, but homeostasis of tissue fluid volume within the bony case has been maintained.

Finally, it may be noted that the fine arterial twigs in bone marrow and cortex are almost certainly end-arteries. Because of this, a possible risk of wide pressure differences between neighbouring sinusoid masses is introduced. The central venous sinus uniting in one venous chain the diaphyseal and metaphyseal sinusoids, and also the large transverse collecting sinuses found in epiphyses, possibly represent local mechanisms for the rapid equalization of pressure between neighbouring groups of sinusoids supplied by end-arteries.

Physical factors influencing flow rates

Some of the variables which may influence the rate of flow in a generalized microcirculation are collated at this point. A more detailed analysis of factors affecting flow rates may be gleaned from Wiedeman *et al.* (1981), Greger & Winhorst (1996) and Guyton & Hall (1996).

The two principal factors controlling the rate of flow of blood through any haemodynamic system are the pressure gradient driving the blood through the vessels and the resistance offered to the movement of the blood; thus:

$$F = \Delta P / R$$

where ΔP is the pressure difference between inlet and outlet and R is the resistance. The latter factor can be expanded, as in the Poiseuille–Hagen equation:

$$F = \Delta P \,.\, 8\pi r^4 / \eta l$$

where r is the radius of the vessel, l its length and η is the viscosity of blood. That is, the resistance to flow is proportional to vessel length and blood viscosity but inversely proportional to the fourth power of the radius. With regard to the latter factor, it has been noted that cortical capillaries have much the same calibre as medullary sinusoids, and hence cortical blood flow will not differ on this account from the flow in the marrow. However, cortical capillaries are unusually long, a factor which acting alone would increase the hindrance to flow in compact bone.

The viscosity of the blood is a measure of the shear force impeding the sliding of one layer of blood over another. If blood were a Newtonian fluid – that is, of a uniform structure throughout – then its viscosity would be constant. In fact, the suspended cells render blood non-Newtonian in its behaviour, so that the viscosity is apparently reduced as vessel diameter diminishes, providing that the vessels are of small calibre. Hence, the viscosity factor and its apparent fall would tend to increase the rate of flow in the cortical capillaries as they narrow towards the periosteal surface. On the other hand, several factors besides vessel calibre affect the viscosity of blood, and amongst these must be reckoned the haematocrit. The greater the proportion of red cells per unit volume, the greater the shear forces impeding movement of the blood column through the vessel. A high haematocrit for marrow blood, for example, would tend to impede the circulation there.

It should also be borne in mind that a low flow rate in itself will raise the viscosity of the blood. This is probably the result of rouleaux formation, that is, the clinging together of red blood cells which occurs when they are not agitated by movement of the suspending plasma. In these circumstances, the larger red cell masses tend to fall away to the sides of the vessel and there create greater shear stresses. Usually, in a fast-moving blood column, the individual red cells develop spin and tend to aggregate in the axis of the vessel. This phenomenon, known as axial streaming, is an important characteristic of haemodynamic systems. It normally operates to reduce the viscosity of blood flowing in small vessels by allowing cell-free plasma to slide over the vessel wall. Hence in the medullary circulation, where a high haematocrit is probable, axial streaming would tend to promote the circulation by reducing the effective viscosity of the blood, providing that rates of flow were high.

Sinusoid dilatation and hyperaemia

It is clear that an increase in the pressure of incoming blood will raise the flow rate. In a living circulation the effect is greater than in one composed of inert tubes, because a rise in intravascular pressure tends to dilate the capillaries. The resulting increase in vessel radius raises the flow rate even further. Now it has been observed by direct intravital microscopy (Brånemark 1959) that marrow sinusoids dilate and contract slowly and rhythmically but not synchronously with the heart beat. It is possible that this phenomenon indicates an independent contractility of sinusoid endothelium as Brånemark suggests. In other microcirculations, however, the balance of evidence is against such a capability of vascular endothelium (Ham & Leeson 1964). It seems likely, therefore, that variability of sinusoid calibre simply reflects variation in intravascular pressure. The latter can be brought about by adjustment to the vasomotor tone of either afferent or efferent vessels in bone marrow. It follows that sinusoid dilation could indicate either a local rise or a local fall in the flow rate, corresponding to an increased pressure gradient due either to arteriolar dilatation or to venous constriction. In both cases, transmural pressure is raised and dilatation results. The rhythmic change in sinusoid calibre observed by Brånemark was not correlated with arterial pulse, so that it probably does not reflect changes in arterial input pressure. Hence it would appear that normal sinusoid dilatation and contraction probably stem mainly from changes in the venous outlet, dilatation corresponding to venous constriction.

A prolonged dilatation of intra-osseous sinusoids and capillaries is known to occur in a variety of pathological conditions associated with changes in radiodensity of the bone. Such hyperaemic conditions may have haemodynamic features in common with the above phenomena. Direct measurement is required, however, to ascertain whether hyperaemia denotes an increased or a decreased flow rate. We have seen how venous constriction can reduce the flow rate and be accompanied by dilatation of the sinusoids. Arteriolar constriction can also reduce the flow rate. But, as already pointed out in the discussion on autoregulation of the microcirculation, a fall in input pressure automatically impedes filtration and promotes absorption – a consequence which, in the special case of bone marrow, would tend to dilate the sinusoids in order to conserve the constancy of tissue fluid volume. Furthermore it is known that, in general, a low oxygen tension results in dilatation of systemic venules and presumably of collecting sinuses in bone marrow. On both counts, therefore, chronic sinusoid dilatation in bone marrow may indicate in certain conditions a reduction in the rate of blood flow. *In fine*, hyperaemic states may occur in bone pathology in the presence of either venous or arterial constriction. Such hyperaemia, evinced by vascular dilatation and demonstrated by perfusion methods, does not necessarily indicate an increased flow rate: on the contrary, it may possibly denote ischaemia.

Chapter 16
Measurement of bone vascularity

The concept of bone vascularity has tended to be rather ill defined. Different writers have used it to refer to the type of vessels present in bone, the density of capillary beds, the length of capillaries, the volume of blood contained in all the vessels, the amount of blood in arterial channels only, and the blood flow rate.

Capillary density, in the sense of the number of capillaries per unit volume of bone, is a particularly awkward quantity to measure because in any capillary bed it is difficult to define where one capillary ends and another begins. The same objection can be raised against estimates of the capillary length. Paraffin histology and electron microscopy have imparted much valuable information, of both a qualitative and a quantitative nature, with respect to the structure of bone blood vessels, while the vascular patterns shown by perfusion preparations still remain hardly touched by quantitative methods. Fortunately, the measurement of bone blood volume provides a convenient approach to the estimation of bone vascularity.

The volume of blood in bone

Perfusion methods

Methods are now available for the accurate measurement of this important haemodynamic quantity. An early suggestion was that blood vessels might be perfused with a Prussian Blue suspension, and the amount of iron in the ferric ferrocyanate particles present in bone estimated by chemical methods. The values obtained would very much depend on the efficiency of the perfusion, but in the hands of any one investigator they might be sufficient to indicate changes in bone vascularity in different experimental situations. An extreme version of iron quantification is applicable in the case of the cortex, where iron estimation can be carried out without prior perfusion; marrow haemoglobin being normally absent from the cortex.

Perfusion with plastics was used quantitatively by Wray & Lynch (1959) in order to detect change in the vascularity of callus during fracture repair. The method demands a perfusion which passes beyond the small artery level and subsequent corrosion of bone specimens, leaving only the vascular cast which may then be weighed. Although the principle is sound, in the writers' experience vascular perfusion with Neoprene latex and similar preparations has proved exceptionally difficult to accomplish when quantification of the capillary bed is aimed at. Recently, electron microscopists have used intra-arterial perfusion of low viscosity methyl methacrylate to visualize the vascular domains within bone. After polymerization, the bone is decalcified and then macerated in a sodium hydroxide solution. The resulting high resolution cast is examined using scanning electron microscopy. The technique has been successfully employed to examine the skeletal microvascular anatomy of normal bone, especially bone marrow (Irino *et al.* 1975; Draenart & Draenart 1980; Ohtani *et al.* 1982), and to examine the pathological changes in an animal model of osteoarthritis (He *et al.* 1990).

Red cell volume in bone

The total content of red cells in a selected bone circulation can be accurately determined by a labelled red cell dilution technique (Brookes 1965), which offers a far less laborious and more fruitful way of measuring bone vascularity than methods based on coloured perfusates and plastics. In effect, a natural perfusion of an experimental animal's own isotope-labelled blood was employed to quantify the vascularity of rat femoral and tibial tissues such as cortex, inferior metaphysis or superior epiphysis in youth and senescence.

Essentially, red cells are obtained by bleeding a large heparinized rat, decapitated under deep general anaesthesia. About 10 ml of blood, easily collected by this procedure, is diluted ten times with mammalian saline and then centrifuged at 1000 rev min^{-1} to obtain a working quantity of packed erythrocytes. Centrifugation at higher speeds tends to produce some red cell fragmentation. The supernatant is discarded and radiochromium in the form of sodium ^{51}Cr-chromate is added to the packed cells in a dose equivalent to 100 mCi ml^{-1} whole blood gathered. The use of chromium-labelled red blood cells was described by Grey & Sterling (1950a), for measuring circulating blood volume in dogs and man (Grey & Sterling 1950b; Sterling & Grey 1950). The anionic hexavalent form ($Na_2{}^{51}CrO_4$) is highly specific for erythrocytes, and injected labelled cells retain their activity, without significant loss to plasma, for at least 24 hours. Following ^{51}Cr labelling, excess chromate is removed from the red blood cells by repeated centrifugation and washing with heparinized saline. The original volume of whole blood drawn from the donor rat is finally reconstituted by adding heparinized saline to the washed, labelled and packed cells.

Radioactive red cells are introduced into the circulation of an experimental animal through a suitable vein, for example the jugular, or the superficial epigastric vein. The dose recommended is 0.3 ml of packed labelled red cells in younger rats, or 0.5 ml for older and larger animals, which amounts to 10–50 μCi 100 g^{-1} rat body weight. The donor radioactive cells are allowed to circulate for 10 minutes to facilitate complete mixing with the host cells. After this time, the tip of the anaesthetized animal's tail is rapidly amputated, and a drop of mixed arteriovenous blood collected on a glass slide. This allows at least three 0.005 ml samples to be collected and transferred to counting vials, and a haematocrit to be obtained. The anaesthetized animal is then killed by rapid freezing in liquid nitrogen to bring the circulation to an abrupt halt.

Table 16.1 Typical raw data work sheet for calculating the circulating red cell volume in regions of bone

Tissue	Count	Count less background	Tissue weights (g)	Radioactivity (counts g^{-1})	Red cell volume (ml 100 g^{-1})
Femur					
Superior metaphysis	413	248	0.0194	12 783	1.151
Cortex	745	580	0.0718	8 077	0.729
Marrow	469	304	0.0240	12 666	1.142
Inferior metaphysis	1335	1170	0.0686	17 050	1.538
Tibia					
Cortex	636	471	0.0611	7 708	0.695
Marrow	269	104	0.0102	10 196	0.919

Rat no. 12
Haematocrit: 43.4%
Rat weight: 110 g Date: 27.11.63

Background count: 165
Count 0.005 ml^{-1} blood = 2571
Count − background = 2406

The bones are then removed, fixed in 10% formol saline for 36–48 hours, and cleaned manually of all soft tissue. Several regional samples of tissue may be taken from a selected bone, for example, the superior and inferior metaphyses, the inferior epiphysis, the middle third of the cortex and the marrow. Bone sampling is facilitated by a low speed dental drill with a circular saw blade attachment. The samples are weighed to the nearest milligram and their net weight recorded. For each rat, the radioactivity of the bone and blood samples is measured using a well-type scintillation counter. After subtraction of the background, the reading is used for estimating the radioactive ^{51}Cr concentration of the various tissues.

Table 16.1 shows a typical raw data sheet. The measure obtained is red blood cell space, and the calculation of whole blood volume requires an estimate of the haematocrit. Because of the difficulty of obtaining direct regional haematocrit measurements from the rat, in practice the mixed arteriovenous haematocrit from the tail vessels of each animal is used. Any error is assumed to be insignificant. In any case, if the regional interior haematocrit distribution is assumed to be similar for bones of both hind limbs, the method offers scope for comparing the effects of experimental procedures performed on one limb with the contralateral unoperated control. This within-animal comparison methodology will be repeatedly advocated throughout the 'methods' section. Because the haematocrit is known (commonly 43.4%), it follows by simple proportion that the circulating red cell volume (CRCV) is:

$$\text{CRCV (ml 100 g}^{-1}) = \frac{\text{radioactive concentration in counts g}^{-1} \times \text{haematocrit (\%)}}{\text{counts 0.005 ml}^{-1}\text{ mixed tail blood} \times 200}$$

Some results obtained by the use of this method are give in Tables 16.2 and 16.3 and Figs 16.1–16.4 (*overleaf*). The plasma space is not measured, in any case this is an equivocal assay (Tøndevold 1983), and no correction is made for trapped plasma. This technique of bone blood volume has been used with little modification to the present day (e.g. Brueton *et al.* 1993a; Brookes *et al.* 1993; Revell & Brookes 1994). It offers the advantages of simplicity, particularly when used for investigations in small animals. Splenectomy is not required in small animals; erythrocytes are

Table 16.2 Summation of raw data for calculating absolute and relative values of circulating red cell volume in various parts of the femur and tibia in 2-month-old rats

Tissue	Number of rats	Σ	Σ^2	s	x[a]	s.e.	Red cell volume relative to value for inferior metaphysis (*P*<0.05)
Femur							
Superior metaphysis	21	25.263	31.514	0.237	1.203	0.053 (4.4%)	64%
Cortex	15	14.052	13.354	0.113	0.937	0.029 (3.1%)	50%
Marrow	21	34.923	61.201	0.395	1.587	0.088 (5.5%)	85%
Inferior metaphysis	21	39.360	76.460	0.367	1.874	0.082 (4.4%)	100%
Inferior epiphysis	21	23.595	28.038	0.293	1.124	0.066 (5.9%)	60%
Tibia							
Cortex	14	10.642	8.407	0.157	0.760	0.042 (5.5%)	
Marrow	18	24.780	36.188	0.346	1.377	0.082 (5.9%)	

Femoral/tibial cortex: 123% (*P*<0.01).
Femoral/tibia marrow: 115% (*P*<0.2).
[a]Absolute red cell volume, ml $100g^{-1}$.

Table 16.3 Variation with age in red cell content of bone tissues of rat (ml 100 g^{-1})

	Age of rat			
Tissue	1 month	2 month	8 month	24 month
Femur				
Superior metaphysis	1.409 ± 0.138	1.203 ± 0.053	0.657 ± 0.050	0.202 ± 0.021
Cortex	1.332 ± 0.088	0.937 ± 0.029	0.303 ± 0.025	0.112 ± 0.005
Marrow	2.110 ± 0.177	1.874 ± 0.082	1.145 ± 0.084	0.458 ± 0.030
Inferior metaphysis	2.110 ± 0.177	1.874 ± 0.082	1.145 ± 0.084	0.458 ± 0.030
Inferior epiphysis	1.330 ± 0.129	1.124 ± 0.066	0.685 ± 0.047	0.262 ± 0.020
Tibia				
Superior epiphysis	1.284 ± 0.136		0.637 ± 0.057	0.254 ± 0.019
Superior metaphysis	2.109 ± 0.218		1.169 ± 0.091	0.534 ± 0.042
Cortex	1.245 ± 0.103	0.760 ± 0.042	0.342 ± 0.044	0.134 ± 0.020
Inferior metaphysis	1.037 ± 0.160		0.543 ± 0.044	0.209 ± 0.017
Inferior epiphysis	1.389 ± 0.081		0.448 ± 0.041	0.248 ± 0.016

robust and survive labelling without significant damage, and in small animals there is no problem counting representative regions of bone. However, large animals such as the dog present problems. Canines require concurrent splenectomy as the arterial haematocrit may be reduced by up to 50% in intact animals (Dietz *et al.* 1979). Furthermore, the canine erythrocyte is particularly fragile, readily undergoing haemolysis (Tøndevold 1983) during even mild manipulations. One should also mention that experimental work utilizing canines is discouraged in the UK, perhaps rightly. For all of these reasons, we continue to advocate the use of small animals, especially the rat, wherever possible in animal investigation.

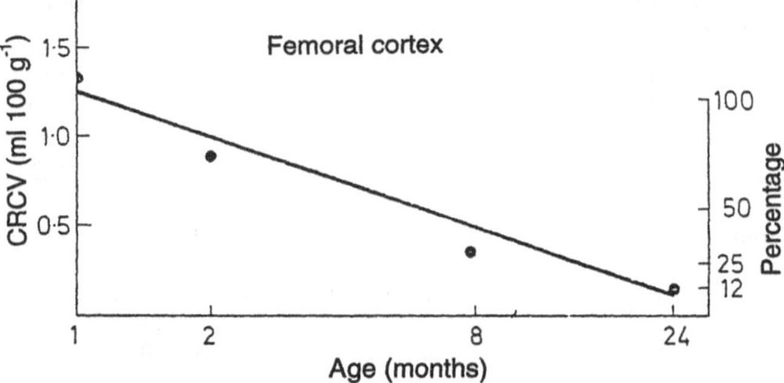

Fig. 16.1. Exponential decline in the red cell volume of rat femoral cortex with age.

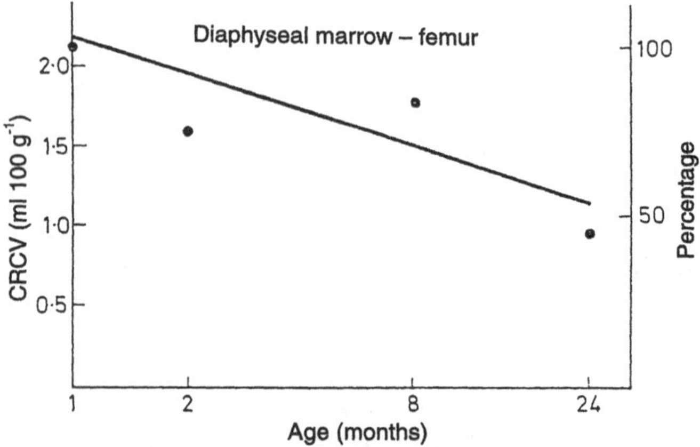

Fig. 16.2. Decline with age in the circulating red cell volume of rat femoral marrow.

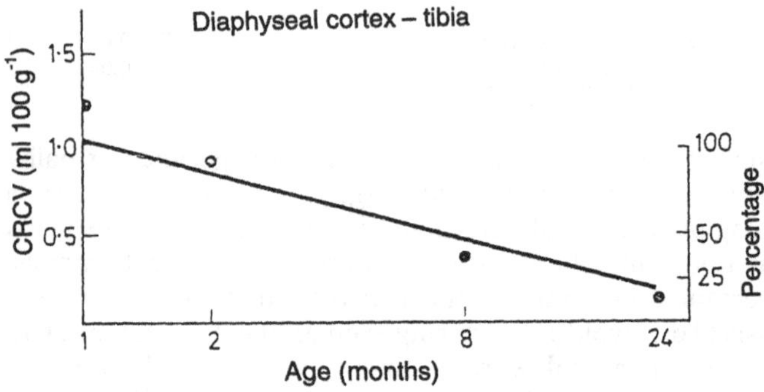

Fig. 16.3. Decline with age in the cortical red cell volume of the rat tibia.

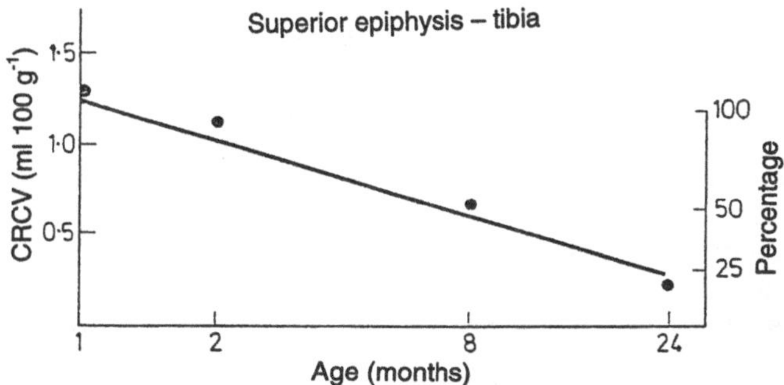

Fig. 16.4. Decline with age in the circulating red cell volume of superior metaphyseal tissue in the rat tibia.

Measurement of the vascular mesh

Parameters related to capillary volume in bone may be obtained by lineal analysis after the method of Loud *et al.* (1965), and discussed in Williams (1985). This involves projecting a regular array of lines or dots across the section and measuring the total number of dots or length of line overlying the feature of interest. The method is based on the Delesse/Sorby principle (Delesse 1887; Sorby 1856) which asserts that on average the fractional area of a feature on sections taken through a solid body, is directly proportional to the fractional volume of that feature in the original solid. In practice, a series of equally spaced parallel lines are superimposed upon the image and the length of intercepts falling on the feature of interest is measured. The total length of intercepts (L_i) is expressed as a fraction of the total line length (L_t) crossing the diameter of the field. Thus an index of the fractional volume (V_i/V_t) may be estimated by L_i/L_t providing that sufficient random sections are taken. In modern times this type of analysis is routinely accomplished with the aid of the ubiquitous computer. However, 'image analysis' is, in spite of extravagant claims by the purveyors of such systems, not without its difficulties, as many practitioners will affirm. The use of a computer, luckily, is by no means obligatory for obtaining useful results.

Brookes has used the principles described above to make an assessment of cortical bone vascularity. India ink-perfused material was embedded in celloidin, and cut into 250–400 μm sections to allow observation of the minimal areas in bone cortex which are completely bounded by capillaries. An eyepiece graticule enabled a regular pattern of dots in the form of a square lattice to be superimposed on the image of the perfused section, as viewed with a microscope. The number of dots occupying several vascular meshes was counted and the mean calculated (= n). The scale of the graticule was selected so that 10–20 dots covered a single mesh, and about 25 meshes were counted in serial sections of bone cortex. If the distance d between adjacent dots in the graticule is known, the absolute area of the vascular mesh equals nd^2. However, for comparative purposes it is necessary only to select homologous pieces of bone throughout the series investigated, and the lattice dimension can then be neglected.

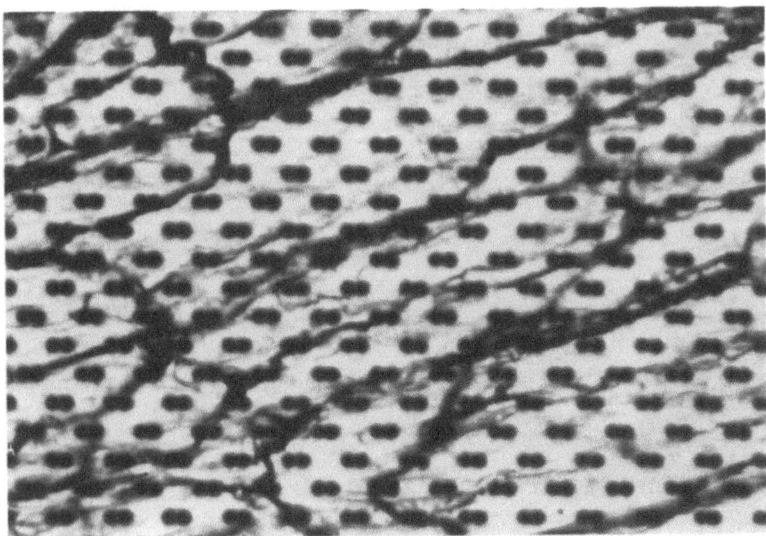

Fig. 16.5. The dot graticule in use. The square root of the mean number of dots occupying clearly focused mesh areas in India ink preparations gives a measure of the mean diffusion distance to any cell. Alternatively, the number of dots lying on the capillaries may be counted to get a measure of the total capillary length irrigating unit volume of tissue.

Fig. 16.5 shows the appearance of the dot graticule in use. A ratio of 1 : 6 was found between the mean number of dots occupying the meshes of cortical vessels in a 1-month-old rat and that in a 2-year-old animal. That is to say, the mean mesh area in the cortex of an old rat 2 years of age was six times greater than that present in a young rat. Hence the mean distance of an osteocyte from the cortical capillary was $\sqrt{6}$ times as great as that obtaining in the young animal. In effect, the cortical diffusion pathway had increased nearly two and a half times ($\sqrt{6} = 2.47$) with the advance of senescence.

Chapter 17

Bone blood flow measurement – 1: Indicator dilution

Introduction

Interest in bone blood flow measurement includes its certain involvement in normal bone growth and decay, and fracture repair, as well as incorporating the entire spectrum of bone disease. It is only now, after 60 years of trial and error, that bone haemodynamic parameters can be quantified in bone with any degree of reliability. Unfortunately, however, skeletal flow values reported from different laboratories, even when using comparable methods, often show considerable diversity. To some extent therefore it seems that the results of skeletal haemodynamic investigations demonstrate some operational dependency. In spite of this cautionary note, it is now possible with confidence, using the very few methods which have withstood the test of time, to investigate the linkage between the osseous circulation in normal bone growth and metabolism and the often profound pathological changes which occur concurrently with a disturbed circulation. Although contemporary research tends to focus on the metabolic cellular and biochemical controlling factors associated with bone vascular status, it is worth bearing in mind that a change in the rate of blood perfusion through a bone, reflecting an alteration in the balance of arterial input and venous outflow, has *direct* and significant effects on the biophysical environment of bone cells; thus pH, $P\text{CO}_2$, $P\text{O}_2$ and interstitial fluid flow may all be affected, with concomitant effects on cellular function.

There are more than 200 bone elements in the body, roughly classified into flat, long, short and irregular groups, each possessed of its own morphological individuality; and not one of them, let alone the entire skeleton, is endowed with a readily accessible vascular hilum. The measurement of bone blood flow has therefore always demanded skill, and is nowhere carried out as a routine classroom exercise. Nevertheless, a review of the principal attempts at measuring blood perfusion rates in bone will serve to illustrate the methodological problems involved, and encourage the diligent investigator to renewed attempts at non-invasive solutions.

Direct methods

The anatomical diversity of the arterial supply to bone, and the even greater diversity of venous drainage routes, ensures that direct quantitative measurement of bone blood flow by methods such as venous effluent collection or even the more simple option of electromagnetic flow-meters is difficult or even impossible. Thus, the work of Drinker *et al.* (1922) and Cumming (1962) who measured blood flow through the femur using venous outflow measurement techniques, although influential, must remain of historical interest only. The results, however, are worth noting because of the direct nature of the measurement.

Venous effluent collection

Drinker *et al.* (1922) isolated a dog's tibia and perfused it via the nutrient artery with oxygenated Ringer's solution from a constant pressure pump. The effluent fluid was collected in a beaker placed beneath the tibial preparation (Fig. 17.1). Previous experiments using India ink perfusion had convinced them that normally the periosteal contribution to the arterial supply was negligible. The vast numbers of capillaries draining the blood from the tibial cortex into the overlying periosteal and muscle veins were possibly left undisturbed, but no consideration was made to the numerous arteries which enter the cancellous epiphyses. The values obtained, 3.5–41 ml 100 g^{-1} min^{-1}, suggest an average whole bone perfusion of 20 ml 100 g^{-1} min^{-1}, but this would be susceptible to wide variation in response to changed physiological conditions. The authors, indeed, showed that low values were obtained under the influence of vasoconstrictor adrenaline, high ones when vasodilator acetylcholine was administered.

Cumming (1962) ligated all of the branches of the femoral artery and vein of the rabbit, except the diaphyseal nutrient vessel. The venous effluent from the cannulated femoral vein produced a wet marrow flow of 52 ml 100 g^{-1} min^{-1} (range 20–100 ml 100 g^{-1} min^{-1}). This value was surprisingly high, but may well be appropriate to the experimental conditions; effectively, the femoral nutrient artery was the sole remaining channel open to the blood normally destined for the posterior limb. Regardless of the fact that this experimental design takes account only of the inflow and outflow from the cannulated vessels (thus effectively ignoring the anatomy of the bone circulation), the technique was adapted by others using isotopic tracers and the Fick principle (see later).

Venous plethysmography

Multiple routes of venous escape also confound the use of venous occlusion plethysmography to determine blood flow rate to a limb. Edholm *et al.* (1945) used this method to show increased flow in patients with Paget's disease, assuming that the initial rate of increase in limb volume distal to a venous tourniquet was correlated with arterial inflow. Errors, however, resulting from venous drainage via the periosteum proximal to the tourniqet, and shunting through other intra-osseous routes, were ignored. They concluded that the rate of flow in the humerus was 1 ml 100 g^{-1} min^{-1}. These workers made the point that the figures of Drinker *et al.* (1922) "are obviously inapplicable to man, as acceptance of the higher value would mean that more than half the systemic flow would be through the skeleton". Nevertheless the most recent data available, using tech-

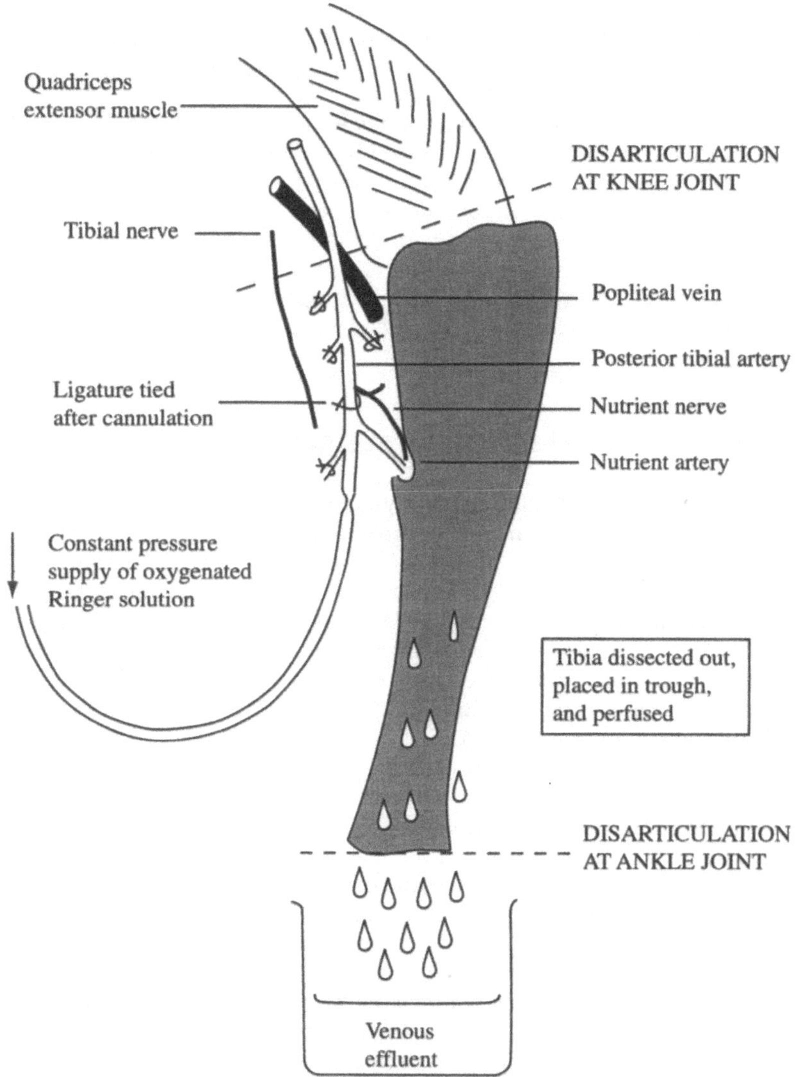

Fig. 17.1. Venous effluent collection in the isolated canine tibia.

niques based on more methodologically robust principles, suggest that high flow rates are normal in the bones of both man and animals.

Red cell velocity

Brånemark (1959) used an even more direct approach, observing red cell movements at the interface between bone marrow and cortex. Again, the method was highly invasive; the results were difficult to interpret and could only be related to the results of other measurement systems with difficulty. It remains, however, an impressive technical achievement. The cortex of the rabbit fibula was carefully pared down until red cells, illuminated by a traversing light guide, could be observed and recorded cinematographically *in vivo*. Red cell velocities of 0.1–0.8 mm s^{-1} were reported. The smallest measured red cell volume for rat bone cortex is 0.9 ml 100 g^{-1}. Converting Brånemark's lowest red cell speed into 1.2 cm min^{-1} it follows that the red cell flow rate is 1.2×0.9 ml 100 g^{-1} min^{-1}. Knowing the haematocrit in rat bone cortex is 0.42, the overall perfusion rate in Brånemark's preparation becomes 2.6 ml 100 g^{-1} min^{-1}. Similarly the upper velocity of 0.8 mm s^{-1} corresponds to a perfusion rate of 10.3 ml 100 g^{-1} min^{-1} in the cortex or 12.8 ml 100 g^{-1} min^{-1} in the marrow. It should be borne in mind that the normal centrifugal blood flow in the fibula was abolished while blood cell velocities were being measured.

Pressure, heat and electromagnetism

In the past, investigators of bone haemodynamics often attempted to obtain an estimate of bone blood flow by means of intramedullary manometry. The recordings were often highly variable and bore no relation to flow. Although stable intramedullary pressures can now be recorded with electromanometers and large bore (>4 mm) cannulae (Arnoldi *et al.* 1972; Bunger *et al.* 1983), the fact remains that manometry has never yielded a bone perfusion rate. In any case, any assumption of a relationship between intra-osseous pressure and flow rate based on Poiseuille's law cannot be sustained because of the anatomical multiplicity of feeder and exit routes (Kofoed 1993).

Thermocouples introduced into bone marrow also give an unstable record. The influence of metabolic processes on the local temperature can be overcome by the use of heated thermocouples and the principle of heat clearance (Hensel & Ruef 1954; McPherson *et al.* 1961). Although a correlation between heat clearance and blood flow has been described in some organs, a suitable probe has yet to be devised for reliable intramedullary flow measurement. Intra-osseous thermometry may contribute to progress in clinical diagnosis, but it has not yet succeeded in quantifying bone blood flow.

The large group of appliances comprising mean-flow recorders, phasic-flow meters and ultrasonic flow meters, which have been used successfully for flow determinations in single large arteries, are not suitable for bone blood flow measurement. Even the largest nutrient artery is really too small for their application. Electromagnetic flow (EMF) meters are much more promising. Blood is a conductor of electricity, so Faraday's law of induced EMF is operative; blood flowing in bone in an applied magnetic field will induce an electric field in a direction mutually perpendicular to the magnetic field and the direction of blood flow. The induced field is then proportional to the product of blood velocity and magnetic field strength (Wyatt 1977).

While standard apparatus is available for flow measurement in a single coronary artery, for example, the anatomy of bone vascularization is not so easy to overcome. Perhaps the development of an encasing sheath, composed of a large number of micro-electromagnets, for a limb bone, followed by computer analysis, might resolve the problem and place an entirely non-invasive, isotope-free method of bone blood flow measurement at the disposal of the clinician.

Laser Doppler flowmetry

A useful qualitative method of assessing bone blood flow has been the introduction of laser Doppler flowmetry, largely by Swiontkowski *et al.* (1986) and also Notzli *et al.* (1989), following its first use as a method of continuously monitoring skin perfusion (Nilsson *et al.* 1980). The method depends upon the fact that light reflected from a moving blood cell undergoes a frequency shift that is dependent upon the relative difference in velocity between the light source and the travelling cell. The technique does not give an absolute flow, but is useful to monitor changes in perfusion rates, for instance before and after an operative procedure. The bone must be exposed and the probe securely clamped in place; a shift in position during a procedure would invalidate comparison. Measurement is localized to the region immediately beneath the probe, and restricted to a depth of 2.9 mm in cortical bone or 3.5 mm in cancellous bone, which must be approached by drilling through the compactum (Notzli *et al.* 1989).

In view of the difficulties of these direct methods, modern studies of bone blood flow in the laboratory have relied upon vascular tracers, using deposition techniques, utilizing either completely extracted tracers (indicator fractionation) or clearance of partially extracted tracers; and techniques of intravascular indicator dilution. Intravascular indicator dilution will be discussed in this chapter, clearance methods in Chapter 18 and indicator fractionation in Chapter 19. Indicator fractionation has become the laboratory method of choice - the "gold standard" of the bone haemodynamic investigative armamentarium. This is most often referred to as the "microsphere" technique, one of the few instances where the proprietary brand of a *material* has given its name to a *method.* The term arteriolar blockade (Brookes 1970) will be used throughout this text, which is a more pertinent description reflecting its crucial characteristic as a technique. In view of its current importance, a later chapter (Chapter 19) has been devoted to blood flow measurement by arteriolar blockade.

In interpretation of bone blood flow investigations it is important to be aware of the limitations inherent in the use of all of these methods. Those reviewed below are mainly concerned with animal studies, which allow the use of terminal procedures. Our own studies have often used the laboratory rat for reasons of economy and convenience, and with normal care most manipulations can be successfully performed. Often, however, techniques that have been shown to be inappropriate for bone blood flow studies in experimental systems have had to be used for evaluation of skeletal haemodynamics in the human patient. Medical investigations often, and rightly, necessitate compromise between robustness and confidence of result, and ethical and safety considerations; these compromises do not need to be considered in the laboratory.

Intravascular tracer dilution

If a freely diffusible tracer is introduced into a tissue, either intra-arterially or by local injection, then its rate of disappearance from a particular site is proportional to blood flow. In the absence of concentration gradients in the tissue surrounding a capillary, the removal of tracer may be regarded as flow dependent. If recirculation of the isotope back to the site does not occur, Kety (1949) showed that the isotope disappearance curve may be considered as a single term exponential, the slope of which represents the ability of the local circulation to "washout" the tracer

$$C(t) = C_o e^{-kt} \qquad (1)$$

where $C(t)$ is the concentration at time t; Co is the initial concentration of the tracer, and k is the rate constant. The rate constant may be determined from a semilogarithmic plot of the disappearance curve, or more usually now, by a computer calculated log/linear regression.

$$k = (\ln C_1 - \ln C_2) / (t_2 - t_1) \qquad (2)$$

where t_1 and t_2 are arbitrary times and C_1 and C_2 are the corresponding concentrations. The rate constant k is related to the blood flow F, and to the combined volume V of tissue and blood for the organ, by the partition coefficient λ, which is the ratio of tissue to blood concentration of tracer at equilibrium:

$$k = F / \lambda V \qquad (3)$$

therefore the blood flow rate F per unit volume of perfused tissue is given by:

$$F = k\lambda \qquad (4)$$

In an early application of the principle (Cumming & Nutt 1962), a small amount of ^{24}Na was injected directly into the femoral marrow of a rabbit and its washout monitored by a collimated gamma-ray detector. Without correcting for losses for diffusion of the tracer away from the observed site in tissue fluid, local cell metabolism and fixation by extravascular plasma proteins, a value of 41 ml 100 g^{-1} min^{-1} for marrow perfusion rate was obtained, thus concurring with the high marrow flows obtained from venous effluent collection (Cumming 1962).

Iodoantipyrene washout

Ideally the chosen tracer must be highly permeable, if not infinitely diffusible, and equilibrium with tissue should occur rapidly, within the length of a capillary. Washout of iodoaminoantipyrene (Kelly *et al.* 1971; Semb 1971; Kelly 1973; McElfrish & Kelly 1974) has been advocated, the isotope being administered through the cannulated nutrient artery of the dog tibia. This direct route into the bone is chosen so that the presence of extra-osseous labelling may be reduced; otherwise the presence of general tissue activity will confound measurement of the osseous label. However, Cofield *et al.* (1975) have pointed out that cannulation of the nutrient artery can decrease perfusion to the tibial diaphyses by up to one-third. McElfrish & Kelly (1974) attempted to circumvent this problem by introducing iodoantipyrene into the anterior tibial artery, but measured an unacceptably high reduction of tracer transport into the canine tibia, compared with the direct nutrient arterial route.

Examination of the results of iodoantipyrene washout experiments have raised the possibility of a two-phase perfusion in marrow; an initial fast washout correlating with a perfusion rate of the order of 100 ml 100 g^{-1} min^{-1}, and a secondary slower phase of about 20 ml 100 g^{-1} min^{-1}. What these components represent is an unresolved problem, but it may perhaps be associated with the presence of parallel supplies, or different compartments within the diaphyseal marrow domain. External counting integrates washout curves from marrow, cortical bone and surrounding muscle, and this tissue heterogeneity may contribute to the observation of the observed biexponential washout curves. Semb (1971) attempted to measure the washout of ^{133}Xenon, the radioactive form of the normally chemically inert gas. This is administered by inspiration of a gas/air mixture and thus removes the problems of invasive dissection. However, the gas was shown to be avidly soluble in marrow fat and the method largely abandoned. However, Lahtinen *et al.* (1982) have used ^{133}Xe washout to measure femoral head flow in humans, obtaining a value of 7.4 ml 100 g^{-1} min^{-1}. Iodoantipyrene also dissolves in fats, but its solubility is less than 10% that of xenon (Kelly 1973). Its use, however, does not resolve the problem of heterogeneity of tissue activity sampling.

Hydrogen washout

Washout of the inert gas freon was used by Kiær *et al.* (1993) in combination with an intra-osseous mass spectrometry probe to obtain a direct measure of declining tissue concentration in dog femoral condyles. The value for blood flow obtained corresponded quite well with simultaneous measurement by microspheres (see Chapter 19). This rather elaborate technique, however, may be regarded as an adaptation of the simpler method using washout of inhaled hydrogen gas developed by Aukland *et al.* (1964) for use in soft tissue, and subsequently used for measurement of bone blood flow rates in the rabbit (Whiteside *et al.* 1977a,b; Kita *et al.* 1987; Revell & Heatley 1990) and the dog (Weiland & Berggren 1981; Weiland *et al.* 1982). Hydrogen is a very small highly diffusible molecule, which is rapidly transported across cell membranes. Washout in bone marrow was found to be biexponential, again suggesting parallel circulation, whilst cortical bone was largely monoexponential. In this technique the decay of hydrogen gas concentration in the tissue is monitored by measuring the oxidation current produced by the dissolved hydrogen at the surface of a platinized platinum electrode. In a low impedance circuit with a calomel reference electrode, the oxidation current is linearly related to hydrogen concentration (Hyman 1961). The value of λ for bone (about 0.75 for cancellous bone; 0.45 for diaphyseal compactum) is readily obtained by measuring equilibrium concentrations of hydrogen in small samples of tissue placed in solutions of the tracer *in vitro* (Aukland *et al.* 1964; Whiteside *et al.* 1977a). As a control, Whiteside *et al.* (1977a) showed that implanted pieces of bone did not take up hydrogen from surrounding muscle *in vivo* in the absence of a blood supply.

Hydrogen washout has its problems, not least the instability of the platinized electrodes; however, they are not expected to "poison" because of an imposed voltage, as in the oxygen polarograph (Ingebrigsten *et al.* 1963). The probes must also, in acute experiments, lie in a pool of extravasated blood which somewhat militates against the utility of the method without adequate controls. Similar comments also apply to early attempts to use thermal "washout" techniques (e.g. Kelly *et al.* 1959; Shaw 1963). The area of measurement is also very localized, making extrapolation to whole bone or larger regional parameters difficult. Also, the presence of strongly electronegative platinum stimulates bone formation around electrodes placed in the marrow. Given favourable circumstances however, Revell & Heatley (1990) have shown that this technique may be adapted to allow repeated measurement over a period of time. With the aim of following the long-term flow sequelae of experimental orthopaedic interventions, electrodes placed bilaterally in the rabbit femoral marrow (Fig. 17.2) were shown to respond to administered hydrogen for periods up to 12 weeks in the same animal (Fig. 17.3). Paired identical electrodes were used so that procedures in one limb could be compared with changes in the unoperated contralateral limb. This is an important control as the platinum electrode must be placed into a hole bored into the bone; as mentioned earlier, this has the effect of adding an extra

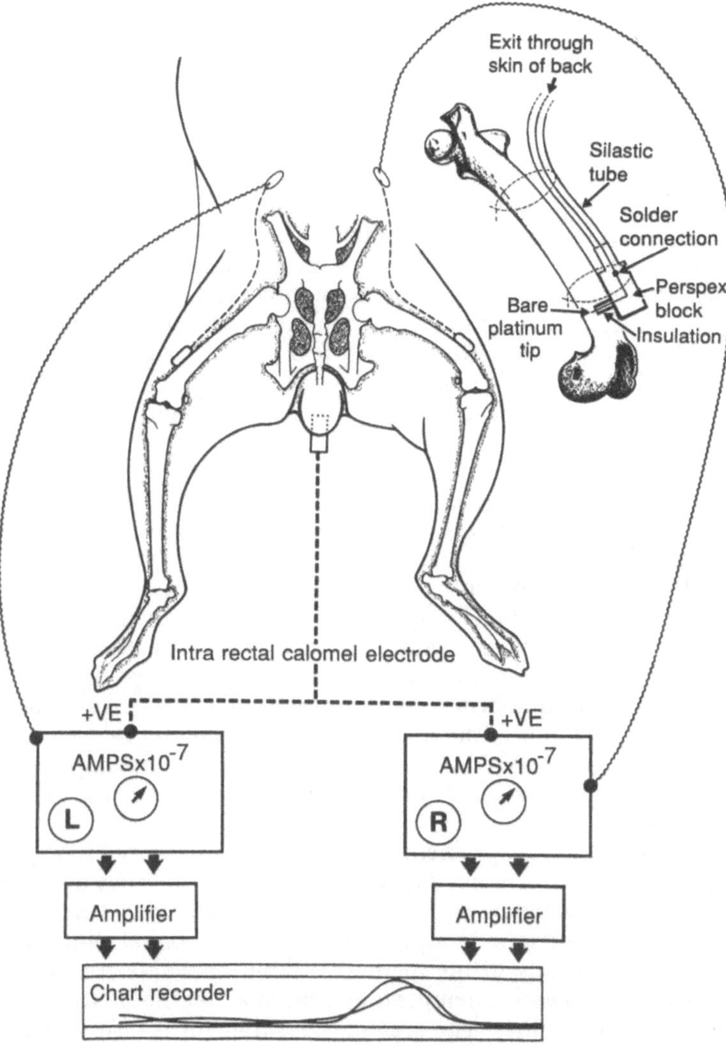

Fig. 17.2. Experimental arrangement for long-term recording of marrow blood flow by hydrogen washout.

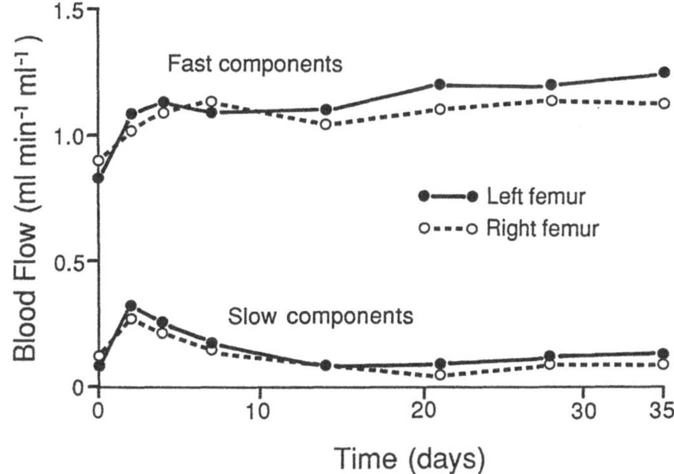

Fig. 17.3. Simultaneous flow recordings from both femoral marrow cavities of a single rabbit for 5 weeks after electrode implantation. Solid line, left femur; broken line, right femur.

compartment of extravasated blood which is not connected directly to the circulation. This may introduce an artefactual reduction in the measured flow rate which becomes significant at higher blood flow rates (>150 ml min^{-1} 100 g^{-1}; Aukland *et al.* 1964). However by assuming similar conditions of electrode implantation in contralateral limbs, the effect of a procedure on one of the limbs may be evaluated relative to the unoperated control (Fig. 17.4, *overleaf*).

A further problem with all washout methods is that of recirculation of tracer; any residual concentration of tracer in arterial blood will result in a diminished, *measured*, flow rate. In the case of hydrogen, femoral *arterial* concentrations of tracer took 40 seconds to clear in the dog, and flow rates measured in kidney cortex by hydrogen washout only corresponded to direct venous effluent measurement after this time had elapsed (Aukland *et al.* 1964). Whilst this time was halved in the rabbit (Whiteside *et al.* 1977a), the presence of a residual arterial tracer concentration in the early stages of washout is still a significant interfering factor. Again, this effect may obscure more rapid components of the washout.

Zierler (1965) demonstrated theoretically that blood flow measurement by washout of a freely diffusible tracer could be considered as a subcategory of the Stewart-Hamilton dye dilution method for determining cardiac output. White *et al.* (1964) used a modified indicator dilution technique to estimate blood flow through the rabbit tibia by analysis of a step response. This measures the activity resulting from tracer entry into the tissue, infused at a presumed constant rate, uptake by the tissue being determined at frequent short intervals. This is the reverse of measuring the residual function at intervals following the introduction of a bolus injection; the resulting 'build-up' curve was assumed to be exponential, but very few rabbits were used, and a clearly insufficient number of points used for curve construction. The authors calculated the rate constant k by measuring activity resulting from influx of ^{51}Cr-labelled red blood cells to a previously tourniquet-isolated lower limb, and calculated blood flow from an indirect

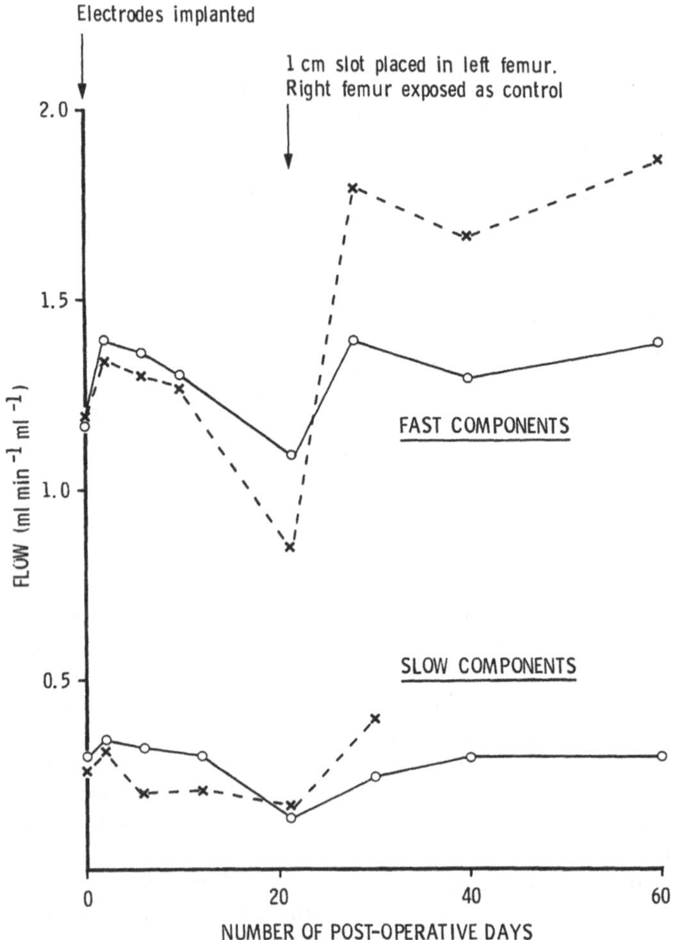

Fig. 17.4. The effect of creating a unilateral 1 cm defect in the cortex of the femur opposite the electrode site. Solid line, left femur; broken line, right femur.

measure of the red cell volume of distribution V per unit weight of bone, by using a modified form of Equation (3).

$$F = \mathrm{k}V \tag{5}$$

The problems of reactive hyperaemia resulting from prolonged tourniquet use must contribute to the errors of the method. However, they obtained a very acceptable value of 16 ml 100 g^{-1} min^{-1} for rabbit tibial flow.

Red cell dilution and follow-through curves

Brookes (1967) also used an indicator dilution method to measure blood flow rate through different regions of the rat femur. In this comprehensive investigation a large number of rats were used with ensuing statistical robustness. The method is not practical for routine laboratory purposes, involving large numbers of animals and considerable labour to calculate each value. Certainly it has yet to be repeated. However, it was based on well-established principles and for the first time allowed computation of a variety of haemodynamic parameters: perfusion rates, transit times, red cell velocities, flow coefficients and haematocrits for regional parts of the rat long bone. Although Brookes' experiment is now largely of historical interest, the flow rate values obtained from this study remain essential reference points for all subsequent haemodynamic investigations in the rat. Because the method facilitates discussion of many important factors in the study of bone haemodynamics, this pioneering investigation is presented in some detail.

Stage 1 A direct measurement of circulating erythrocyte volume in regions of the rat femur was determined by haemodilution of ^{51}Cr-labelled red blood cells introduced into the venous system; bone red cell volume being calculated by comparison with radioactivity counts obtained from a known volume of mixed tail blood, after adequate mixing in the circulation (see "Red cell volume in bone" in Chapter 16).

The method assumes that the circulation in any part of the bone can be represented by the dynamic equilibrium in a tank (Fig. 17.5). A radioactive isotope (or dye) introduced into the tank at time t_o will have a concentration C_o. The relation of F, the flow rate, is given by:

$$\log_e C = \log_e C_o{}^{-kt} \qquad (6)$$

where k = a constant = F/V, therefore

$$F = Vk \qquad (7)$$

To measure F, both V and k were required. V was determined in a separate animal, as described in Stage 1.

Stage 2 To measure k, intravenous bolus injections of ^{51}Cr-labelled erythrocytes were injected into 140 rats. Each rat was subsequently killed at precise intervals post injection, and the circulation abruptly halted by rapid freezing. The femora were then removed, divided into anatomical regions, and activities of cortex, marrow, metaphyses and epiphyses determined. Haemodynamic curves were then constructed relating bone activity to time following bolus injection

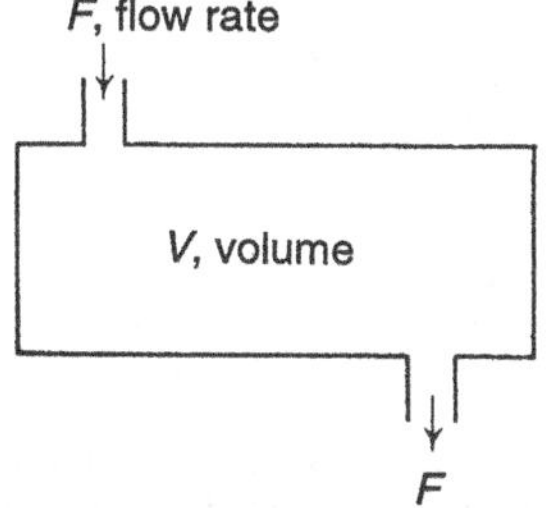

Fig. 17.5. Diagram of single compartment flow.

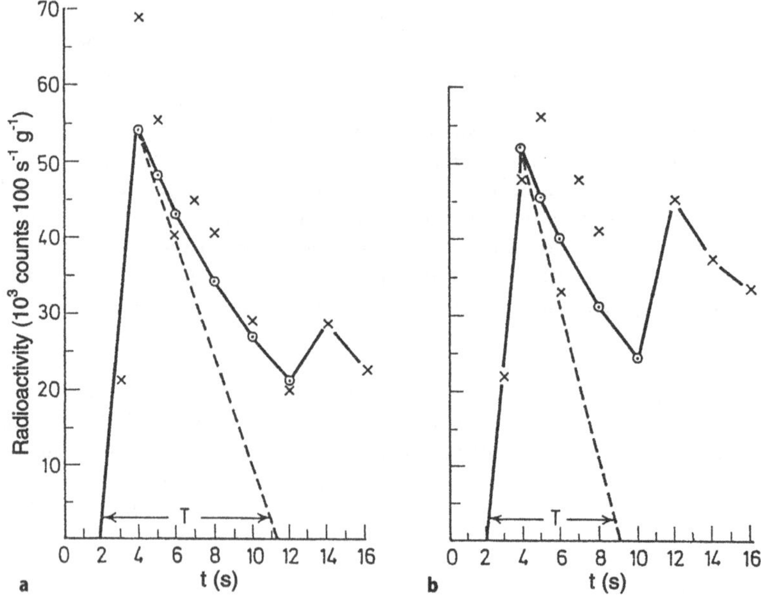

Fig. 17.6. Cartesian plots of: **a** marrow radioactivity; **b** inferior metaphyseal radioactivity. ×, Observed mean values; o values calculated by regression; T, transit time, i.e. the time for a red cell to traverse 1 g marrow.

(Figs 17.6, 17.7). The amount of tracer per unit weight of bone increased for the first 3–4 seconds and then declined as labelled cells were washed out by unlabelled red blood cells.

Recirculation of marked cells was shown by a later increase in activity (≅14 seconds) marking the end of the useful washout phase. Regression of the logarithm of ^{51}Cr activity against time yielded the value of factor k (Table 17.1).

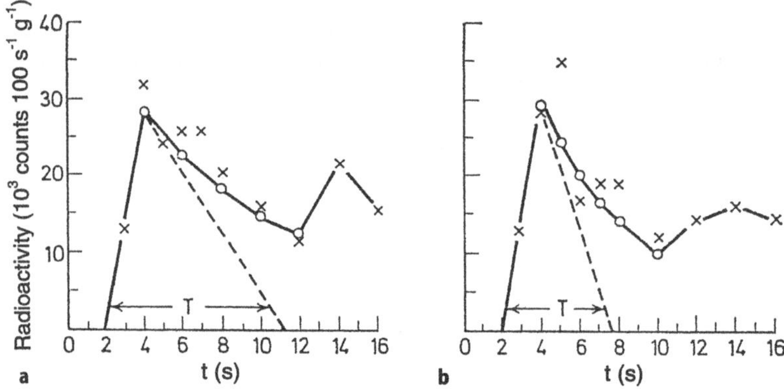

Fig. 17.7. Cartesian plots of: **a** cortical activity; **b** inferior epiphyseal radioactivity. ×, Observed mean values; o, values calculated by regression; T, transit time, i.e. the time for a red cell to traverse 1 g marrow.

Table 17.1 Regression constants in different parts of the rat femoral circulation

Tissue	C_o	k	s.d.
Superior metaphysis	49.7	0.14	0.03
Cortex	43.6	0.11	0.02
Marrow	85.2	0.12	0.03
Inferior metaphysis	85.1	0.12	0.04
Inferior epiphysis	61.8	0.19	0.04
Mean		0.133	0.031

The flow rate was then calculated for erythrocyte velocity ($F = Vk$); not for that of whole blood, because the passage of red cells alone through the bone tissue was observed in this experiment. Furthermore, V as calculated, is the red cell mass, not the whole blood volume. By extrapolating the tangent (Figs 17.6, 17.7) to the beginning of the fall-off curve down to the abscissa, the value of T, the transit time through unit weight of bone tissue, was gained.

Validation of the method

The above method assumes that each femoral tissue investigated can be treated as a simple open compartment system such that a small bolus of red cells enters at time t_0 a circulating space V contained by innumerable capillaries. The radioactive cells are found at t_0 at a maximum concentration of C_0 in the specified tissue. Thereafter the bolus is washed out, exponentially by unlabelled blood following on the bolus. However the large bolus originally injected into the whole animal has had to pass through the heart and lungs before reaching the arterial system, and hence has undergone some dilution. Nevertheless, the radioactivity of arterial blood on entering the selected tissues is the same in all cases. Further dilution of the radioactive red cells occurs in the circulatory space of each tissue. At t_0, the degree of dilution of the red cells should be the same for all tissues investigated.

Now C_0 can be found from the regression line for each tissue (Table 17.1). The graphs were constructed for 1 g of tissue, and the red cell bolus injected into each rat had a standardized radioactivity of 100 000 counts 100 s^{-1} 0.005 ml^{-1} packed red blood cells (Brookes 1967b). It follows that: $C_0/100\,000 \times 0.005 \times 100 = V_1$ where V_1 is the apparent volume of red cells in 100 g of tissue at time t_0. The actual volume, V, has, however, already been measured independently (Stage 1). Hence, for each tissue an initial dilution factor for the bolus on entering it can be

Table 17.2 Calculated dilution factors for a radioactive bolus on entering various femoral vascular compartments

Tissue	V	V_1	Dilution (%)
Superior metaphysis	1.2	0.24	21
Cortex	0.9	0.22	23
Marrow	1.6	0.43	27
Inferior metaphysis	1.9	0.43	23
Inferior epiphysis	1.1	0.31	27

Table 17.3 Haemodynamic data for the rat femoral circulation (see text for explanation)

		Superior metaphysis	Marrow	Cortex	Inferior metaphysis	Inferior epiphysis
Red cell volume (V ml 100 g^{-1})		1.2	1.6	0.9	1.9	1.1
Red cell flow rate (F ml 100 g^{-1} min^{-1})		10	13	7.5	15	9
Transit time (T s)		7	9.2	9.2	7	6
Red cell velocity ($S \propto (\sqrt[3]{V})/(T\sqrt[3]{100})$ mm s^{-1}		0.327	0.274	0.226	0.381	0.371
Haematocrit (h)		0.39	0.6	0.42	0.5	0.31
Plasma flow rate (P)		16	8	10	15	20
Whole blood flow rate (Q)		26	21	18	30	29
Rate of flow per unit vascular space (Qh/V)		8.4	7.9	8.4	7.9	7.9
Data as percentage of inferior metaphyseal value (=100%)	S	86	72	59	100	97
	Q	86	72	60	100	97
	V	64	85	50	100	60
	F	64	85	50	100	60

calculated (= $V_1/V \times 100\%$). Table 17.2 gives these calculated dilution factors for the five tissues studied.

Considering the wide variation in the haemodynamic data readings to be expected under these experimental conditions, it is all the more remarkable that the five tissues treated separately and independently, should indicate that the bolus of radioactive red cells, as it reaches them for the first time on the first circuit round the body, dilutes to approximately the same extent, namely 1 in 4; a test which suggests that the method of flow measurement adopted here is valid.

Haematocrit and red cell velocity

The values of some haemodynamic characters in the rat femoral circulation obtained by this method are given in Table 17.3. The rates of whole blood flow through various parts of the bone were originally calculated by applying an arbitrary haematocrit of 43.4%, that of "mixed" arteriovenous tail blood following amputation of the tip (Brookes 1965). There is every probability however that haematocrits, like other haemodynamic characters, are not the same in all anatomical domains of the long bone.

The haematocrit for rat marrow blood is fairly easily obtained by sampling from the principal nutrient vein using a heparanized micropipette, followed by centrifugation at 1000 rev min^{-1}. Taking rat femoral marrow blood thus obtained to be 60%, the other regional haematocrits can be calculated. Consider a quantity of blood drawn as a quadrangular solid and plotted three-dimensionally (Fig 17.8). Let the vertical axis OH represent the haematocrit scale, the point H being the maximum of 1. OU is unit linear depth. The area UO . HX is one unit of cross-sectional vascular area. Let the horizontal axis OS represent the distance travelled by a red cell, and Os the distance travelled in 1 second, that is, the red cell velocity. Let the shaded part of the solid represent the packed red cells; above it lies the plasma. The height h is the haematocrit of that whole blood which has travelled s cm in 1 second. The volume of the red cells represented in Fig. 17.8 is F, the red cell rate of flow. Then, $F = h \times s \times 1$ cm^3 . s^{-1}

In particular:

$$\frac{F\text{ marrow}}{F\text{ cortex}} = \frac{h\text{ marrow}}{h\text{ cortex}} \times \frac{s\text{ marrow}}{s\text{ cortex}} \tag{8}$$

By transposition:

$$h\text{ cortex} = \frac{F\text{ cortex} \times h\text{ marrow} \times s\text{ marrow}}{F\text{ marrow} \times s\text{ cortex}} \tag{9}$$

Now, the term *s*, velocity, has the dimensions length per unit time, cm s^{-1}. The volume of red cells traversed by a red cell in time *T* seconds in a living bone is given by *V*/*T* cm^3 s^{-1}. It follows that the units of $\sqrt[3]{V/T}$ are cm s^{-1}, and that this therefore may be taken as a valid expression of red cell velocity;

$$S \propto \sqrt[3]{V/T} \tag{10}$$

Substituting Equation (10) in (9) above:

$$h_c = \frac{F_c \times h_m T_c \times \sqrt[3]{V_m}}{F_m \times T_m \times \sqrt[3]{V_c}} \tag{11}$$

where the subscripts c and m, stand for cortex and marrow respectively.

The mean red cell velocity can be calculated if the red cell volume *V*(ml 100 g^{-1}) is reduced to ml g^{-1} to correspond to the graphs from which *T* was derived (Figs 17.6, 17.7). Then red cell velocity:

$$S = \frac{\sigma \quad \sqrt[3]{V}}{T\sqrt[3]{100}} \text{ cm s}^{-1} \text{ (where } \sigma \text{ is a constant)} \tag{12}$$

The right side of the Equation (12) has been used in Table 17.3 to gauge relative red cell speeds in various parts of the femur. All values on the right of the Equation (11) are now known. In particular, the haematocrit for cortical blood is:

$$h_c = \frac{7.5 \times 0.6 \times 9.2 \times \sqrt[3]{1.6}}{13 \times 9.2 \times \sqrt[3]{0.9}} = 0.42$$

By substituting the data (Table 17.3) for other tissues into the Equation (11), it can be calculated that the haematocrits for the inferior and superior femoral metaphyses, and the inferior epiphysis, are 0.5, 0.39 and 0.31 respectively. Table 17.3 also gives whole blood and plasma flow rates which can be estimated because the haematocrit and the red cell flow rate are now known. In addition,

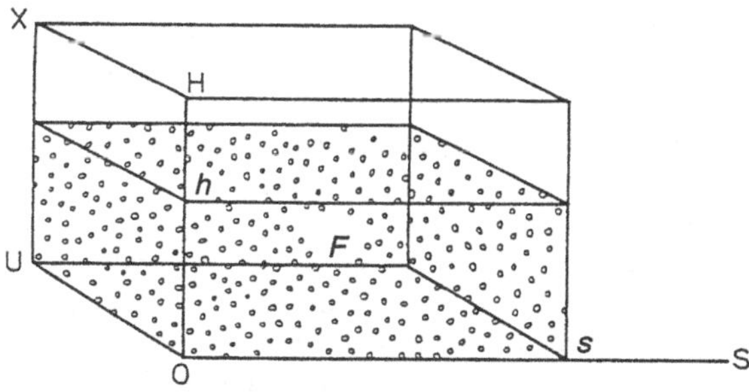

Fig. 17.8. Three-dimensional axes for calculating blood haematocrit in the osseous circulation.

certain haemodynamic parameters relative to the values obtained in the inferior metaphysis, which are taken as 100%, are also shown.

To summarize the sources of the numbers in Table 17.3: V was estimated directly (Stage 1 above); F was estimated by constructing follow-through curves (Stage 2 above); h was measured directly in the case of marrow blood and calculated subsequently for other tissues; Q and P were derived from known values of F and h; and the relative red cell velocities were obtained after both numerator and denominator in the expression $^3\sqrt{V/T}$ had been measured directly (Stages 1 and 2 above).

Flow rate and driving pressure

The relative data given in Table 17.3 indicate that the speed of a red cell passing through the vascular lattice of unit weight of bone tissue is proportional to the whole blood flow rate, that is, $s \propto Q$. These two parameters of the osseous circulation have been calculated from different sets of observations in quite different experimental situations. Because it is difficult to conceive how red cell speed in a bone compartment can be otherwise than in proportion to the whole blood flow rate to it, it follows that the close linear relationship between s and Q shown in Table 17.3 provides an internal check on the validity of all calculations. Furthermore, the linear relationship between s and Q indicates that in the osseous circulation at any rate, variation in the diameter of sinusoids in the vascular bed are not important in the control of blood flow rate; otherwise the r^4 factor in the Poiseuille equation might have been expected to disturb the linearity of proportion between s and Q. As a matter of fact, the calibre of the sinusoids and capillaries of bone appears to be much the same in all parts (see Figs 8.8, 9.3, 9.24), although red cell speeds and rates of blood flow differ markedly from one region to another in the same bone.

The length of a sinusoid, which linearly affects the resistance and therefore might be held to be important in the control of blood flow rate through bone, is difficult to define in practice and therefore awkward to measure. Nevertheless in one situation, the cortex, we can be sure that we are dealing with unusually long vessels (see Fig. 8.8). It may be noted from Table 17.3 that red cell speeds are lowest in the cortex (only 60% of those recorded from the growing metaphysis). The total flow rate through the cortex is similarly reduced. However, a *variation* in the flow rate in the cortex, as indeed elsewhere in a bone, cannot be due to a *change* in vessel length. Nor is it reasonable, as argued above, that a change in calibre is the basis of a change in flow rate. Indeed, there is no firm observational evidence of variability in vascular calibre in normal bone cortex, whose capillaries are as wide as medullary sinusoids. Discounting changes in viscosity, it follows that the important variable affecting blood flow rate is the driving pressure across its vascular bed.

In the case of the upper and lower metaphyses, the vascular patterns and calibres are identical. The factors affecting the vascular resistance, vessel length and calibre, cannot therefore account for the observed difference in the flow rates through these two territories. Nor is it likely that the viscosity should differ markedly in two regions showing such close vascular similarities. It follows that, as for the cortex, it is the driving pressure that chiefly regulates the flow rate in metaphyseal tissue in normal circumstances, a concept which may well apply to the osseous circulation as a whole.

Vascular stress in bone

A simple calculation permits us to gauge the rate of blood flow in bone per unit vascular space. This quantity, arrived at by simple proportion, may be expressed as Qh/V. It is noteworthy that this quantity is much the same in the five different parts of the rat femur investigated (see Table 17.3), and amounts to about 8 ml per unit vascular space per minute, although differences may exist within the same bone. Diaphyseal marrow and the epiphysis and metaphysis at the growing end of the femur all appear to be regions where the vascular lattice is subjected to the same amount of stress, and yet they exhibit marked differences in structure, bone content and rates of bone metabolism. The cortex and the superior metaphysis are localities which differ radically in bone structure, and yet their blood vessels are stressed by the flowing blood to the same amount.

Three conclusions can be drawn from this finding. The first, already borne out by direct observation, is that the basic character of the osseous vascular lattice is much the same everywhere insofar as factors such as vessel structure and calibre do not radically differ, if only because everywhere in bones, including the cortex, sinusoids are the overwhelming constituent of the vascular bed. The second conclusion that follows from the general uniformity of the rate of flow per unit vascular volume of bone is that the osseous vascular lattice is everywhere physically stressed to much the same extent. On the other hand, the rate of blood flow, Q, varies markedly when measured with respect to unit weight of tissue, and reflects the different metabolic levels at which disparate parts of a bone function as well as differences in degree and type of ossification.

Flow rate and bone formation

The red cell flow rate, F, in the cancellous bone of the inferior femoral epiphysis is low compared with that in the adjacent metaphysis. The 3 : 1 preponderance of the metaphyseal over the epiphyseal red cell flow provides further evidence that it is not the latter which is so important for the nutrition of the growth cartilage as a whole; rather it supports especially the cells of the germinal layer (see "Epiphyseal subchondral vessels", Chapter 11). Presumably a red cell flow rate in a microcirculation gives an indication of the aerobic metabolic activity of the corresponding tissue. Table 17.3 shows that there is a 3 : 2 relationship in the flow rates F through the inferior and superior metaphyses of the rat femur. It is noteworthy that this is the same as the ratio found to exist between the rate of growth in length at the "growing" end and the "non-growing" end of long bones (Digby 1916; Payton 1934).

It is also appropriate to utilize red cell flow data to gain a relative estimate of the amount of bone formation, an aerobic process, that is taking place in selected sites. On this assumption, the rates of flow given in Table 17.3 indicate that bone formation is maximal in the "growing" metaphysis and minimal in the cortex, the two quantities being in the proportions 2 : 1. By the same token, the rate of bone formation in the inferior epiphysis is much the same as that occurring in the superior metaphysis of the femur. Relative bone formation rates have been compared in various parts of different long bones in dogs by Amprino & Marotti (1964). These Italian investigators utilized a method involving tetracycline feeding and moving spot densitometry. Their results also indicate a preponderance of bone formation in the growing metaphysis and a sharp fall-off in the epiphysis and cortex.

Plasma shift and synovial water

Table 17.3 indicates the presence of markedly different haematocrit values of blood flowing in the vascular lattice in various parts of a bone. It should be mentioned that there remains some controversy over regional variation in the interior haematocrit of bone. It has been known for many years (Fahraeus 1929) that when blood flows through tubes of small calibre the haematocrit varies linearly with the diameter of the conduit. Thus the haematocrit from blood flowing in the mucosa of the small intestine is only 50% of that found in the afferent arteries (Jodal & Lundgren 1970).

Tøndevold & Eliasen (1982) calculated haematocrits from separate measurements of plasma and erythrocyte volume in different regions of the femora and tibiae of dogs, obtaining values of 50–70% of the arterial haematocrit. Interestingly, they reported that the lowest haematocrits were found in regions with the fastest flow rates. The authors acknowledge that their result differs from that expected from the predictions of Fahraeus, implying a divergence from normal flow physiology in bone; this requires further investigation.

In our experiments reported here (Brookes 1967b) blood collected from the femoral vein yielded a haematocrit of 0.6, allowing a calculation of 0.42 for the cortical haematocrit; the arterial haematocrit in the rat is 0.33. This near doubling of the haematocrit in the nutrient femoral tibial vein could be correlated with the escape of bulk fluid from bone marrow exiting through the cortex as shown by Montgomery *et al.* (1988). In bone many channels are available to facilitate interstitial fluid movement; junctional clefts between capillary endothelial cells, canaliculi, Haversian and Volkmann's canals (Kelly 1983). Various labels have been used to determine fluid movement through the capillary clefts, osteocyte lacunae, and the canalicular system (ferritin, Dillaman 1984; horseradish peroxidase, Lorenz & Plenk 1977; Thorotrast, Seliger 1970). Montgomery *et al.* (1988) clearly demonstrated an anatomical pathway from capillary to matrix and thence into the general circulation, by examining ferritin transport haemodynamics in conjunction with histology. They argued that the rapid movement of the label was not consistent with the view held by Hughes *et al.* (1977), that the mechanism of exchange between blood and interstitial fluid was by passive diffusion. They argued instead that the pattern of label movement suggested bulk interstitial fluid flow influenced by hydrostatic pressure.

Mammalian bone capillaries in the dog show similar anatomical characteristics to those of soft tissues (Cooper *et al.* 1966). Hughes & Blount (1979), however, found that a basement membrane was not present in cortical bone capillaries from rat ribs and fibulae, and is also absent from the cortical capillaries of human fetal bones (Brookes 1971). Nevertheless it is usually assumed that the capillary wall will behave similarly in man and dog with regard to the transport of ions, molecules and water (Kelly 1983), and be subject to Starling's Law. One formulation of this states that increased capillary pressure increases transudation. Increased capillary pressure in soft tissues can result from venous obstruction or arteriolar dilatation. This results in a net fluid efflux which collects in the tissue spaces causing oedema, until the interstitial fluid pressure rises high enough to balance the elevated capillary pressure (Guyton & Hall 1996).

Diaphyseal marrow has a haematocrit of 0.6; the growing metaphysis, 0.5. Peripheral mixed blood in the large bony and tendinous tail of a rat has a smaller haematocrit, 0.43. Lymphatic channels are absent in bone. Since all parts of the bone are supplied with arterial blood, with the same characteristically low haematocrit of 0.33 in the rat, it would appear that plasma water rapidly leaves the marrow vessels, and escapes from the bone elsewhere.

It is unlikely that a massive shift of plasma water takes place from the marrow through the fundamental bone substance of the cortex, to be absorbed by periosteal lymphatics. The fact that living bone hardly drips water after periosteal elevation suggests that if transcortical transfer does occur in this way, it is not considerable. On the other hand, the evidence suggests that sinusoid plasma water leaves the marrow cavity at the endosteum and is gradually absorbed by the cortical capillaries, thus reducing the capillary haematocrit. Nevertheless, the fact that this at 0.42 approximates to that of mixed blood suggests that the haematocrit for the cortex as a whole is brought about by the mixing of medullary sinusoid and cortical arteriolar bloods. Both of these pass centrifugally from the marrow towards the periosteal surface.

It is also noted that the haematocrit in both metaphyses is lower than the high marrow value, particularly in the case of the non-growing end. In the one epiphysis examined, it is lower than that of arterial blood. If the inferior epiphysis were a sealed hydrodynamic chamber, then, on the principle that "what goes in must come out", it would be expected that the epiphyseal vascular lattice would show a purely arterial haematocrit. Whilst this principle certainly applies to the red cells circulating through the inferior epiphysis of the rat, it probably does not apply to the epiphyseal plasma water and its solutes.

The permeable articular and growth cartilages separate the epiphyseal circulation from the synovial fluid and the metaphysis respectively. It has been shown above (see Chapter 13) that there is still some uncertainty as to the origin of synovial fluid and its constituents, and as to whether the joint cartilage absorbs synovial water or passes it out into the joint cavity during joint movement. The source of the materials used in the production of a growth cartilage is also a matter of dispute, as is the direction of flow of nutrient substances, including water, through it. From the evidence of intra-osseous haematocrits which diminish as one approaches articular cartilage, it would appear that plasma water shifts along the marrow cavity and passes through the growth cartilage into the epiphysis. The looped metaphyseal subchondral sinusoids (see Figs 8.6; 11.5) suggest a filtration mechanism (compare the renal glomerular tufts). The epiphyseal vessels (see Figs 8.33, 11.25) suggest an absorbent arrangement. Water, on this interpretation, could pass from the marrow cavity into the epiphyseal circulation.

The data in Table 17.3 may be utilized to give some indication of the magnitude of the plasma water that could possibly be made available to the epiphysis by this occurrence. The inferior metaphysis weighs very roughly the same as the inferior epiphysis, and both are much heavier than the diaphyseal marrow, which can be neglected in this equation for the time. If the metaphysis were a closed hydrodynamic system with respect to plasma water, then the haematocrit should be arterial, about 0.33. The plasma flow rate P should therefore be 30 ml 100 g^{-1} min^{-1}, not 15 as calculated on the basis of a haematocrit of 0.5. Likewise, the epiphyseal plasma flow should be 18, not 20 ml 100 g^{-1} min^{-1}. If in fact 15 ml of metaphyseal water were lost to the epiphysis each minute, our data would allow only 2 ml of this to be drained away by the epiphyseal veins. The rest might possibly be transuded through the articular cartilage. Taking the weight of the whole epiphysis in a 250-g rat to be about 0.5 g, then the 13 ml 100g^{-1} min^{-1} (water) which must be accounted for, are transformed into the much more credible 0.026 ml min^{-1} water displaced into the joint cavity from the whole inferior femoral epiphysis, and easily accommodated in a hydrodynamic squeeze film during joint movement.

It is known that the passage of various minerals from the joint cavity into the synovial membrane is very rapid. Hence the possibility of water shift from the marrow cavity to the joint space, indicated by haematocrit and haemodynamic observations, would not seem to tax unduly the absorptive capacities of the subsynovial circulation. Only about 50 μl of water per minute are required by the above considerations to be absorbed from the synovial fluid by the joint membrane in order to preserve the homeostasis of synovial fluid volume in the resting knee joint, the largest in the rat skeleton (see also, Chapter 13).

In the light of the above analysis, it may be concluded that haemodynamic investigation suggests, and is capable of, quantifying what has for too long been ignored in many studies on growth and articular cartilages, namely the possibility that nutrient fluid passes through them from the metaphyseal and articular circulations respectively. As far as a *growth* cartilage is concerned, it is unfortunate that destruction studies of epiphyseal vessels have led many into believing that its nutrition is confined to the epiphyseal subchondral circulation (see Epiphyseal Subchondral Vessels in Chapter 11). The subarticular contribution to *joint* cartilage deserves a much needed re-emphasis (see "Articular nutrition of joint cartilage" in Chapter 14).

Chapter 18

Bone blood flow measurement – 2: Clearance of bone seeking tracers

This important group has a large literature. Whilst several of the method assumptions have now been criticized, the use of bone seeking tracers is of importance in the clinical measurement of human skeletal haemodynamics. Whilst our emphasis in this book is on the experimental bases of skeletal vascular study, aspects of clinical investigation will be introduced and discussed.

The Fick principle was originally developed for measuring cardiac output, assuming that all gaseous exchange between the body and the surrounding atmosphere took place at the lungs (and none for example at the skin surface). It follows that a knowledge of the O_2 consumption per minute, together with a measurement of the arteriovenous difference in the mean volumetric concentrations of this gas in pulmonary arterial and venous bloods, provides sufficient data to calculate the total pulmonary circulation, and hence the cardiac output (Fig. 18.1, *overleaf*). In effect the Fick principle is often stated as "what goes in is equal to what comes out; plus what is retained or excreted". More formally:

$$Q_a = Q_i + Q_{nv} + Q_v + Q_m \quad (1)$$

where Q_a = the mean radioactive concentration of indicator accumulating in tissue, usually determined by arterial sampling;

Q_i = amount retained by the tissue;

Q_{nv} = amount excreted by non-venous routes; e.g. the lymphatics; negligible in bone;

Q_v = amount of isotope in venous effluent blood;

Q_m = amount metabolized in the tissue; may be ignored if metabolically inert tracer used.

The difficulty in this model situation lies in obtaining an accurate assessment of the radioactive concentration in total bone venous effluent (Q_v). A femoral vein sample has often been deemed sufficient in spite of the mixing of bloods, from the femur itself and its related muscles and soft tissues. Due to the complexity of the venous drainage route, bone-seeking isotopes are used where a 100% single passage extraction is *assumed* to occur. If this assumption is allowed, then:

$$Q_a = Q_i \quad (2)$$

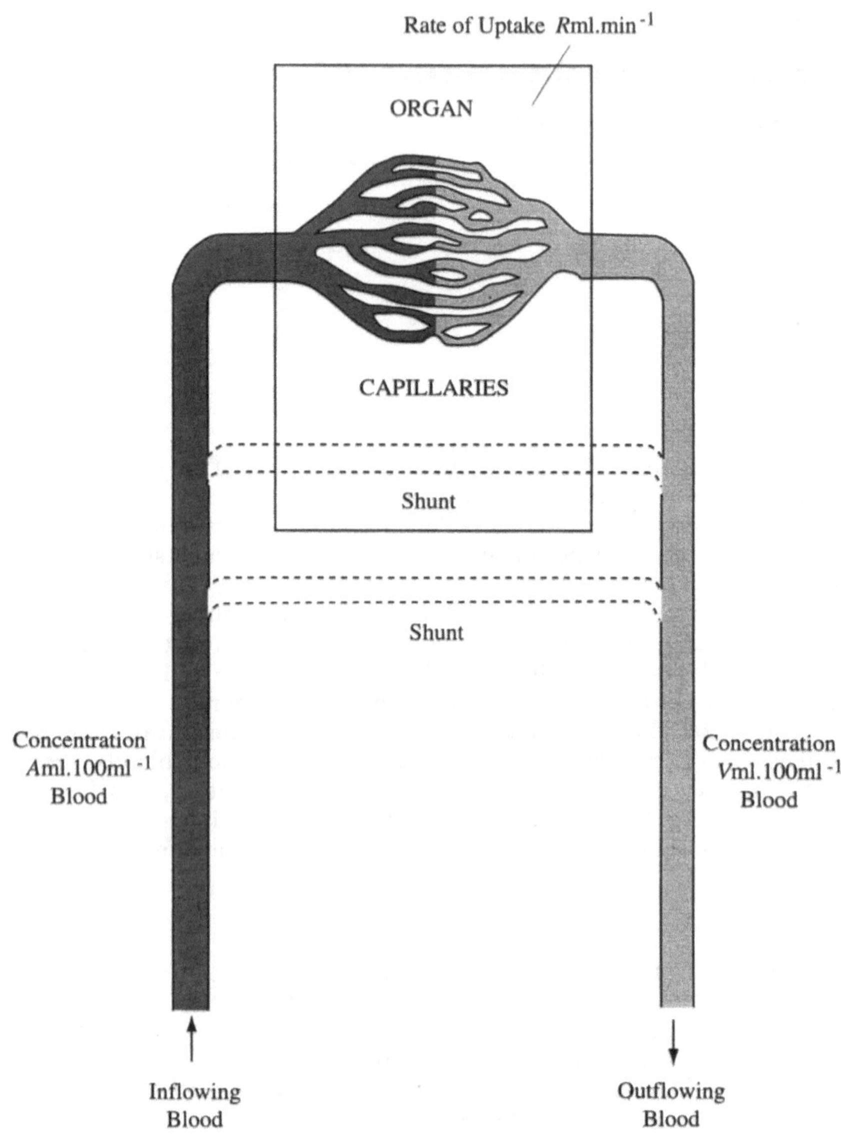

$$\text{Organ blood flow rate} = \frac{R}{A - V} \times 100 \text{ ml.min}^{-1}$$

Fig. 18.1. The Fick principle. The presence of arteriovenous shunts between blood sampling sites invalidates the calculation.

The amount of tracer entering the tissue during time t is the product of the flow during time t and the mean tissue concentration; i.e. tissue flow equals Q_i divided by the integral (between t and zero) of the arteriovenous difference in indicator blood concentration across the tissue.

$$F = Q_i / \int (C_a - C_v)\, dt \tag{3}$$

where F = tissue blood flow per unit volume; Q_i = tissue concentration of indicator; C_a = arterial concentration of tracer; C_v = venous concentration of tracer.

Clearance is defined as the minimal quantity of blood entering an organ per unit time that could supply the amount of indicator removed in unit time *t* during its passage through the organ. It is the product of extraction and flow, and has the same units as flow. Extraction is the fraction of tracer removed from blood during a single passage through an organ, and therefore *cannot* exceed unity.

$$\therefore \text{Flow} = \text{clearance} / \text{extraction} \tag{4}$$

and

$$Cl = Q_i / \int C_a\, dt \tag{5}$$

where Cl = clearance of tracer in tissue per unit volume; C_a = arterial concentration of tracer; Q_i = tissue concentration of indicator.

It is to be emphasized that use of the desired simple calculation is dependent on the total removal of the isotope during a single passage through bone (usually by bone salt, but possibly by living cells or even bone substance). If tracer extraction is 100%, then venous concentration becomes zero after transit and clearance is equal to blood flow. If extraction is not equal to 100% then the extraction ratio must be measured and the flow rate corrected as in Equation (4). This, in fact, has not always been done; many investigators often only *assume* a sufficiently high extraction rate. Furthermore, any return of the isotope to the circulation vitiates the foundation of the method by reducing the uptake, resulting in an underestimate.

Frederickson *et al.* (1955) reported the first use of a clearance method using the bone-seeking isotope ^{45}Ca, to measure bone blood flow in the rat. Assuming complete extraction, they calculated values of 10–30 ml min^{-1} 100 g^{-1} bone, which are similar to the values obtained by Brookes (1967b) using labelled red cell washout. Since then, the use of many bone-seeking isotopes have been reported, including those of calcium, rubidium, fluorine and strontium. For all of these trace nuclides, the extraction ratio has, in fact, been shown to be less that unity.

Copp & Shim (1965) measured an extraction ration of 0.764 during the first 5-minute clearance of ^{85}Sr in the dog tibia by comparing the fractional amount of ^{85}Sr in the venous outflow, with that of the intravascular tracer Evan's Blue. Venous outflow concentration was measured in the femoral vein, which is *not* the total venous outflow, and the figure obtained must therefore be treated with caution. However, in a later paper (Shim *et al.* 1968) the same group produced a figure of 9.6±0.47 ml 100 g^{-1} min^{-1} for blood flow to the rabbit femur, using ^{85}Sr clearance but assuming total extraction. If the same extraction ratio applies to the rabbit as in the dog (0.764) then the flow rate can be adjusted upward to 12.6 ml 100 g^{-1} min^{-1}. Using a perfused canine tibia and ^{125}I-labelled albumen as an intravascular tracer, McCarthy & Hughes (1990) determined a maximum value of 0.48 for the 5 minute net extraction of ^{85}Sr. This value was similar to that found by Weinman *et al.* (1963), who measured 10-minute extraction ratios of 0.43 in the canine femur, for both ^{85}Sr and ^{47}Ca, when the isotopes were injected into the nutrient artery. Kane & Grim (1969) assumed complete single passage extraction of ^{86}Rb in an attempt to measure bone blood flow in dogs; they obtained a value of 13 ml 100 g^{-1} min^{-1} for perfusion rate through the canine femur. Subsequent measurement, regrettably, has shown that the 5-minute net extraction of ^{86}Rb is only 0.38 (McCarthy & Hughes 1990) and the blood flow figure needs to be substantially revised upward. Considerable recirculation of ^{86}Rb in and out of cells occurs during the first few seconds following injection; a unitary extraction ratio is therefore fallacious, and the Fick principle cannot be applied under these circumstances.

These examples show that there can be great variance in reported extraction ratios, and an assumption of 100% extraction using tracer clearance measurement for bone blood flow can introduce considerable error. To calculate an extraction ratio it is now usual to measure the cardiac output at the time; this is usually done by the reference flow method (see Chapter 19), whereby a 5-minute blood sample (for instance) is gathered by means of a constant flow pump from a convenient artery. The pump flow rate divided by the mean arterial concentration as a proportion of the injected dose of a radionuclide, yields the cardiac output. Next, the clearance is calculated, that is, the minimum arterial blood flow rate which could account for the observed uptake of the isotope in the bone under investigation, assuming that all the isotope is leeched from the blood (Tothill 1984). Finally, the blood flow rate in the observed bone must be available, but measured in a different way from the uptake, usually by indicator fractionation. Flow is proportional to clearance and if extraction is unitary, the two are equivalent. If not, the extraction ratio for the radionuclide may then be given by the clearance divided by the perfusion rate. The dimensions of both are the same; the ratio is a number.

What the number means is debatable. On the face of it, it has something to do with the isotope concentration in the blood perfusing bone, and is possibly a complex function of isotope diffusion, exchange and uptake in the metabolism of bone substance. Extraction ratios have been shown to be dependent upon flow rate and other factors which influence exchange dynamics. Increasing blood flow rate shortens the transit time through a capillary, and may eventually become less than the minimum time required for the tracer to diffuse through the capillary wall. It has been reported (Hughes *et al.* 1977; McCarthy *et al.* 1980) that transcapillary solute transport into bone mineral is normally by free passive diffusion, being flow limited at low perfusion rates, but becoming diffusion limited as the flow rate increases. Diffusion limitation of extraction has been further verified using ^{99}Tc-methylene-diphosphonate (^{99}Tc-MDP)in dogs (McCarthy *et al.* 1980; McCarthy & Hughes 1983; Riggs *et al.* 1984) . Interestingly, Hughes *et al.* (1979) showed that ^{85}Sr instantaneous and net extraction (5 minutes) did not alter during the increased blood flow phase of a healing osteotomized tibia in the dog. The authors suggested that in this pathological situation the exchange surface area or capillary permeability had increased; presumably by vasodilatation of the vascular bed and/or vessel recruitment. In normal bone increased surface area of exchange does not occur with increasing blood flow (McCarthy & Hughes 1983).

Schoutens *et al.* (1979) artificially manipulated flow rates in the rat hind limb by varying the ambient temperature, and compared flow rates measured with 15 μm microspheres, with extraction of ^{45}Ca. In the tibia, extraction varied from 0.77 to 0.27 as the blood flow rate changed from 6 to 12 ml min^{-1} 100 g^{-1}. Similarly, Tothill *et al.* (1985) demonstrated that the ^{85}Sr net extraction ratio over a 5-minute period, in canine hind-limb bones, fell from 100% at low flow rates (approaching zero) to approximately 40% at flow rates greater than 10 ml min^{-1} 100 g^{-1}. Similar results were shown using ^{18}F and ^{99}Tc-MDP. Tothill's group concluded that the variation in extraction ratio of several tracers with flow rate "preclude the use of bone-seeker clearances to measure bone blood flow". Unfortunately, other factors also cast doubt on the utility of the clearance method.

Wootton (1974) determined the extraction ratio of ^{18}F in rabbit femora and tibiae. The technique assumed a single passage of the tracer, and was conducted by comparing bone activities resulting from a mixture of ^{18}F and ^{51}Cr microspheres (extraction assumed to be 100%; see Chapter 19) injected into the rabbit aorta, and killed 10 seconds later. The mean ratio of activities was close to 1, which was used to claim 100% extraction of ^{18}F in a single passage through bone. No account, however, was taken of the avidity of bone mineral for the bone-seeking isotope, which would not be reflected in the distribution of the microsphere tracer. Using a multiple indicator dilution technique, Davies *et al.* (1979) found a maximum extraction ratio of only 65% for ^{18}F, measured in the canine tibia. An intrinsic error of the microsphere/clearance method for determining extraction ratio is that microspheres will label bone marrow as well as cortical and trabecular bone, whilst ^{18}F uptake will be confined to bone mineral. Tothill & McPherson (1980) used a similar procedure to Wootton (1974), and obtained largely the same result, but also noted that some measured extraction ratios significantly *exceeded* unity; a severe, if not entirely fatal, test for the method.

The length of time the isotope spends in the circulation is an important, and potentially confounding, factor. Both Wootton, and Tothill's group assumed that the time between introduction of tracer and sacrifice of the animal did not exceed the minimum recirculation time; it is also important for the validity of the method that the time between injection and sacrifice is greater than the maximum time required for passage through the bone. If ^{18}F remained in transit through the vascular domain for longer than the arbitrary 10-second period, the assumptions of the technique cannot be met; non-extracted isotope will remain in conjunction with that taken up by the bone, thus inflating the extraction ratio. Davies (reported in Davies *et al.* 1979) found that the transit time in bone for ^{18}F was considerably greater than 10 seconds in the dog, but generously conceded that this may be less in rabbits. However, using rats and rabbits, Tothill & Hooper (1984) injected bolus injections of the "intravascular" tracer, albumen, into the heart and measured the time for activity in hind limb bone to disappear before recirculation activity produced a second peak. They reported that "at no time between 5 and 60 seconds did the activity fall to negligible levels". Again, they concluded that single passage techniques were invalid for measurement of extraction ratios.

The minimum recirculation time in the dog skeleton is under 1 minute (Kane & Grim 1969). Compare this with the reported 2–4 minute albumen washout time following a bolus injection into the tibial artery of the dog (Cofield *et al.* 1975; Lemon *et al.* 1980). Calculation of extraction ratio, from arterial sampling during the time "window" before recirculation occurs, must therefore introduce errors when inferring blood flow rates from clearance measurements. Furthermore, efforts to eliminate recirculation effects by experimental manipulation must introduce severe and ultimately unacceptable perturbations of the system under investigation.

One final complication of clearance methods is that tracer diffusion occurs post-mortem. Bone-seeking tracers continue transferring to bone, at least until the bones have been safely removed and stripped of soft tissue; a procedure which in practice is often delayed. Tothill & MacPherson (1978) found that the bone content of the common bone-seeking isotopes ^{85}Sr, ^{47}Cr and ^{18}F, following *in vivo* injection in rats and rabbits, continued to increase for at least an hour after sacrifice. Charkes *et al.* (1979b) noted that isotopes diffuse into bone from blood vessels within 2 minutes following death, and Wootton & Doré (1986) found that the calculated ostensible extraction ratio of ^{18}F in rabbit bone continued to rise post-mortem at the rate of 0.01 min^{-1}. Uptake, therefore, is present when blood flow is absent, again pointing to the limitations of the clearance method to predict bone blood flow rate.

For all of these reasons, including the avidity of bone-seeking isotopes, difficulties in establishing accurate and meaningful extraction ratios, variations in extraction ratio in response to physiological change and recirculation artefacts, clearance of bone-seeking isotopes has proved a difficult technique to use, and even more difficult to interpret. The methods have perforce, however, formed the basis of mathematical models which have been utilized for clinical skeletal blood flow measurement.

Mathematical modelling

Skeletal tracer uptake

Van Dyke *et al.* (1965) introduced a method of bone blood flow suitable for clinical use, which depends on estimating the fractionation of an injected dose of ^{18}F between the skeleton and the kidneys. This was done by collecting the urine output over 3 hours post-injection, during which time the venous concentration of ^{18}F was continuously monitored from an arm vein. Uptake is rather slow, and it takes an hour or so after intravenous injection of sodium radiofluoride to obtain a well-delineated scintillation scan of the normal skeleton. A three-compartment mathematical model was postulated to describe ^{18}F kinetics. The model contained an initial mixing volume, and as in models of calcium kinetics, this was larger than the blood volume. At first this was linked irreversibly to the bone uptake compartment. In order to provide a reasonable fit with observed blood sample data, the analogue computer solution required the addition of a mammillary compartment, the slowly exchangable fluoride pool, whose anatomical nature remains undetermined. Nevertheless, a curve showing total skeletal uptake with time was generated, from which the mean flow rate for bone could be calculated.

On general anatomical grounds it might be supposed that the fluoride ion F^- would diffuse from the bone capillaries through the extravascular space to reach bone substance, where it substitutes for the hydroxyl ion in the hydroxyapatite of the mineral phase. This and other models like it which ignore the individuality of bone substance, distinct from extracellular fluid, have given values for mean bone blood flow considerably lower (e.g. 2 ml 100 g^{-1} min^{-1} or 3% of the resting cardiac output in man) than those obtained using methods based on indicator fractionation (see Chapter 19), or indicator dilution methods (e.g. Table 17.3). Using a positron camera to scan patients with myelofibrosis, an enhanced contrast in regions of interest, compared with normal control bone, was found in 15-minute post-injection scans. This was attributed to increased flow. Calculation then yielded a raised flow rate of 8.7 ml 100 g^{-1} min^{-1} in these abnormal circumstances; and yet still below the *normal* values calculated by other methods. Scanning alone will not resolve whether an increased bone uptake results from increased cardiac output, bone perfusion rate or bone extraction, because each process can produce the same effect. As might be expected an ^{18}F extraction ratio of 1.0 was assumed (Wootton 1974) in calculating blood clearance, by dividing the uptake in a given initial time by the mean blood concentration in that time, in order for the Fick principle to apply. The experimental inconsistencies of this assumption, have already been discussed at length, although Wootton's group maintains that the use of more advanced techniques confirms a 100% extraction for ^{18}F (Wootton & Doré 1986).

Another assumption of the skeletal tracer uptake method (van Dyke *et al.* 1965) is that the bone crystal is not saturated with respect to the tracer. Although the non-linearity of uptake of several commonly used tracers suggests that this is a real hazard, it is made more likely by the failure to register increasing uptake with increasing blood flow. It is unlikely that this is because of blockade of binding sites in bone crystal, since a second injection of tracer increases the counting rate of bone. Rather, it reflects an adaptive isotopic equilibrium which is inherent in the blood, bone extravascular fluid and the calcified matrix of bone, which provides a basic homeostatic mechanism conserving the constancy of blood calcium with increased cardiac output during exercise.

Deconvolutional analysis

Recognizing that there is an anatomical extracellular fluid compartment in bone (ECF), visible in paraffin histology (Fig. 9.24), Wootton *et al.* (1976) redesigned the human skeletal tracer uptake method using ^{82}Br-bromide or ^{51}Cr-EDTA as a marker for the ECF alone, and ^{18}F-fluoride for the combined bone substance and ECF of bone. By deploying a governing integral equation incorporating a unit input-response function, it was believed possible to transform the skeletal uptake of ^{18}F in bone substance to what it might look like if there had been an instantaneous uptake of the bone marker, before all the recirculation had occurred. The value of this deconvoluting function at time zero multiplied by the skeletal blood volume yielded the skeletal blood flow per minute, 11% of the cardiac output at rest. Basic to the mathematical analysis is the linearity of the deconvoluting function. In practice this assumption appears to be unfounded.

The Claude Bernard model

This was devised to permit a mathematical analysis of a five compartment model of ^{18}F kinetics (Charkes & Brookes 1976; Charkes *et al.* 1978). The model (Fig. 18.2, *overleaf*) takes note of a rapid fall in ^{18}F blood concentrations to 30% of the initial values, suggesting a rapid dispersion of fluoride into a larger compartment exterior to the blood, namely the ECF. Thereafter the slow decline in blood concentrations is clearly a correlate of bone uptake and urinary excretion. Since the bone ECF space is demonstrable in a histology slide, it requires no special defence to include it in the model. Renal tubular re-absorption is also provided for, and

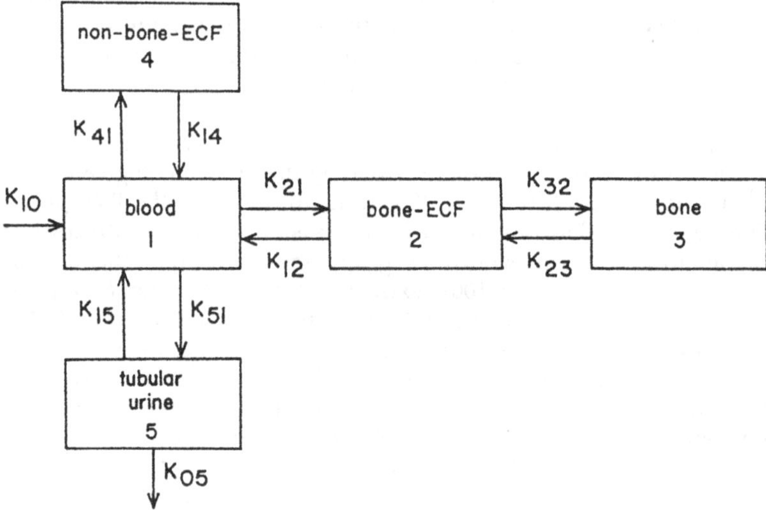

Fig. 18.2. Five-compartment model of fluoride kinetics.

the compartments are reversibly linked to acknowledge bidirectional ionic flux. Although there is no *a priori* reason why a five-compartment model should better explain data than any other number of partitions, the model was based on recognizable physiological principles, and hence dedicated to Claude Bernard. Furthermore, the model was tested in Brookes' laboratory, where experimental confirmation of the theoretical assumptions were obtained (Charkes *et al.* 1979a,b).

Radiobromide ^{77}Br and radiofluoride ^{18}F were injected intravenously into rats, and the animals investigated at repeated intervals up to 2 hours post-injection. Ten minutes before injection, a bolus of radiochromated red blood cells was injected to allow blood volumes to be calculated (see Chapter 16). The data, duly processed on a two-channel scintillation counter, were entered into a digital computer programmed to generate the rate constants of the differential equations linking the compartments. A least-squares fit was obtained to the observed blood and urinary data in both rat and man, and curves for ^{18}F uptake in bone substance, and bone and non-bone ECF were constructed (Figs 18.3, 18.4). Maximal uptake in rat bone is about 90% of the administered dose (in man, about 60%). The direct measurement of skeletal ^{18}F uptake is not possible in man, but was carried out in the rat, confirming the computer-predicted curve for bone and its ECF. In particular, the forward rate constants out of blood were found to be extremely valuable. From them, and knowing the blood volume, it was possible to calculate the cardiac output, the fractional skeletal flow, and therefore the overall skeletal perfusion rate (rat 19.3 ml 100 g^{-1} min^{-1}; man 11.7 ml 100 g^{-1} min^{-1}; Charkes *et al.* 1979b).

Dynamic uptake

Methods are currently being developed which allow skeletal haemodynamic parameters to be measured *in vivo* by the use of advanced imaging apparatus

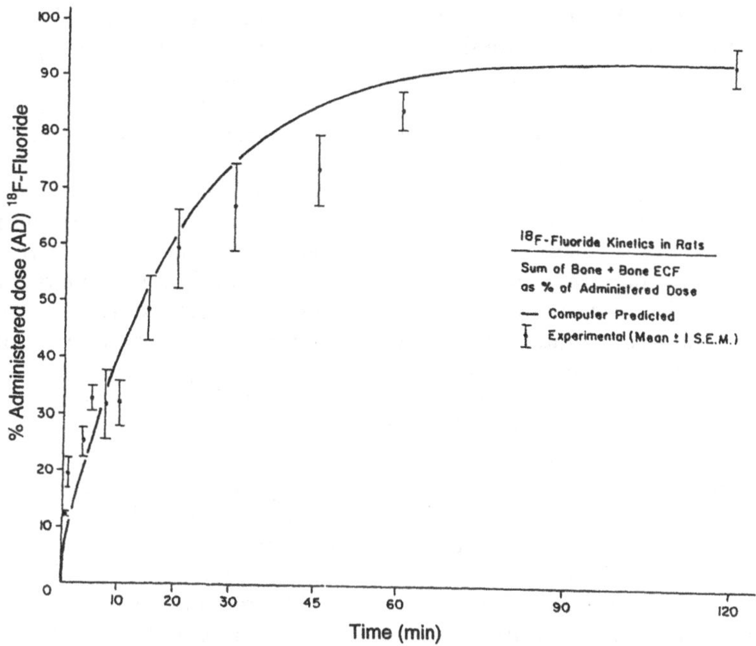

Fig. 18.3. Computer-generated curve of fluoride kinetics for five-compartment model (Fig. 18.2), based on computer-generated rate constants, and observed rat flow data.

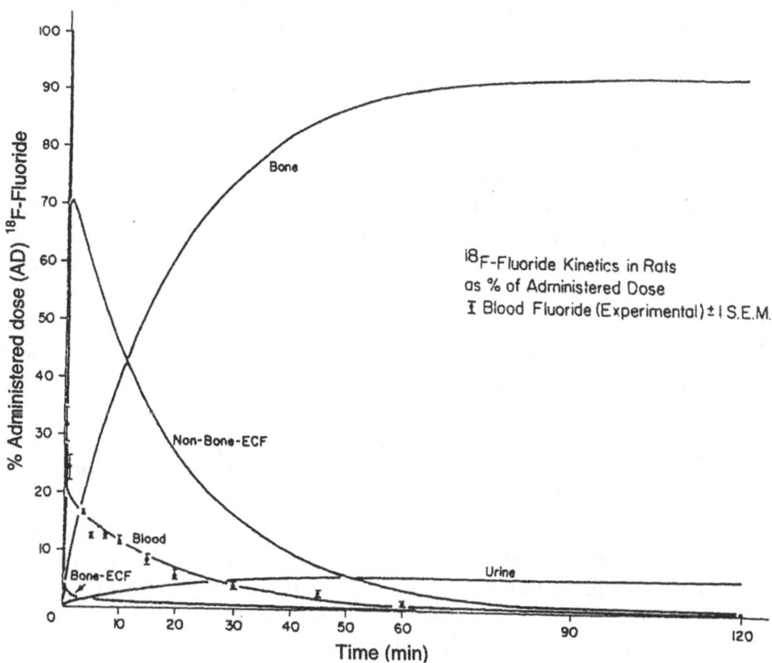

Fig. 18.4. Computer-generated curve of ^{18}F-fluoride kinetics for the sum of "bone ECF" and "bone" compartments of Claude Bernard model derived from blood data only.

(Schiepers 1993). For instance, using positron emission tomography (PET) in combination with a composite three-compartmental model it is now possible to estimate with some confidence ^{18}F input and output functions. By solving the differential equations linking the compartments, regional bone haemodynamic parameters may be determined by non-linear regression. The calculations are again dependent on knowledge of extraction ratio, and the current PET spatial resolution does not permit precise regional differentiation. Ashcroft *et al.* (1992) have also used $^{15}O\text{-}H_2O$ in combination with PET imaging to determine relative skeletal flows, and methods are being developed using magnetic resonance imaging. With modern computer technology it is surely only a matter of time before reliable, and comparatively non-invasive, techniques are routinely available to determine quantitative haemodynamic parameters in the human.

The recent advances in instrumentation and computerization also allow quantification of the standard orthopaedic "technetium bone scan"; dynamic uptake curves can now be plotted during the first few seconds following injection of ^{99}Tc (Deutsch *et al.* 1981). The uptake curves are reminiscent of Stewart–Hamilton dilution curves for cardiac output, and prima facie are susceptible to analogous mathematical treatment. However, while differences in tracer uptake in regions of interest may usefully be compared with uptake in control areas (Nutton *et al.* 1984), the cumulative evidence discussed in earlier sections suggests that the clearance concept/tracer uptake method has consistently been insecure for the quantification of blood flow rates in bone. It remains to be seen to what extent reliable bone blood flow measurements can be derived from these new dynamic images, based on the uptake of radionuclides, which demonstrably have been so troublesome in interpretation and unreliable in the past. The solution would seem to lie in observing the first passage of a single bolus of a subject's own radiochromated red cells through bone. In this way the use of a diffusible radionuclide of very short half-life would be replaced by the deployment of a very small dose of non-diffusible labelled erythrocytes, thus following in the pathway of haemodynamic perfusion of rat bone pioneered by Brookes, some 30 years ago (Brookes 1967b; described in Chapter 17).

By whatever means bone blood flow is measured, the results show large variation. Wootton (1993) examined the results of seven different estimates of skeletal flow rates in the human, concluding that skeletal blood flow is contained within a range of 3.5–9% of the cardiac output. The *mean* skeletal perfusion calculated from these figures was 3.5 ml 100 g^{-1} min^{-1}. This range discounted the much higher value, produced by the Charkes five-compartment analysis, of 16.8% of the cardiac output, although high figures for skeletal flow have also been reported using other methods in animals. Wootton's review produced an average figure, but as these values were obtained from rather different clearance techniques it may be inappropriate to combine them in this way. Each method may have their own intrinsic methodological inconsistencies, some of which have been identified in previous sections of this book, and the numbers produced may therefore be to some extent operationally dependent; to use a simile from psychology, the result obtained may be due to the method chosen for investigation. In spite of this caveat, clearance methods will continue to have a place in *clinical* skeletal haemodynamic studies for the simple reason that investigation does not necessitate tissue destruction to follow the nucleotide flux; the result, however, will likely be an underestimate.

In order to circumvent the problems inherent in bone-seeking isotope clearance methods (including recirculation of non-extracted isotope, and the mobility of extraction ratios depending upon flow rate and transit times), a method is required that utilizes tracers which are fully extracted in a single passage; tracers which enable the different anatomical domains to be identified, including the marrow, and which do not migrate from the soft tissue vascular tree post-mortem. These requirements are met by the use of an alternative form of skeletal tracer deposition; indicator fractionation. This is otherwise known descriptively as the "microsphere" method, or more informatively as arteriolar blockade. This technique has become the "gold standard" of haemodynamic measurement techniques; a technique against which other methods must be compared to claim veracity. Arteriolar blockade is discussed in the next chapter.

Chapter 19

Bone blood flow measurement – 3: Arteriolar blockade

Arteriolar blockade depends upon the fact that appropriately sized particles introduced into the circulation, usually the left ventricle of the heart or the aorta, will be distributed throughout the tissues in proportion to the cardiac output perfusing that tissue. Assuming an appropriate size in relation to afferent arterioles of the capillary beds, it is assumed that total extraction occurs in the first passage. The concept was originally introduced by Saperstein (1958), who suggested ^{42}K as a completely extractable tracer for clinical use. Kane & Grim (1969), however, later applying this technique to bone, found that ^{42}K was not removed in a single passage. In the same study they introduced the use of glass microspheres labelled with ^{24}Na as a quantitative vascular tracer. Glass microspheres are much heavier than erythrocytes, and hence subject to rapid sedimentation in the circulation. Brookes (1970) used ^{59}Fe-labelled cationic exchange resin particles to measure blood flow in rat hind limb bones, using the term arteriolar blockade for this technique. In the same year Lunde & Michelson (1970) introduced the use of labelled Dextran microspheres for measurement of bone blood flow in bone, using a reference artery method (see below) to determine absolute flow rates. Arteriolar blockade allows flow rates to be measured in tissues which are otherwise inaccessible to direct measurement.

The fundamental equation for arteriolar blockade is as follows;

$$F = CO \,.\, (N_t/N_{inj}) \quad (1)$$

where F = flow per unit volume of tissue;
CO = cardiac output;
N_t = number of particles in tissue;
N_{inj} = number of particles injected.

Usually, quantification of the number of particles is simplified by labelling them with an isotope. However, microsphere tracer particles have recently been introduced that are dye-marked, their concentration in tissues being measured spectrophotometrically (Kowallik *et al.* 1991). Coloured microspheres were first used to determine cardiac coronary flow parameters, but they have now been used to determine blood flow in knee ligaments (Bray *et al.* 1996), and it is surely only a matter of time before their use is extended to bone. The tracer conveniently eliminates the use of radioisotopes, which is an important consideration in this "health and safety" conscious age.

In the event that particles are marked isotopically, then N is replaced by counts:

$$F = CO \,.\, (\text{counts}_t/\text{counts}_{inj}) \qquad (2)$$

For many investigations the proportion of the cardiac output perfusing a given tissue is sufficient, and often a constant cardiac output may be inserted to describe the flow in absolute rather than relative terms. Thus Brookes (1987b) has recommended a value of 200 ml kg^{-1} body weight as being an appropriate cardiac output for the rat or other small rodent, which would enable an absolute value to be quickly determined for bone blood flow with little error. Cardiac output may be determined separately, for instance by dye dilution, or by the use of a reference flow, sometimes known as a "surrogate organ". If blood is withdrawn at a known rate from an artery during injection of labelled particles, then the reference flow F_{ref} is given by:

$$F_{ref} = CO \,.\, (\text{counts}_{ref}/\text{counts}_{inj}) \qquad (3)$$

and, in terms of CO:

$$CO = F_{ref} \,.\, (\text{counts}_{inj}/\text{counts}_{ref}) \qquad (4)$$

If this expression for CO is substituted in Equation (2), then:

$$F = F_{ref} \,.\, (\text{counts}_t/\text{counts}_{ref}) \qquad (5)$$

Note that in using this relationship the total number (or radioactive counts) of particles injected need not be known, only the counts in the reference flow and the counts in the tissue. It is usual to express the result as a specific flow; that is the flow rate per unit weight of bone, usually ml 100 g^{-1} min^{-1}.

Important criteria must be met before the results of blood flow measured with arteriolar blockade may be treated with confidence (Heymann *et al.* 1977). These considerations are now well known amongst practitioners of blood flow measurement, being repeated, almost as a mantra, in the introduction to many publications. Tracer particles must be homogeneously mixed, both prior to injection, and subsequently in passage through the circulation, so that all arteries receive the same vascular concentration of indicator. Rheological properties of tracer particles, usually microspheres, should approximate to those of blood, and sufficient numbers injected to ensure statistical confidence (Buckberg *et al.* 1971; Dole *et al.* 1982). However, too many particles injected may interfere with the normal circulatory dynamics of the target organ, and these limits should be ascertained for particular circumstances. Furthermore, as already noted, the tracer particles should be removed in a single pass through the circulation. Apart from the numbers of particles injected, factors which affect homogeneity of tracer distribution include the site of injection, and the presence or absence of significant arterial streaming or "skimming".

Mixing of tracer particles

Many studies have demonstrated adequate mixing of tracer particles in the circulation, both by comparing measured flows to paired contralateral organs such as the kidneys, and by assaying microsphere concentrations from different arteries.

Thus, homogeneity of tracer distribution has been confirmed in circulations of the rabbit (Neutze *et al.* 1968; Warren & Ledingham 1974; Gregg & Walder 1980; Bray *et al.* 1996), the rat (Mendel & Hollenberg 1971; Sasaki & Wagner 1971; Malik *et al.* 1976; Kirkby & Berg-Larsen 1991) and the dog (Morris & Kelly 1980; Moore *et al.* 1981; Jones *et al.* 1982).

Site of injection

In order to achieve adequate tracer mixing in the region of interest, it is necessary to inject particles some distance proximal to that point. It has been advocated that particles should be introduced into the left atrium (Kaihara *et al.* 1968; Buckberg *et al.* 1971; Archie *et al.* 1973), and this was found to be the preferred injection route when determining myocardial blood flow measurements in anaesthetized rats (Wicker & Tarazi 1982a,b). No advantage, however, was found between left atrial and left ventricular injection in myocardial flow determinations in the *conscious* rat (Kobrin *et al.* 1984). The latter observation may relate to statistical difficulties in making the comparison; Neutze *et al.* (1968) found standard deviations of blood flow rates to some regions in conscious animals to approach 50% of the mean, attributing this to the presence of functional autonomic reflexes in the absence of anaesthesia. Left ventricular microsphere injection, however, has been shown to be quite satisfactory for determinations of blood flow to more peripheral structures (Buckberg *et al.* 1971; Sasaki & Wagner 1971; Hales 1974).

Left ventricular injection has the advantage that the chest wall does not need to be opened, catheterization being effected via the carotid artery/aortic system. In fact, for muscles (Laughlin & Armstrong 1982), and for bones of the hind limb (Aalto & Slätis 1984; Gregg & Walder 1980; Triffit & Gregg 1990 (rabbit); Kirkby & Berg-Larsen 1991 (rat)), injection into the aorta has given satisfactory results. Furthermore, Maki *et al.* (1993) reported that microsphere injections into the distal aorta of the rabbit produced no significant differences in calculated hind limb muscle and skin blood flows, from values obtained following simultaneous injection into the left ventricle. The use of a *local* tracer injection is particularly important for flow measurements in peripheral structures with low perfusion rates; in these cases left ventricular injection may result in very few tracer particles entering the tissue. Willans & McCarthy (1991) injected microspheres separately into both femoral arteries of the dog to obtain comparative data on sphere distribution in the tibia, specifically to obtain high tracer representation.

However in small animals such as the rat, left ventricular injection offers the advantage of simple and positive location of the injection catheter, which may be introduced via the right carotid artery. Malik *et al.* (1976) found no significant difference in microsphere concentration in blood samples simultaneously withdrawn from the left carotid and femoral arteries of the rat during left ventricular injection. Similarly Laughlin *et al.* (1982) found equivalent microsphere distributions in simultaneously withdrawn samples from the thoracic and abdominal aorta. Sasaki & Wagner (1971) further confirmed adequacy of mixing in the rat by observing that two different labelled batches of microspheres injected a few minutes apart produced equivalent patterns of distribution; and similar results have been shown for other species (e.g. Kaihara *et al.* 1968 (dogs); Neutze *et al.* 1968; Warren & Ledingham 1974 (rabbits)).

Size and density

The size and density of particles also affect the precision of the method. Whilst these may not significantly affect the measurement of distribution of blood flow to major organs, local measurements within organs require that tracer distribution to the microvasculature is similar to that of circulating erythrocytes (Heymann *et al.* 1977). Commercially available microspheres have a higher density than red blood cells, and therefore sedimentation and streaming phenomena will differ from those obtained from normal erythrocytes. Phibbs & Dong (1970) reported the use of a rapid freezing technique to examine the distribution of different sized microspheres in the rabbit femoral artery. They found no evidence of sedimentation of particles in the size range 7.5–80 μm diameter, but with decreasing size the microsphere distribution within the artery more closely approximated the normal distribution of blood cells. The largest spheres (60–80 μm) were shown to concentrate centripetally, whilst 10 μm microspheres were evenly distributed across the total cross-sectional area of the artery. Axial streaming of large microspheres may result in smaller branching arteries, with proportionately lower flow rates, receiving a disproportionately lower microsphere representation for that flow.

Size may also affect the distribution of particles in another way, unrelated to flow velocity; a phenomenon which Mϕrkrid has termed steric hindrance (Mϕrkrid *et al.* 1976). For instance, Katz *et al.* (1971) found that different flow rates were obtained at different sites in the kidney, depending upon the size of microsphere used. Differential entrapment resulted in 15 μm spheres lodging in the glomeruli, whilst 35 μm spheres were judged unrepresentative, becoming trapped in afferent vessels, sometimes outside of the kidney. Gregg & Walder (1980) showed that 15 μm microspheres distributed equally between the two ends of the rabbit femur and the upper and lower parts of the diaphyseal shaft, whilst 50 μm spheres were found predominantly in the upper metaphysis of the femur and the lower shaft, and with a greater percentage "filtered" out in the marrow. Thus, steric hindrance may be an important determinant of the distribution of larger sized microspheres *within* the various vascular domains of bone, and invalidate the assumption that particle distribution is determined by flow rate.

Size is therefore a matter of great importance. If the tracer is too large, compared with the diameter of the capillary feeder vessels, then the distribution of tracer may only represent the largest afferents. Certainly, it is now recognized that the 50 μm-sized microspheres used by some early investigators are too large for representative labelling. In cortical bone, Haversian vessels vary between 15 and 30 μm in diameter (Brookes 1993), as shown in Fig. 9.24. It is now accepted that medullary arterioles are the most important resistance vessels controlling the flow through bone, and that representative blockade of these arterioles will give the most stringent estimate of blood flow to the tissue. Their size extends from 30 μm down to metarterioles of only 5 μm diameter (Brookes 1993). On these anatomical grounds most advocates of arteriolar blockade now use 15.5 μm microspheres, although Triffit & Gregg (1990) found no significant difference between flow rates in the rabbit tibia measured with spheres of this size, and with those obtained from the use of slightly smaller, 11 μm, microspheres. As these authors point out, the use of a smaller size enables considerable cost benefits! This is an important point which we shall discuss further.

The use of 11 μm microspheres must be reaching the practical minimum effective size. Whilst it is attractive to consider a tracer approaching the dimension of an erythrocyte, it is obvious that such a particle would pass through the capillary exchange beds unhindered, thus removing at a stroke both theoretical assumption and practical convenience of single passage extraction and, of course, ignoring the flexibility of red blood cells which allows them to squeeze through the smallest capillary vessel. The problem of tracer recirculation therefore becomes increasingly significant as size diminishes. The use of microsphere sizes below 10 μm have produced apparent flow rates up to only half those achieved with larger sizes (e.g. Gross *et al.* 1979; Niv & Hungerford 1979) and their use must be questioned. Tothill *et al.* (1987) examined non-entrapment of 15±5 μm microspheres in the dog, following injection into the tibial nutrient artery. The percentage of administered activity found in femoral venous blood (n=10) was 0.86±1.24% (s.d.), again arguing for the general utility of the 15 μm microsphere.

Another question related to particle size results from arteriovenous shunting, but this only really becomes problematical if recirculated particles are not extracted by the pulmonary circulation. Mendel & Hollenberg (1971), using 34 μm microspheres, found that 1% of spheres injected into the left ventricle were found in the lungs, which reduced to 0.04% following introduction into the descending aorta. Sasaki & Wagner (1971) measured 0.4% of 50 μm spheres in the lungs of the rat following injection into the abdominal aorta. When spheres of this size were injected *intravenously* in the rat, Sasaki & Wagner (1971) found that virtually 100% extraction occurred in the lungs with no detectable counts being obtained from the kidneys; they concluded that particle tracers of this size were not subject to pulmonary shunting. However, using 9 μm spheres Fan *et al.* (1979), found pulmonary shunting to reach 3.5% in the dog, compared with less than 1% for 15±1 μm spheres. In a sense, arteriovenous shunting should not be considered as a non-physiological "artefact" of the measuring technique, but rather to be seen as representing a pertinent feature of the system to be characterized. Again, amelioration, if not elimination of the difficulty, lies with the selection of an appropriately sized tracer particle.

Arteriolar blockade: nature of particle tracer

It appears that the assumptions of arteriolar blockade as a method of bone blood flow measurement may be met, and the technique used with some confidence. Many of the problems associated with other types of measurement procedures are eliminated, and the lack of interference with the measurement sites clearly adds utility. Of all the methods of bone blood flow measurement, with the exception perhaps of hydrogen washout, it remains the only technique which can be used to measure blood flow repetitively in the same animal (Kaihara *et al.* 1968; Hoffbrand & Forsyth 1969; Launder *et al.* 1981; Jones *et al.* 1982; Davis *et al.* 1990; McGrory *et al.* 1994). By using different isotope tracers, for instance, this capability enables measurement to be carried out over extended periods of time using in-dwelling catheters, or before and after a surgical procedure. For acute experiments, however, McGrory *et al.* (1994) have drawn attention to the decline in bone blood over the period of an extended anaesthetic; a fact which clearly should be borne in mind when carrying out sequential labelling procedures. Although the technique of arteriolar blockade is well established, the most commonly used tracer particles remain the ubiquitous microspheres. Modern microspheres have a narrow size distribution and are resistant to isotope leaching in physiological fluids. Their specific gravity is still more than that of red blood cells. It is often argued that the properties of commercial microspheres, combined with the theoretical considerations outlined, make their use a *sine qua non*. They are *very* expensive however, and this factor may deter smaller laboratories from undertaking haemodynamic studies. On the other hand, cationic exchange resin particles as introduced by Brookes (1970) are very cheap and easily labelled in the laboratory. The aim at the time was to provide a method of blood flow measurement in bone with the laboratory advantages of simplicity and economy, dispensing with expensive counting equipment (to which the author at that time did not have access), and to enable investigators to engage in bone circulation experiments outside specialized centres. At least in the authors' laboratory, this philosophy still prevails. Resin particles have been used in many studies (Brookes 1970; Singh & Brookes 1971; Brookes & Gallanaugh 1975; Tothill & McCormick 1976; Brueton *et al.* 1993; Revell & Brookes 1993a,b, 1994), often and ideally in situations where isotope activities in a limb, following a surgical procedure, are compared with the contralateral unoperated limb. Whilst microspheres undoubtably possess aesthetic attractions, we would argue that in practice simpler, cheaper products may still offer great utility for providing useful and valid haemodynamic measurements.

The authors recently had the opportunity to compare blood flow rates in whole bones and bone segments measured with ^{59}Fe-labelled cationic exchange resin, and commercial microspheres labelled with ^{85}Sr (Revell & Brookes 1993a,b). In order to facilitate evaluation of previous reports of investigations utilizing resin particles, the exchange resin used was from the *same original batch, and prepared in the same way*, as previously used by Brookes and his associates. Because this investigation enables a practical discussion of many of the points mentioned in the introductory review, space has been devoted to this study and it is hoped that the details given here will be useful to the novice investigator.

Resin particles versus microspheres: a practical digression

Common laboratory exchange resin particles (Amberlite CG120; BDH Ltd, UK) were prepared according to the method of Brookes (1970) by a process of "differential sedimentation" in a cylinder of water, and labelled with ^{59}Fe-ferric chloride. Finally, they were suspended in 5 ml of distilled water to which 0.1% of Tween 80 was added. Injections of 0.5 ml of this suspension were made into each rat. The resulting resin particles are shown as seen by the polarizing microscope in Fig. 19.1 (*overleaf*). The particles are irregular in shape; the size distribution was 32.28±15.15 μm, measured along the long axis (Fig. 19.2, *overleaf*). The dry weight of particles in the total injectate (5 ml) was approximately 14 mg, and as 0.5 ml of this suspension was injected into each rat, it follows that each animal received approximately 1.4 mg of particles. The number of particles in the

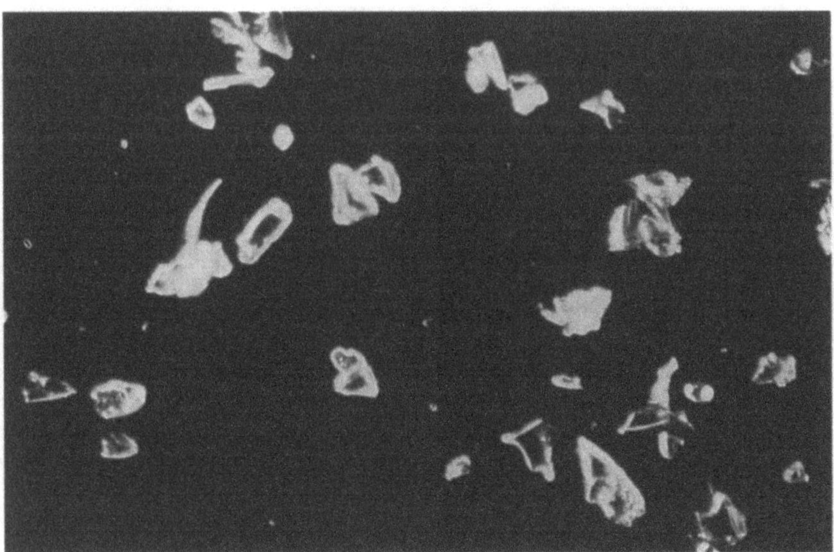

Fig. 19.1. (*See also Colour Plate section*) Polarized light view of prepared resin particles. The mean length along the long axis is 32.28 μm.

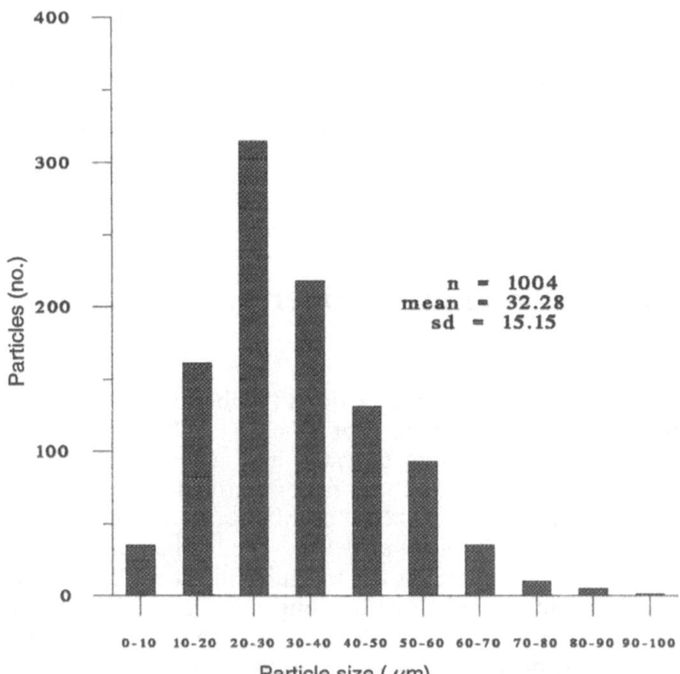

Fig. 19.2. Resin particle size distribution.

prepared suspension, measured on a Coulter analyser, was around 800 000 particles ml^{-1}, in the size range 10–70 μm; each rat therefore received in the order of 400 000 particles per injection.

^{85}Sr microspheres

These were NENTRAC (Dupont) microspheres, 15.5±0.1 μm in size, resin coated after ^{85}Sr labelling, to minimize isotope leaching. They were suspended in 0.9% mammalian saline to which 0.01% Tween 80 was added to minimize aggregation. Two batches were used to determine blood flow; 1 mg per rat, and 3 mg per rat, equivalent to 350 000 and 1050 000 microspheres per animal respectively; suspended in 0.5 ml saline/Tween 80 for each injection. A plot was made of the specific activity per sphere, in order to estimate the number of microspheres residing in tissue samples.

Blood flow measurement

Eleven-week-old male Wistar rats (weight 270±18 g) were used, 10 in each group. Anaesthesia was by intramuscular Hypnorm, followed by an intraperitoneal injection of diazepam. In the original method (Brookes 1970), resin particles were injected into the right carotid artery, towards the heart. In fact, this method results in a large proportion of particles being swept into the right humerus, therefore drastically reducing the numbers available for labelling the vascular beds of the hind limb. Tracer particles were therefore introduced directly into the left ventricle.

The left and right carotid arteries were exposed by sectioning the overlying sternomastoid and omohyoid muscles. A flexible nylon catheter was introduced into the right carotid (Fig. 19.3, *overleaf*). The catheter was connected via a three-way tap to a transducer, which enabled intra-arterial pressure changes to be monitored. The catheter was advanced until the tip was positioned in the left ventricle, the location being unequivocally identified by the characteristic change in pressure waveform on entering the heart. A further catheter was placed in the left carotid artery and connected to a pump, calibrated to withdraw a reference flow sample at a rate of 1 ml min^{-1}. Particle suspensions were ultrasonicated at 40°C for 30 minutes and then agitated on a vortex mixer just before injection. The withdrawal pump was started and allowed to run for 10 seconds, at which point blood was seen to enter the syringe. Injection of particles was then made over a 20-second period, followed by a 0.5 ml saline flush, again taking 20 seconds. Withdrawal continued for a further 10 seconds. The total withdrawal period therefore was 1 minute, during which 1 ml of blood was taken, and a total of 1 ml of particles/saline suspension injected. The animal was then killed by an injection of barbiturate through the intracardiac catheter. Tibiae and femora were removed from both limbs, weighed, stripped of soft tissues, and placed separately in scintillation counting vials. The activity of the contained ^{59}Fe or ^{85}Sr in reference blood samples and bones were measured on an automatic scintillation counter. After subtracting the background count, and correcting for height in the tube (Heyman *et al.* 1977), the measured activities were used to calculate the absolute flow rate through the bone specimens. The distal femoral epiphysis and meta-

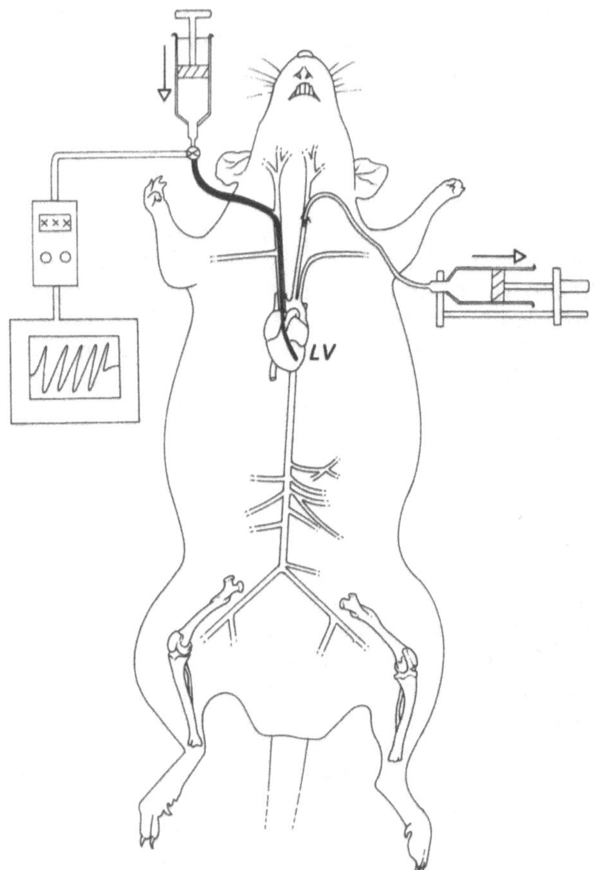

Fig. 19.3. Experimental arrangement for bone blood flow measurement using arteriolar blockade.

physis and the proximal tibial epiphysis and metaphysis were then separated from each of the paired bones. A segment of diaphysis was also isolated; the marrow was extruded using a blunt probe and the cortical bone cleaned with a pressurized water jet. All samples were weighed, and their activities counted.

One of the assumptions of the method is that tracer particles in a sample drawn from the reference artery is representative of tracer delivery to the region of interest. In a further series of rats, simultaneous withdrawals were made at a rate of 1 ml min^{-1}, from the left carotid and femoral arteries, following injection of ^{85}Sr microspheres into the left ventricle. The activities in the two arterial samples were compared.

Blood flow determinations

Blood flow values were calculated for the following three categories of tracer:

1. ^{59}Fe-labelled cationic exchange resin (1.4 mg/400 000 particles per rat).

2. ^{85}Sr-labelled microspheres (1 mg/350 000 spheres per rat).
3. ^{85}Sr-labelled microspheres (3 mg/1050 000 spheres per rat).

As there were no significant differences between left and right samples of whole bones or regions of bone, these values were combined to compare whole bone and segment flow rates in each group. The results of these comparisons are shown in Fig. 19.4 for the femur and Fig. 19.5 (*overleaf*) for the tibia (note that the error bars show standard deviations to emphasize the considerable range of values found within each group). There was no significant difference between blood flows of whole femora and tibiae measured with resin particles and microspheres (1 mg rat^{-1}), or between measured blood flows using 3 mg and 1 mg microspheres per rat.

When segment results obtained from the use of resin particles were compared with those from the 1 mg dose of microspheres, no significant difference was found between the metaphyses and epiphyses of femur or tibia. In both femoral and tibial marrow, however, the flow measured with resin particles was reduced

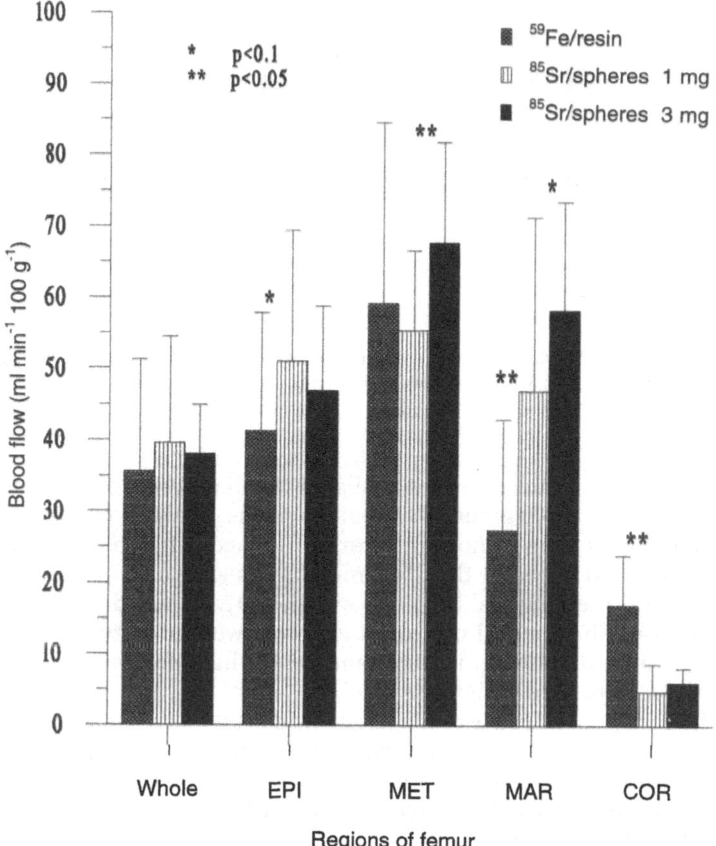

Fig. 19.4. Blood flows to whole femora and femoral segments; summary of data from all groups. EPI, Epiphysis; MET, metaphysis; MAR, marrow; COR, cortex.

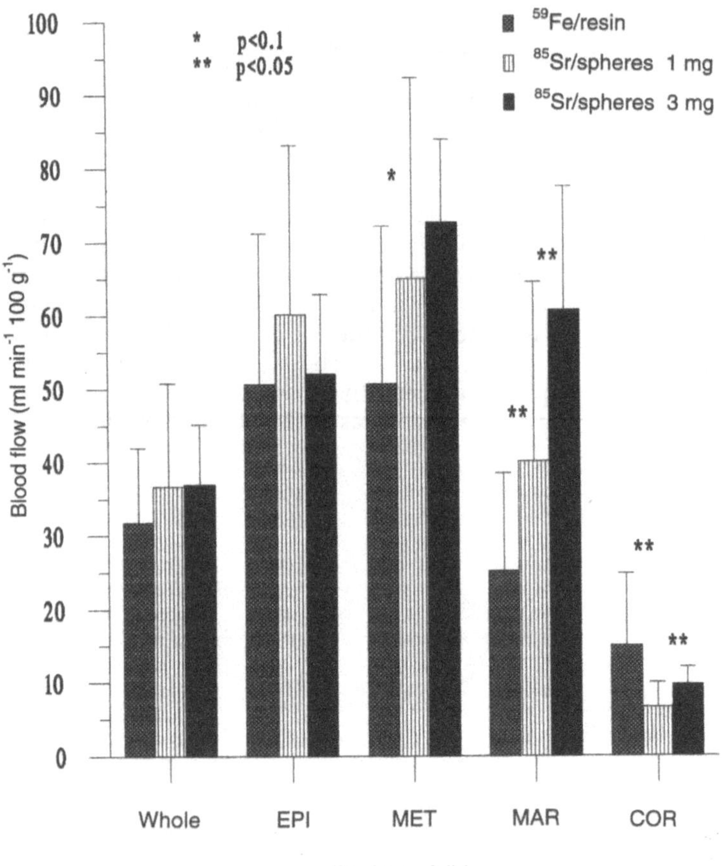

Fig. 19.5. Blood flows to whole tibia and tibial segments; summary of data from all groups. EPI, Epiphysis; MET, metaphysis; MAR, marrow; COR, cortex.

compared with 1 mg microspheres, whilst in the diaphyseal cortices the flow was significantly elevated. Segment flow comparisons between the 1 mg and 3 mg microsphere doses showed no significant difference between epiphyseal flows in femur or tibia, and flows for the tibial metaphysis were also not significantly different. Femoral metaphyseal flow was significantly elevated using 3 mg microspheres per rat. The femoral marrow and cortex were not significantly different. In the tibia, both diaphyseal marrow and cortex had elevated flows in the 3 mg dose animals, compared with those receiving only 1 mg.

In order to validate the use of the left carotid artery as a reference sampling site for calculating blood flow in the lower limb, simultaneous and identical blood reference samples were taken from the femoral and carotid arteries of ten rats. After injection of ^{85}Sr-labelled microspheres, counts obtained from the two sites were compared (Table 19.1).

A scatter diagram is shown in Fig. 19.6, with a simple regression line fitted. Pearson's correlation coefficient for the two data sets was 0.91.

Table 19.1 Simultaneous femoral and carotid counts following intracardiac injection of ^{85}Sr microspheres

	Femoral	Carotid
Mean counts	24 045	24 622
Standard deviation	4 342	3 600

t test (matched pairs): $P = 0.35$.

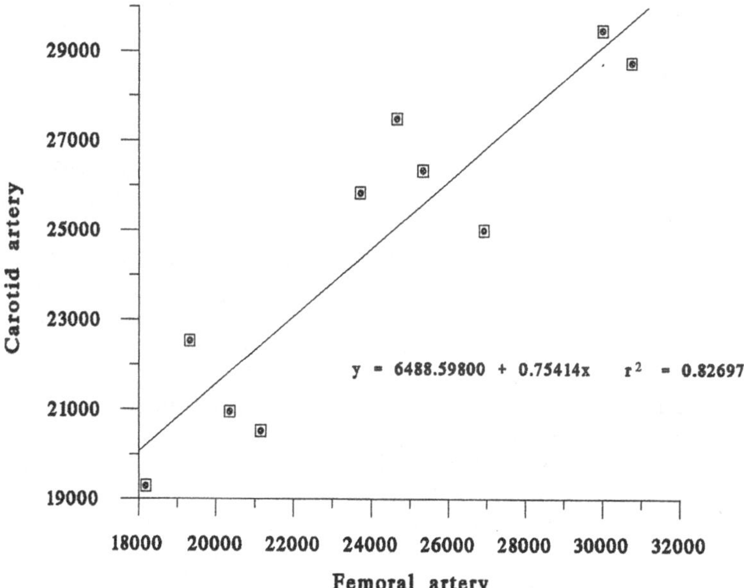

Fig. 19.6. Radioactivity, counts per minute, recorded from simultaneous carotid and femoral reference samples.

Estimates of the number of microspheres in various bone samples are shown in Table 19.2 (*overleaf*). A substantial elevation of sphere numbers was obtained using 3 mg batches (>1 000 000 spheres) injected into each animal.

Discussion and conclusions

The rat is widely used in experimental biological research; its cheapness and small size enable large numbers to be used, thus facilitating statistical validity; furthermore, the radioactivity of whole organs or component parts can conveniently be counted, to obtain estimates of regional blood flow. Arteriolar blockade, combined with reference artery sampling in order to determine absolute organ perfusion rates, has been extensively utilized for soft tissue measurement (Malik *et al.* 1976). Surprisingly, however, comparatively few haemodynamic investigations of rat bones have been performed. The results of this study, like

Table 19.2 Comparisons between microsphere numbers found in whole bones and segments, using 1 mg and 3 mg doses.

	Microsphere numbers			
	1 mg dose	s.d.	3 mg dose	s.d
Whole femur	254	98	1382	429
Femoral epiphyses	86	41	332	118
Femoral metaphyses	95	64	413	140
Femoral marrow	20	10	157	72
Femoral cortex	7	6	50	18
Whole tibia	223	143	1200	337
Tibial epiphyses	51	24	216	60
Tibial metaphyses	102	71	514	195
Tibial marrow	12	8	129	53
Tibial cortex	8	4	73	24

those of Brookes (1967a,b, 1970), Gross *et al.* (1979), Okubo *et al.* (1979), Charkes *et al.* (1979a,b) and Kirkby & Berg-Larsen (1991), produced high values for regional blood flow, which may be related to the high red marrow content found in young rats. Red marrow is associated with the richest vascularity and high blood flow rates. Schoutens *et al.* (1979) determined plasma flows in rat femora and tibiae, which, adjusted to whole blood flow rates, are about 20 ml min^{-1} 100 g^{-1} for the femur, and 19 ml min^{-1} 100 g^{-1} for the tibia. Interestingly, Schouten's group reported that roughly equivalent numbers of microspheres were found in epiphyses and metaphyses of the rat after intraventricular injection (Schoutens *et al.* 1979), also supporting the findings here of high flows in cancellous bone. Tothill & McPherson (1986) determined a value of 4.46% of cardiac output going to the whole skeleton in the rat, with 0.57% of cardiac output perfusing the combined contralateral femora and tibiae. This suggests a much lower specific flow rate than measured here. These authors, however, boiled the carcass to aid cleaning of the bones, and it is known that up to half the microsphere radioactivity may be lost as a result of this somewhat harsh treatment (Wootton 1988); a further practical point to keep in mind.

Anaesthesia An important factor that can influence the absolute determined flow rate through bone, and one which is often not considered, is the effect of anaesthesia. Blood flow rates, range and standard deviation are generally elevated in conscious animals, compared with anaesthetized animals (Neutze et al. 1968; Gross et al. 1979; Jones et al. 1982; Davis et al. 1990; McGrory et al. 1994). Bone blood flow rate may decline substantially over long periods. For instance, Davis et al. (1990) reported a 24% mean fall in rabbit skeletal blood flow rate following 1 hour of anaesthesia; this compares with a mean fall of only 7% over a 4-hour period in the conscious rabbit. The decline in blood flow may occur in conditions of respiratory and cardiovascular haemostasis. Pharmacologically, the use of neuroleptic analgesics (e.g. fluanisone, droperiodol) are expected to show less effects on the cardiovascular system than the usual pentobarbitone or halothane agents; the latter anaesthetics can result in significant respiratory and cardiac depression. The current study used hypnorm in combination with droperidol to give some muscle relaxation; the anaesthetic therefore, although effective for pain relief must be considered light when compared, for instance, with the use of a pentobarbitone infusion. The authors have not used arteriolar blockade to

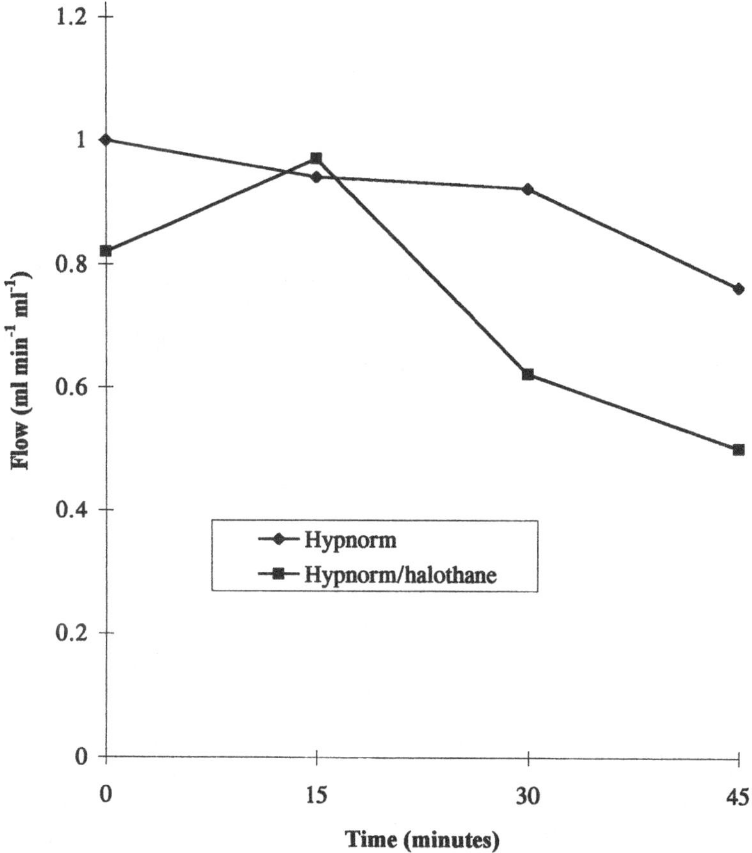

Fig. 19.7. Flow rate recorded from the femoral marrow cavity of a rabbit by hydrogen washout, showing changes in blood flow rate over a 45-minute anaesthetic period. Comparison between the use of hypnorm alone, and hypnorm induction followed by halothane maintenance. Fast components only are shown.

compare blood flows measured with different types of anaesthetic, but femoral medullary flows in the rabbit have been measured following hypnorm induction and maintenance, and compared with hypnorm induction followed by maintenance with halothane (Fig. 19.7). Even from this single experiment (W.J. Revell, unpublished data), the comparative blood flow depression produced by addition of halothane is apparent.

Homogeneity of microspheres Another factor influencing absolute flow values using microspheres, is the assumption of homogeneity of sphere concentration throughout the arterial system. In this study the left carotid artery was used as a reference. The catheter was only inserted about 4–5 mm, and no attempt was made to enter the aorta; the reference sample was therefore collected in its normal flow direction. To determine that the reference activity was representative of blood perfusing the lower limb bones, tracer activity from the left carotid reference sample was compared with an identical and simultaneous sample withdrawn from the femoral artery. The results (Fig. 19.6) show a high correlation (r=0.91) and a matched paired t-test showed the two data sets were not significantly different. Malik et al. (1976) also found close agreement between left carotid and femoral artery reference samples. The technique described here therefore appears to be adequate, thus removing the need to utilize more awkward reference sources such as the brachial or renal arteries. Schoutens et al. (1979) used the tail artery of the rat to collect a reference flow sample, but in the authors' experience, this is by no means a simple procedure.

Variability of measured blood flows The above discussion emphasizes the variability of skeletal blood flow measurement obtained from different laboratories, even when using similar methods and materials. Just as striking is the dispersal of flow values obtained within any particular experiment (McGrory et al. 1994). The coefficient of variance for whole femoral and tibial blood flows using 3 mg microspheres per rat was 18% and 23% respectively; and for the 1 mg microsphere dose the figures were 37% and 38% respectively. The coefficient of variance for whole bone flow, using resin particles, was 44% for the femur and 32% for the tibia.

If the statistical distribution of microspheres in the bone follows Poisson's law, then the expected variance is approximated by the reciprocal of the square root of the number found in any particular bone sample (Dole *et al.* 1982). If there are sufficient numbers of spheres in the reference sample, then the variance in flow measurement should be similar to variance in sphere numbers. The mean number of spheres found in the reference arterial sample was 4600 in the 3 mg dose animals, and 1200 in the rats receiving 1 mg spheres. However, the disparity between these two variances does not vary linearly with the number of spheres found in the reference sample. Dole *et al.* (1982) calculated that for a tissue sample containing 400 spheres, increasing reference sample sphere numbers from 400 to 2000 will decrease relative flow error from 13.9% to 10.7%. An increase in reference sphere number to 10 000 only reduces the relative flow error to 10%. From Table 19.2 it can be calculated that the expected variances in whole bones, *from microsphere numbers*, are 6.2% and 6.7% for femur and tibia respectively in the 1 mg dose category, and 3% for femur and tibia when 3 mg of spheres were injected. These figures suggest that measured variance in blood flow rate far exceeds the expected variance from the numbers of resident spheres, and it is suggested that flow variation may be a reflection of a real dissimilarity, either in a given instance in time in an individual animal, or in different animals in the population.

Microsphere numbers in situ Another consideration gained upon inspection of Table 19.2, is the very low numbers of microspheres found, particularly in the low dose animals. It has been calculated that 400 is the minimum number of spheres required in a tissue sample to give 10% precision at the 95% confidence level (Buckberg et al. 1971), although 100–200 have given acceptable results in low flow rate situations in canine tendon and ligament (Riggi et al. 1990). Other authors, working with low flow rate tissues, have challenged the "Buckberg" number, claiming lower error rates associated with low absolute particle numbers. Li et al. (1989) calculated a relative error of 4.7% for a sample containing 250 microspheres, and where fewer than 50 microspheres were present they suggested an error of only around 14%. Ensuring a minimum 400 particles is not difficult in larger animals. In the rat, tissue size, particularly of bone segments, is a limitation. This study used a maximum dose rate of 3.9×10^6 microspheres per kilogram rat weight and 1.3×10^6 kg^{-1}, for animals receiving 1 mg spheres. The number of ^{59}Fe-labelled resin particles injected per kg rat weight (1.48×10^6) was similar to the 1 mg microsphere dose. Only whole bones and the metaphyses of rats receiving 3 mg microspheres exceeded the statistical minimum requirement of 400 spheres. For animals receiving 1 mg of microspheres, and similarly for the resin particles, the numbers recorded were woefully small, especially in the marrow and cortical samples. The marrow sample it should be noted has a very low weight (0. 05 g is typical), while the cortical sample has a greater mass but a comparatively low flow rate. Kirkby & Berg-Larsen (1991) used a microsphere dose rate of 5.26×10^6 kg^{-1} rat weight, obtaining a minimum tissue number of 200, found in the proximal tibial epiphysis. The diaphysis was not separated into cortical and marrow components and therefore it is not possible to estimate numbers found in these segments, but by extrapolation it is likely that the numbers in the cortex remained small. It is clear that large numbers of particles need to be infused to achieve acceptable confidence levels, and it is equally clear that many studies fall short of the theoretical ideal. The rat, fortunately, is known to tolerate intraventricular catheterization well, and large injections of microspheres are permissible without haemodynamic perturbation (Flaim et al. 1978; Stanek et al. 1983; Kirkby & Berg-Larsen 1991). In this study, detailed physiological parameters were not monitored, but intracardiac pulse amplitude and frequency did not change as a result of injections containing up to 1 050 000 microspheres.

The great variation between individual flow rates makes it desirable to use large numbers of animals to determine the mean flow rate within a population, and with a reasonable confidence interval. This favours the rat as an experimental animal. It is also apparent that investigation of regional bone blood flow requires the injection of large numbers of particulate iontophors, whether resin or spheres, to obtain statistical confidence. The results of the comparison made here between flow values obtained using labelled resin particles and microspheres, are of great practical importance in spreading bone blood flow measurement to non-specialized laboratories. In the whole femur and tibia, and the epiphyses and metaphyses, no statistical difference was found in flow rates measured by the injection of ^{59}Fe-labelled resin particles or an equivalent dose of microspheres.

Only in the cortex and bone marrow were significantly different flow values obtained from the two materials (Figs 19.4, 19.5). Cortical flow was elevated when measured by resin particles, while marrow flows were reduced; both in comparison with microsphere results. This may be related to plasma leaching of some ^{85}Sr from the particle preparation; microspheres, of course, are resin coated by the manufacturers after labelling to prevent isotope leaching. It has been suggested that plasma transferrin has a higher affinity for iron than exchange resin (observation attributed to Dr Veall in Tothill & McCormick 1976), and higher than background levels of ^{85}Sr activity were found in venous blood which was not attributable to particle recirculation. Femoral vein samples from animals injected with resin particles labelled with ^{59}Fe in the presence of *unlabelled* iron, showed no significant activity above background; leaching was thereby effectively eliminated, presumably as a result of competitive binding. Plasma leaching of ^{59}Fe from the resin would have the effect of reducing the counts in areas of moderate flow, but giving more counts in regions of low flow, such as the cortex; in effect, an element of bone blood volume is included in the calculated flow value. The resin used in the comparative study was not treated with unlabelled iron, as it was intended to evaluate published results, where this treatment was not performed. However, the effect of isotope leaching seems statistically insignificant in most cases, given the very large intrinsic standard deviations, and in any case is easily prevented.

Because of the large coefficient of variance found within any single population, comparisons of absolute blood flow between different populations demand large numbers to obtain an acceptable confidence interval for the population means. It must be emphasized, however, that irrespective of the absolute flow rates measured, comparisons between left and right limbs in all animals examined in this investigation were never significantly different. This is remarkable when one examines the very low numbers of microspheres found in bones injected with 350 000 (1 mg) microsphere batches, and must indicate an extremely homogeneous dispersal of the available particles in the perfused arteries. From the findings presented here, therefore, it is suggested that the best strategy for determining haemodynamic effects of orthopaedic procedures is always to compare the operated limb with its contralateral control. If left/right comparisons are taken as an index of haemodynamic change over time, it obviously becomes unnecessary to determine absolute flow rates; counts per unit weight of bone are sufficient for useful comparison. Also, by always incorporating a within-animal control bone the problem of anaesthetic changes associated with absolute flow determinations is obviated.

In view of the considerable theoretical and aesthetic advantages of the microsphere product, it is perhaps remarkable that the use of inexpensive resin particles generates equivalent data, with a not dissimilar variance of results. If care is taken to produce an appropriate particle size distribution; injection is made into the left ventricle to ensure adequate mixing, a sufficiently large dose is infused, and procedures adopted to prevent leaching of the isotope label to plasma, then the results of using cationic exchange resin particles as a tracer in bone blood flow measurement by arteriolar blockade appear to be, in practice, indistinguishable from those produced by the use of microspheres.

Using just such resin particles, Brookes (1970) calculated a mean perfusion rate to mixed skeletal tissue of about 20 ml 100 g^{-1} min^{-1}. This perfusion rate compares with values of 19 ml 100 g^{-1} min^{-1} in the rat and 12 ml 100 g^{-1} min^{-1} in man using ^{18}F uptake with a five-compartment model (Charkes *et al.* 1979b), 20 ml 100 g^{-1} min^{-1} in the rat using chromium-labelled red blood cell dilution (Brookes 1967b; described in Chapter 14) and 18 ml 100 g^{-1} min^{-1} in the dog, also by arteriolar blockade (Bove *et al.* 1977). The proportion of the cardiac output distributed to the entire skeleton formerly calculated (Tothill & McCormick 1976; Brookes 1971) in the range 3–27% is now held to be of the order of 10% in the conscious rat and 17% in resting man by ^{18}F uptake (Charkes *et al.* 1979b); 11% in the unconscious dog (Gross *et al.* 1979b) by arteriolar blockade, and 19% in the monkey (Forsyth & Hoffbrand 1970).

Regional flow differences in long bones, first measured by Brookes (Brookes 1967b, 1970), have been repeatedly confirmed by means of arteriolar blockade (e.g. Gross *et al.* 1979b; Okubo *et al.* 1979; Schnitzer *et al.* 1982; Jones *et al.* 1982; Gregg & Walder 1980; Tøndevold 1983; Revell & Brookes 1993a,b). The rates vary *inter alia* with age, exercise, vasoactive drugs, growth status, presence or absence of medullary haemopoiesis, and direct and reflex neural stimuli. Flows to the different gross regional subdivisions can be clearly associated with functional or metabolic differences. Whiteside *et al.* (1977b) used hydrogen washout to show increased flow rates to regions of elevated osteoblastic activity, supporting the proposition that flow rates are proportional to bone deposition rates (Sim & Kelly 1970; Lavendar *et al.* 1979; Schnitzer 1982; Reeve *et al.* 1988). Osteoclastic activity has also been associated with increased perfusion rates (Sim & Kelly 1970). Willans & McCarthy (1991) have further pointed out that considerable heterogeneity of flow occurs between small segments of anatomically similar domains within the cortex of the tibial shaft of the rabbit. Their data also showed that regionally matched right and left bone samples were similar, suggesting that the heterogeneity of flow distribution along each paired shaft was genuine, probably resulting from localized differences of metabolism. Harris *et al.* (1968) also reported spatial and temporal variations in cortical bone formation, and it may be that the large scale differences between anatomically distinct regions of bone are also reflected in flow heterogeneity within the microenvironment of single-bone domains. These results suggest a remarkably "finely-tuned" autoregulatory flow control mechanism in the skeleton.

Chapter 20
Disturbed osseous circulation – 1: Arterial ischaemia

The disturbed osseous circulation, particularly those events leading to ischaemia, is a matter of concern for orthopaedic surgeons. In the natural world, a fractured bone for instance will heal, if not always in optimal alignment, and delayed or non-union is uncommon. On the other hand, the interventions of the orthopaedic practitioner, with his or her armoury of plates and nails, sometimes seem designed to obstruct the passage of blood to the bone, and in just those circumstances when a proper perfusion is most required. That bones thrive in spite of the application of metal, cement and plastic is testimony to the versatility of the circulatory arrangements in bone. It is difficult, in fact, to keep blood out of a bone, although the application, for instance of an intramedullary nail *in combination* with an external plate may present a severe challenge.

Fracture repair

Ischaemia in a bone may arise from blocking the nutrient artery, or by injuring the marrow cavity, thus removing an important normal afferent supply. Brueton and his colleagues (Brueton & Brookes 1995; Brueton *et al.* 1996; Brueton *et al.* 1993b) have shown that intramedullary reaming of the intact rabbit tibia destroys the marrow circulation completely, although this is partially restored by the end of the first week. Vascular regeneration is accompanied by a pronounced deposit of external callus, supplied by the recruitment of periosteal blood vessels. In the presence of a simulated intramedullary nail, a polyethylene tube blocking most of the medullary cavity, marrow revascularization can be delayed until the second week; the inner cortex is rendered ischaemic during this period. However, a similar florid periosteal vascular response occurs in combination with formation of a substantial external callus. Intramedullary nailing does allow the regeneration of medullary vessels between the diaphyseal endosteum and the nail. In the experimental situation described, the periosteal circulation was spared, thus allowing the cortex to be revitalized. If the shaft is filled with bone cement for instance, then the preservation of the periosteum must be a paramount consideration.

In young and senescent bones the periosteum is an important reserve source of supply to the cortex, and always a route of venous escape for the cortical blood flow. It follows that obstruction of the surface with an orthopaedic plate might also disturb the underlying osseous circulation. Revell and colleagues (Revell *et al.* 1991; Brookes 1993) examined the effects of applying flexible nylon plates to the surface of the intact rabbit femur. By 4 weeks a marked hypervascularity affected the inner two-thirds of cortex beneath the plate, accompanied by the appearance of erosion cavities. Removal of bone from the periosteal cortex was much in evidence, resulting in thinning of the cortex in association with endosteal buttressing deep to the plate. These changes continued unabated for the 12 weeks of the observation period. The consequences of plate application, in circumstances where so-called stress protection cannot apply, are to produce a profound ischaemia in the related cortex with much cell death, followed by a sustained vascular congestion. Removal of dead bone at the periosteum and elsewhere in the cortex leads to a general osteoporosis of the bone. Less obviously then, prevention of venous drainage is also a factor in the production of acute bone ischaemia.

These brief comments are meant to draw attention to the importance of vascular and haemodynamic considerations in orthopaedic practice. Here, the experimental basis for our understanding of the effects of arterial ischaemia is discussed.

Arterial ischaemia

It is well known that experimental ligation of the main arteries of a limb produces only slight evanescent changes in the associated skeleton (Pearse 1928; Benassi 1931). To overcome the potentiality of bones for establishing collateral circulations, and thereby lessen the consequences of reducing their arterial supply, arteries must be obstructed close to, or even in the bone, before ischaemic changes become manifest.

The nutrient artery

Experimental ligation of the nutrient artery of the femur or tibia, principally in rabbits and dogs, has been investigated by several workers (Huggins & Wiege 1939; Bragdon *et al.* 1949; de Marneffe 1951; Brookes 1960b). Their results indicate that in the cortex and marrow of the diaphysis, an ischaemia results which is manifested by the following changes. Haemopoiesis ceases in erythroid marrow, which for a time reverts to a primary marrow type. At first, perfused preparations show that much of the marrow is hyperaemic in the sense that the vessels are abnormally dilated (Fig. 20.1, *overleaf*). Also conspicuous are patches of infarcted marrow whose vessels do not fill with perfusate. These necrotic regions, showing marked sinusoid collapse and loss of staining of the interstitial cells, do not involve the entire cross-sectional profile of the marrow cavity. Some viable marrow, especially in the endosteal zone, always survives the lesion. Thereafter a reactive phase sets in, characterized by the presence of widely dilated vessels and abundant active cellular elements scattered diffusely through the affected areas (Fig. 20.2, *overleaf*). Myelocytes, fibroblasts and multinucleate giant cells are conspicuous in the cellular reaction of marrow to ischaemia, but fibrosis does not go beyond

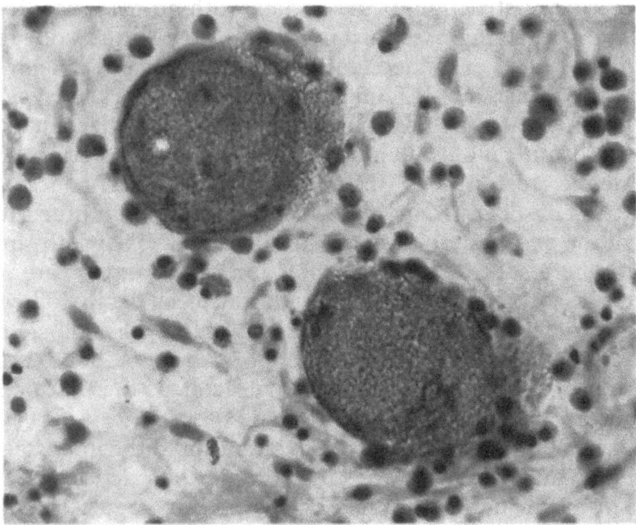

Fig. 20.1. Dilated blood vessels (perfused with Micropaque) in bone marrow 2 weeks after ligation of the principal nutrient artery. (Original magnification ×430)

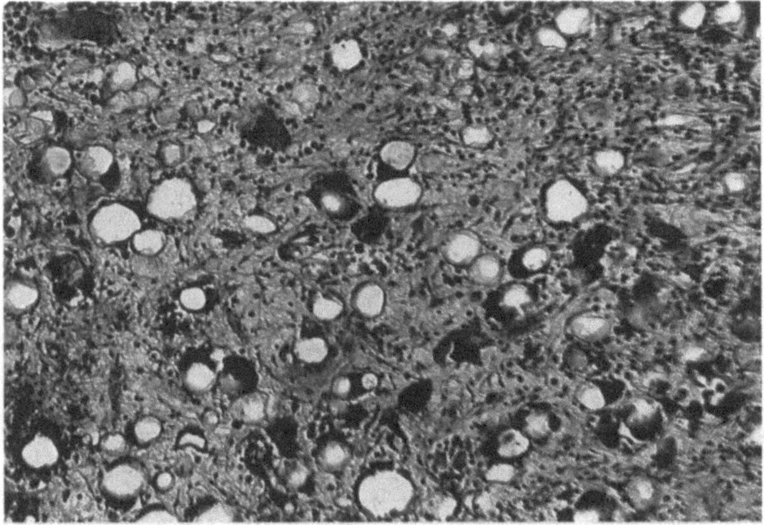

Fig. 20.2. Myelofibrosis after nutrient artery ligation in the rabbit. Haemopoietic tissue has been replaced by fibroblasts, plasma cells and eosinophils. (Original magnification ×110)

the laying down of a loose feltwork of collagen. This phase is followed by one of repair wherein abnormal cells and interstitial fibrous tissue disappear, the sinusoid bed is restored and normal haemopoiesis is resumed.

The cortex of the bone after nutrient artery ligation shows at an early stage an abnormal diminution in radiopacity (Fig. 20.3). This may progress slowly for several months and is not necessarily reversible. Perfused preparations also show

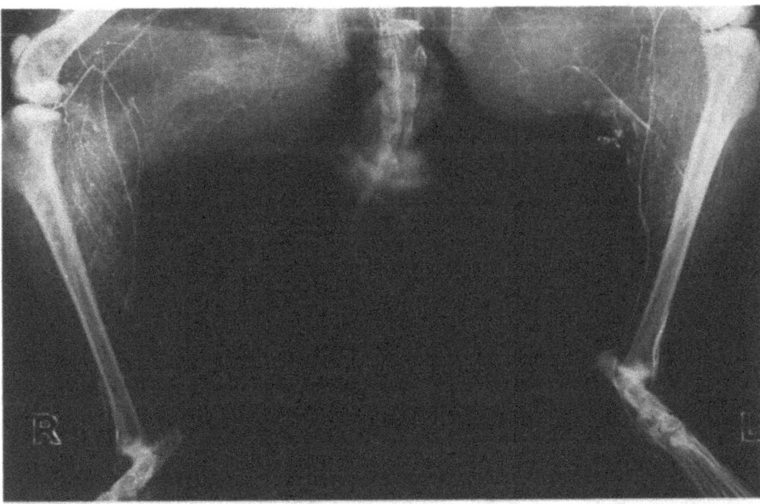

Fig. 20.3. X-ray of the posterior limbs of a rabbit 5 months after nutrient artery ligation on the right side (R). Note the arterial channels which have opened up on the operated side, and the increased radiotranslucency of the bones. (Original magnification ×0.35)

a drastic change in the pattern of vascularization. In the initial acute phase of the experiment, the same centrifugal pattern of arterialization of the cortex is found as in normal material. Thereafter a definite periosteal arterial supply to the cortex of the ischaemic bone can be shown by microradiographic methods (Figs 20.4, 20.5). At first, periosteal arterial pathways into the cortex are fine in calibre and penetrate only its outer half. As repair of the circulation proceeds, however, large anastomoses may form between periosteal and medullary arteries (Figs 9.5, 9.6), while other centripetal arteries may pass right through the cortex and open directly into clumps of medullary sinusoids. While the periosteal arterial supply to cortex and marrow develops, the ischaemic bone also shows enlargement of the metaphyseal arteries, and anastomoses between the medullary branches of these vessels and the terminals of the nutrient artery become conspicuous (Figs 2.24, 2.25). Hence, although the nutrient artery normally supplies both the diaphyseal cortex and the marrow of a long bone, periosteal and metaphyseal arteries form a considerable collateral blood supply which can take over the function of the nutrient vessel.

Furthermore, although a profound ischaemia may be produced in the marrow by ligation of the nutrient artery, it by no means follows that the cortex is thereby rendered ischaemic. On the contrary, in the course of the vascular reaction to medullary ischaemia, many new arterial channels are developed in bone cortex (Figs 9.6, 20.5). This suggests that in these circumstances an abnormally large amount of arterial blood may pass through the cortex of bone from the periosteum, tending to restore thereby the arterial input to the marrow which had been deprived of its normal nutrient supply. It must be emphasized, however, that a periosteal centripetal supply to cortex is an abnormal occurrence before 35 years of age, involving a considerable disturbance to and rearrangement of the circulatory conditions within the osseous circulation. This disturbance of the cortical

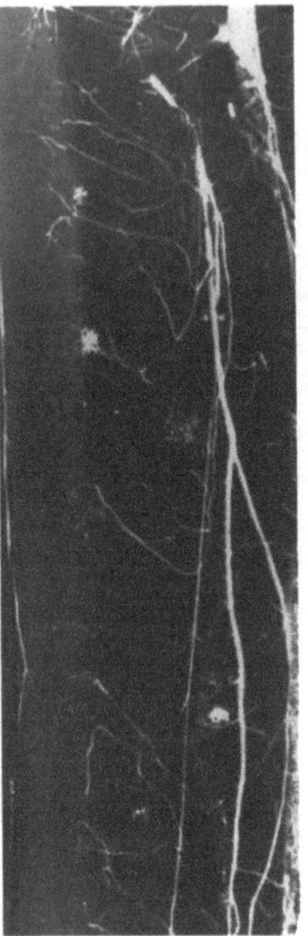

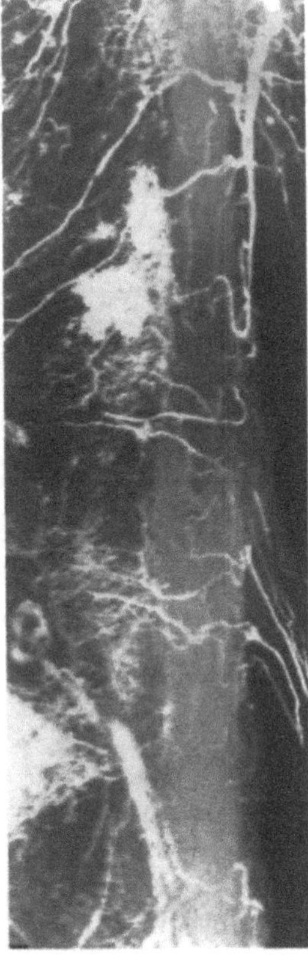

Fig. 20.4. (*left*) Angiograph of a longitudinal section of a normal rabbit tibia control to Fig. 20.5. A periosteal arterial supply to the cortex is absent. (Original magnification ×9.7)

Fig. 20.5. (*right*) Angiograph of a longitudinal section of a rabbit tibia rendered partially ischaemic by nutrient artery ligation 3 months previously. An abnormal periosteal arterial supply to the bone has developed. (Original magnification ×9.7)

circulation is presumably the reason why the cortex of the bone undergoes such prompt and long-lasting changes in response to medullary ischaemia.

Together with the vascular reorganization taking place within compact bone, there occur radical changes in the cellular elements and the fundamental bone substance (Figs 20.6–20.11). Histological investigation of experimental material shows that the characteristic reaction of compact bone to medullary ischaemia is a widening of the cortical vascular canals and the appearance of numerous "bone-forming cells" (Fig. 20.9, *overleaf*). The latter are mononuclear cells which line up in palisade fashion. Although bone removal must considerably exceed bone formation in early phases of experimental ischaemia, few multinucleate osteoclasts (Fig. 20.10, *page 273*) are visible. The predominant type of cell close to the border of an enlarging vascular canal is mononuclear, and is indistinguishable from a bone-forming cell by conventional staining techniques. These specialized cells seem to be derived from the loosely packed mesenchyme cells which fill the canal space, and among which numerous dilated capillaries are found. Massive osteocyte death is not a consequence of nutrient artery ligation in the experimental animal according to the investigators quoted above. Both periosteal and endosteal plaques of new bone may occur, especially the latter, in relation to areas of marrow infarction. Finally, although the marrow may be restored to normal function, the cortex nevertheless tends to show a persistent osteoporosis, evinced radiologically by diminished radiopacity and histologically by the presence of

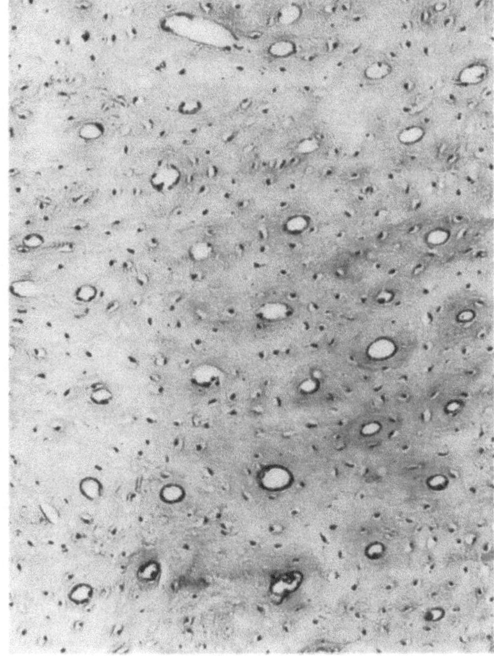

Fig. 20.6. Normal rabbit tibial cortex in cross-section. (Original magnification ×80)

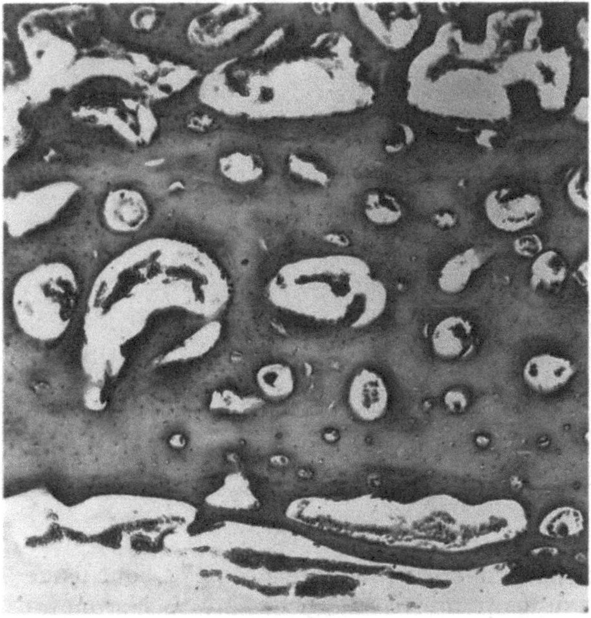

Fig. 20.7. Porotic bone cortex in a rabbit tibia following ligation of the nutrient artery 2 weeks previously. (Original magnification ×60)

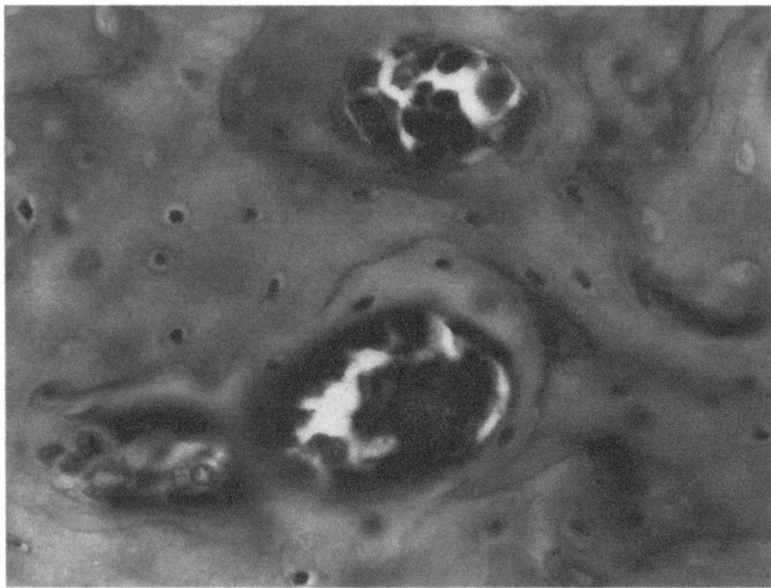

Fig. 20.8. Enlargement of the vascular canals in the cortex 2 weeks after nutrient artery ligation. The osteocytes stain normally. (Original magnification ×500)

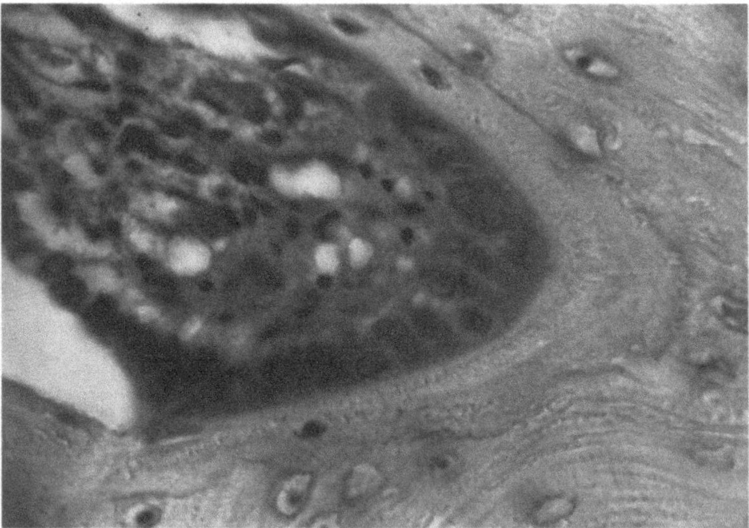

Fig. 20.9. A palisade of mononuclear cells, supported by vascular mesenchyme, in a porotic region of the cortex of the rabbit tibia, 4 weeks after nutrient artery ligation (Original magnification ×500)

large vascular spaces in otherwise normal compact bone tissue. The spaces may not only contain the primitive osteogenic and vascular mesenchyme described above; some may enclose erythroid marrow continuous with that of the originally infarcted marrow cavity (Fig. 20.12, *overleaf*).

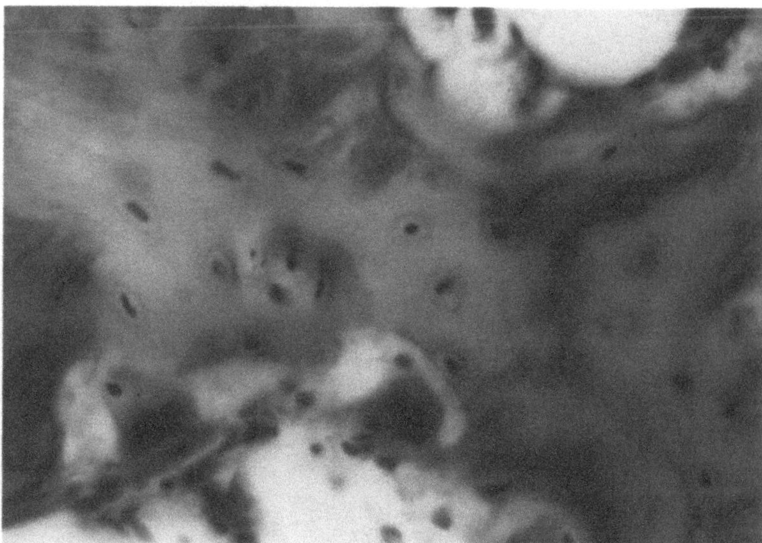

Fig. 20.10. Multinucleate osteoclasts in partially ischaemic bone cortex. Although the bone is undergoing dissolution, the osteocytes appear normal. (Original magnification ×500)

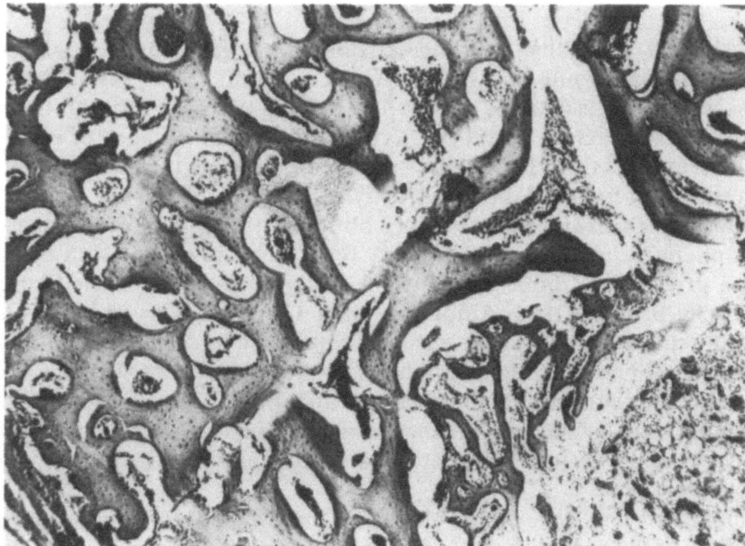

Fig. 20.11. Extensive cortical bone loss, in the presence of a periosteal arterial supply, after nutrient artery ligation 2 weeks previously. Massive osteocyte death has not occurred. (Original magnification ×36)

The mechanisms involved in the various changes described above, particularly those occurring in the cortex, are as yet not clearly understood. It would appear that nutrient artery ligation causes a profound fall in the intravascular pressure of small arteries running in the subcortical zone of marrow. A direct consequence of this would be a fall in the driving pressure of blood entering the cortex. Indeed,

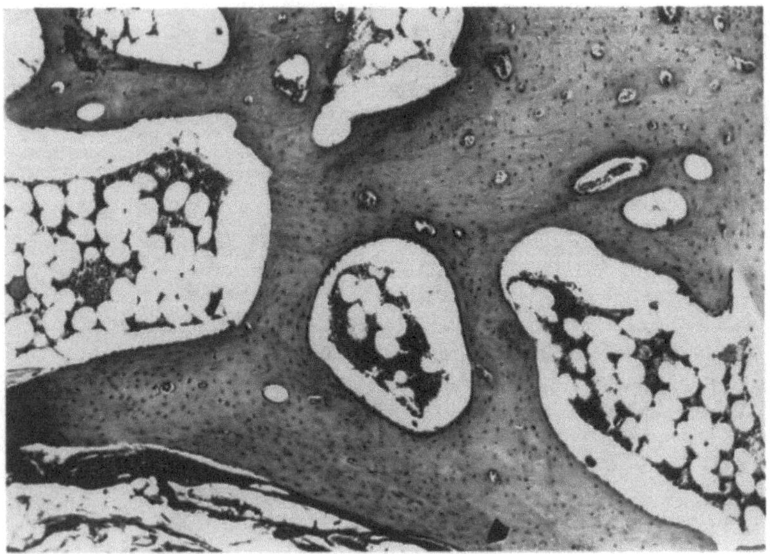

Fig. 20.12. Medullary tissue in the bone cortex of a rabbit's tibia 5 months after the principal nutrient artery had been ligated. (Original magnification ×60)

the experiments show that the normal centrifugal gradient in young animals across the cortical profile is reversed, which accounts for the centripetal blood flow observed in the ischaemic cortex. The driving pressure through the marrow sinusoids is also severely curtailed, accounting for the collapse of sinusoids in central marrow areas and for the hyperaemia in those regions which retain a circulation sufficient to maintain vital reactivity.

The massive excavation of compact bone following marrow ischaemia is a complex phenomenon and may possibly represent an exaggeration of normally occurring processes of bone substitution and vascular neogenesis (Amprino & Bairatti 1936; Brookes 1964; Amprino 1968). The osteocytes in bone substance and the mesenchyme cells in the vascular canals are in continual chemical commerce with the blood flowing through the cortical capillaries. This, as alluded to above, exhibits changed haemodynamic and physicochemical features. The microangiographic evidence of a considerable periosteal arterial supply suggests that the cortical flow rate is raised and that a drift towards alkalinity occurs in the capillary blood.

The increased flow rate might also raise the oxygen tension and depress the carbon dioxide tension of the blood circulating in the cortex. Changes in the gas tensions and pH of the tissue fluid in the canaliculi and vascular canals are to be expected as a consequence. The canal contents respond by cellular and vascular multiplication and differentiation. The osteocytes also participate in the production of the ensuing osteoporosis, at least in the resorption of crystalline matrix from the lamellae (Belanger *et al.* 1963). These local changes in cellular activity are presumably due solely to changed local vascular conditions. It is by a precise specification of these variables that one may be able to determine the causation of the cellular differentiation, growth and intense remodelling that are so conspicuous in compact bone cortex reacting to marrow ischaemia.

Metaphyseal arteries

Experiments carried out on growing animals, in which groups of metaphyseal arteries are ligated or destroyed (Kistler 1935; Trueta & Amato 1960; Fyfe 1964), result in an area of necrotic cancellous bone, the base of which is the growth cartilage. The vessels in the infarcted area do not fill in perfusion preparations, nuclei vanish, and normal staining properties are lost. As pointed out in Chapter 11, the cartilage plate associated with the infarction does not die. Instead, the hypertrophic zone thickens and juts step-like into the metaphysis. Normal invasion of the growing hypertrophic zone is abolished as well as endochondral bone formation. The germinal cells of the growth cartilage related to the infarcted area are probably also affected by the lesion, because growth in length of the bone is no longer balanced evenly, but considerable shortening and distortion occur at the joint. This suggests, therefore, that the metaphyseal nutrition of the growth plate extends at least as far as the germinal zone, because there is presumably a fall in mitotic rate of the cells which give rise to the infarcted growth cartilage. If growth in thickness of the infarcted cartilage were normal, no distortion of the bone extremity would occur (see Chapter 11).

It is not definitely known whether new vascular mesenchyme grows into the infarcted zone from contiguous healthy areas, to what extent the excess of hypertrophic cartilage cells is removed, or whether normal appearances are in fact restored. In the literature, the sequelae of metaphyseal infarction seem to have been followed for an insufficient time to allow any certainty in the matter. Nevertheless, the work of Kistler (1935), Fyfe (1964) and others does indicate that the resulting disturbance is long lasting and that recovery, if it occurs at all, is a slow process.

Epiphyseal arteries

The effects of ligation of the nutrient and metaphyseal arteries confirm anatomical appearances and show that these vessels are end-arteries. The epiphyseal arteries differ from them anatomically in that they form prominent intracancellous anastomoses. However, the arterial subdivisions which feed into the two specialized subchondral circulations, articular and epiphyseal, suggest that, at this level at least, the vessels are end-arteries.

Experiment shows that destruction of a group of epiphyseal arteries while still in an extra-osseous position, or ligation of the large middle genicular artery which is distributed to the lower femoral epiphysis, can lead to massive cancellous infarction (Nussbaum 1923). Revascularization and repair of the epiphysis is, however, vigorous, so that a blood supply to both articular and epiphyseal cartilages may be restored in a week or two following external epiphyseal stripping procedures. Neither of the cartilages died as a result of the ischaemia in Holdsworth's (1966) experiments. Cellular proliferation was reduced or may even have ceased for a short interval, but the integrity of the cartilages was conserved, so that restoration to normal activity was possible after re-establishment of an intra-osseous circulation. On the other hand, intra-osseous destruction of epiphyseal vessels by heat or by mechanical means (Trueta and Amato 1960) often gives rise to infarction of the germinal cells of the growth cartilage. This is then replaced by a bone or fibrous (Holdsworth 1966) bridge uniting the epiphyseal and metaphyseal parts of the bone. The bridge forms in relation to vascular mesenchyme from the metaphysis, whose inroads into the cartilage cannot be checked by fresh chondrocytes spawned from an intact germinal zone. When the growth cartilage is entirely destroyed by severe epiphyseal infarction produced by ultrasonic lesions, growth in length ceases and the entire epiphysis may be replaced by a knot of fibrous tissue.

There is little evidence available to indicate the effects of interrupting the articular circulation alone. Carbon particle blockade (Kistler 1934, 1935) sometimes results in articular necrotic foci in mature rabbits. Similarly, bacterial injections into the blood stream may result in abscesses adjacent to the joint cavity (Robertson 1927), although usually this procedure results in metaphyseal and periosteal abscesses.

In experiments involving segmental infarction of cancellous bone and the overlying articular cartilage (Holdsworth 1966), the metabolism of chondrocytes was undoubtedly depressed, in that initially the cartilage became unusually thin and failed to exhibit metachromatic staining with Toluidine Blue. Synovial fluid, secreted at least in part from large areas of intact joint cartilage, may have kept the chondrocytes alive in these circumstances. Nevertheless, revascularization of epiphyseal infarcts was difficult to abolish in these experiments, so that given time, a return to normality of ischaemic joint cartilage was the typical finding.

Chapter 21

Disturbed osseous circulation – 2: Effects of venous obstruction on bone

It may be thought that a simple venous obstruction of the cortical circulation could be brought about by abolition of the pumping action of surrounding muscles (Brookes 1958b; Brookes *et al.* 1961). The muscle pump can be abolished by local immobilization or by experimental nerve section (Tower 1937a,b; Brookes & Irving 1962). In both instances a loss in cortical radiodensity is a common finding. After nerve section (Brookes & Irving 1962), the femoral cortex of rats showed after an interval of 2 months, a widening of the medullary cavity, a diminution in cortical radiodensity and hyperaemia of the periosteum. Histologically, however, the compact bone tissue appeared normal, and excavation of bone did not occur. The venous effluent would normally have been pumped away by muscular activity, but was now dependent solely on the dynamics of the osseous circulation and tended to linger on the surface of the bone. Abolition of the muscle pump does not necessarily lead to a reduction in the rate of flow in the osseous circulation. Vascular shunts may be developed between the skeleton and the surrounding inactive muscles which may actually raise the flow in the bones, especially the marrow.

The above comments have addressed some of the effects of impeding venous drainage in cortical bone by eliminating the muscle pump. Venous impediment in the broadest sense, however, has been implicated in the stimulation of normal bone formation, the enhancement of fracture healing, as a factor in the aetiology of osteoarthritis, as well as being involved in current views of transduction mechanisms in the operation of Wolff's law. Venous impediment is currently undergoing a renaissance of investigative interest, and has a long history.

Clinical experiences

Interference with the venous circulation can have a profound and potentially therapeutic effect on bones. Empirical observations led to attempts to employ venous impediment in the treatment of delayed fracture union and, more controversially, for leg lengthening in children with limb inequality. According to Bier (1905), the first recorded use of venous engorgement to treat delayed fracture healing was by Ambroise Paré (c.1510–1590), the great French military surgeon, who gained his experience on the battlefields of Europe. In 1875 Nicoladoni

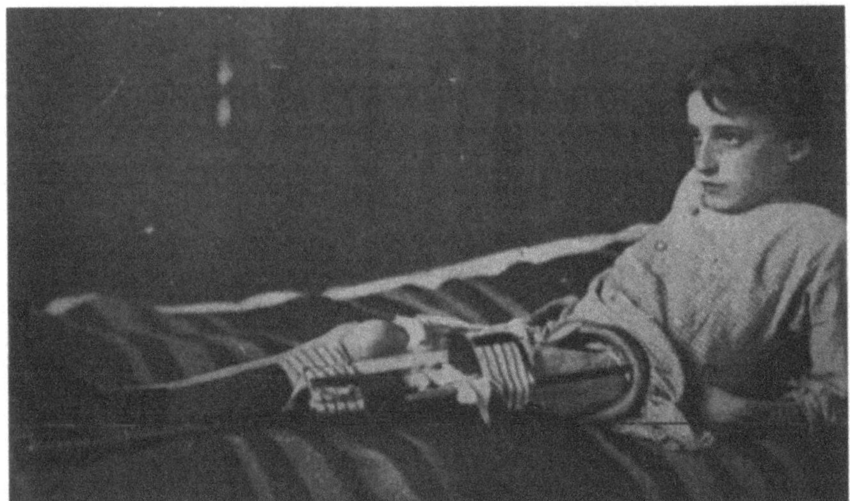

Fig. 21.1. Thomas' splint. Early form of splint, as recommended for tuberculous osteitis.

reported the use of "von Dumreicher's method" of venous hyperaemia as a treatment for delayed fracture healing, and also claimed success in stimulating bone cavities to heal. Venous hyperaemia was achieved by a rubber tourniquet. At the same time (1875), Thomas first described his famous metal splint which stabilized the mechanics of a fracture, and in his book (Thomas 1886) claimed originality for its combined use with venous stasis to stimulate healing of fracture non-unions. It is clear that the Thomas splint was not only an efficient fracture fixation device, but also well suited for the application of a proximal venous tourniquet (Fig. 21.1).

Helferich (1887) and Schüller (1889) used tourniquet-induced venous stasis to produce leg lengthening in children with post-traumatic limb shortening. The treatment, involving the rather unpleasant application of a long-term tourniquet, produced increases in length of up to 2 cm. It was the first deliberate use of venous impediment to stimulate bone elongation. A large body of evidence was accumulating at that time that any disease process which caused long-lasting inflammatory venous congestion would be followed by bone growth (e.g. Stanley 1849; Paget 1867).

Pearse & Morton (1930) cited 31 references, describing accelerated bone growth associated with impeded venous drainage, either resulting from therapeutic intervention, or contingent upon pathological processes. Horton (1932) reported congenital aneurysm of the extremities in 23 cases, with lengthening of the bones in 18 instances. Servelle (1948) described 14 cases of leg lengthening associated with venous varicosities in the lower limb, resulting from traumatic occlusion of the femoral or popliteal vein. Peck (1957), however, reported *decreased* bone growth in a young girl, associated with an incomplete occlusion of the iliac vein on the affected side.

The use of a tourniquet to produce venous congestion required stoicism in the patient, who had to withstand great discomfort for long periods, and it is unlikely that the modern patient would endure it. There is also the possibility of soft tissue damage, arterial obstruction and gangrene (Colt & Iger 1963). Servelle (1948) advocated femoral vein ligation in children with shortened limbs, but did not actually try it out. Rojos (1961) created an obstruction to the osseous venous return in children, by impacting ox horn in the medullary canal, but could only report a temporary increase in leg length.

With the advent of modern methods of internal fixation, utilizing plates and screws, intramedullary "nails" and external bone fixation devices, the use of vascular perturbation to influence bone repair and growth is now largely redundant. It is of interest however that the "Aircast" system of fracture bracing has been claimed to be not only an efficient fixation device, but also to enhance the rate of bone healing. It is suggested that this device, which incorporates pneumatic or hydraulic pressure bags to achieve stiffness, also acts as a venous tourniquet; and it is the *impediment to venous drainage* which produces the increased rate of fracture repair (Dale *et al.* 1989).

Clinical observations of the effect of venous stasis on bone are, however, difficult to interpret, due to the inevitable involvement of other factors. These may be arterial deficiency, soft tissue oedema, impairment of lymph flow or alteration of bone metabolism secondary to trauma (Just-Viera & Yeager 1965). To determine the effect of venous impediment alone, it is necessary to utilize an animal model, with adequate controls.

Effects of venous impediment on bone growth

Grey & Carr (1915) reported a transitory oedema following saphenous vein ligation in dogs, distal to the ligation. No change in the structure of the bone was noted. They concluded that passive hyperaemia in itself brings about little, if any, *atrophic* change. Wu & Miltner (1937) were also unable to find any growth or structural change in femora and tibiae following femoral vein ligation in rabbits. Kishikawa (1936), however, applying a venous tourniquet to the rabbit hind limb claimed an increase in length and width of long bones distal to the tourniquet (i.e. a *hypertrophic* response). The use of a tourniquet is expected to maintain an elevated venous pressure for much longer than the simple femoral vein ligation used by Wu & Miltner (1937), where collateral escape routes reduced the degree of venous congestion (Just-Vierra & Yeager 1965; see below).

Hutchison & Burdeaux (1954) also used a limb tourniquet in growing dogs, finding a general increase in the diameters of the radius and femur distal to the tourniquet, resulting from subperiosteal new bone deposition. Length increases were less constantly achieved. Seeking to avoid the discomfort of long-term tourniquet application, Colt & Iger (1963) used a Teflon tube to produce a stenosis in the femoral vein of puppies, reducing the vessel diameter variously from 25 to 75%. Again, weight, circumference and length were generally increased in the long bones distal to the stenosis; the authors acknowledged, however, that the increases were often trivial.

Dickinson (1953) ligated the external iliac and popliteal veins in puppies. He found no changes in bone length over a period of 3 months, although terminal venograms showed that the venous block had persisted. Just-Vierra & Yeager (1965) examined the effect of resecting the *entire* femoral venous system of puppies; extirpating the femoral vein and its branches, the external iliac vein, and portions of the external pudendal and deep epigastric veins. The effects of this extreme procedure on tibiae and femora were compared with sham operated contralateral bones. Phlebograms performed at regular intervals revealed rapid formation of venous collaterals, providing new pathways for eliminating congestion. The collaterals were resected at intervals, but new, smaller channels were rapidly re-established, sometimes immediately postoperatively. The largest difference in length observed between ligated and non-ligated tibial bones was 0.4 cm, and in femora, 0.7 cm; most differences were in the order of 0.1 and 0.2 cm. The largest gain in extremity length was 2.7%, although negative differentials for both length and volume were reported.

Persistent, longstanding venous stasis is therefore difficult to achieve in dogs, and must be borne in mind when interpreting results of "stasis" investigations in this animal. Nevertheless, venous resection and stasis results suggest a trend towards bone growth, whose extent is determined by the degree of collateral drainage. Keck & Kelly (1965) ligated the femoral vein and resected the iliac vein in growing puppies. No significant difference in tibial and femoral lengths were found 6 months after venous ligation. Again, marked increases in collateral venous circulation occurred, and saphenous vein pressures increased only transiently, returning to normal levels after 9 weeks. Lilly & Kelly (1970), in a similar model, found a significant increase in tibial weights and volumes, but not lengths, on the ligated side.

Kelly (1968) obtained similar results by the use of an elastic tourniquet applied proximal to the knee of growing puppies. Although saphenous pressure remained elevated throughout the period of the investigation, no increase in tibial length was reported. Annan *et al.* (1985) also reported increased periosteal tibial bone formation resulting from a venous tourniquet, in puppies after 40 days. Standing venous pressure was substantially elevated in the treated limb, as well as vascular volume and extracellular fluid space. Similar results were obtained following the application of an Aircast pressure brace to an intact canine tibia (Kelly & Bronk 1990).

Whilst more bone substance seems to be produced distal to a ligation or tourniquet in the dog, reports of increases in length are less frequent. In the rat following unilateral femoral vein ligation, femora and tibiae on the ligated side continue to increase in weight (Figs 21.2, 21.3) for periods up to 24 weeks following the ligation (Singh & Brookes 1971). The percentage *weight* increase in the ligated femur after 24 weeks was 1.24%, and in the tibia, 4.3%; the ligated bone was heavier in every case. The mean *length* of bones in the ligated limb was also greater than their contralateral control, although not all bones increased in length. The percentage length increase for the femur after 24 weeks was 1.1%, and in the tibia, 0.6%. More recently, Revell & Brookes (1994) have confirmed this trend. Following unilateral femoral ligation in young rats, they found a significant relative *weight* gain in ligated femora (+2.9% at 8 weeks; +3.7% at 16 weeks) compared with the contralateral bones. Relative bone *lengths* also showed a small increase but only became statistically significant at 16 weeks following ligation (femur +1%; tibia +0.44%).

Effects of venous impediment on fracture repair

The above review suggests that venous impediment has a hypertrophic effect on intact bone, if not always constant or predictable. The degree of venous occlusion

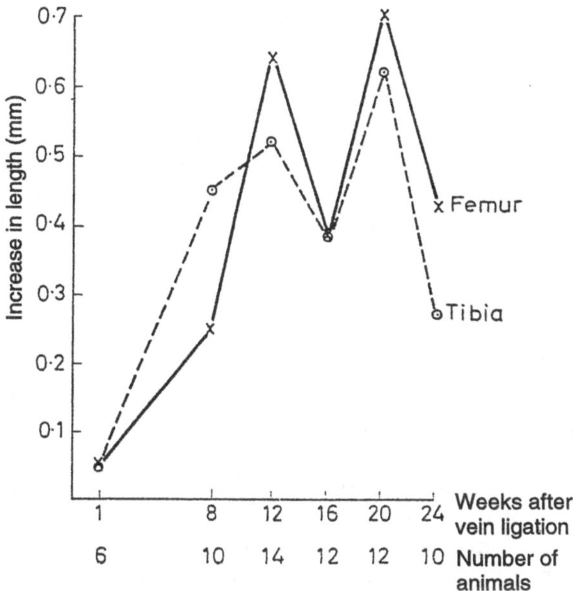

Fig. 21.2. The length of the rat femur and tibia after femoral vein ligation. Bone elongation is increased.

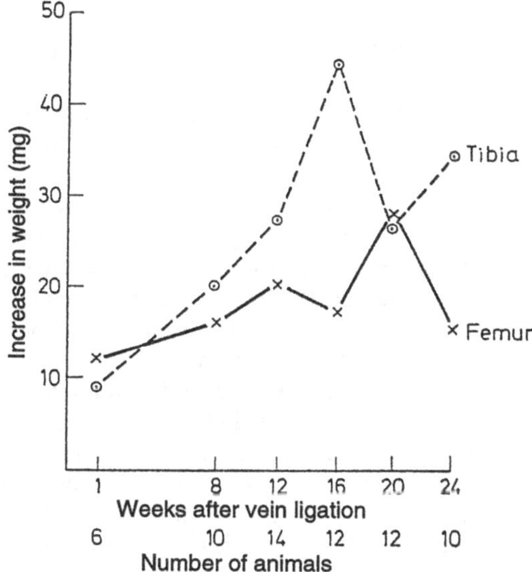

Fig. 21.3. The weight of the rat femur and tibia is increased after femoral vein ligation.

can vary considerably between experimental models, and the control conditions need to be clearly defined. Reports of increased periosteal bone production, however, suggest that venous impediment may favourably influence the healing of fractures.

The results of venous impediment on experimental fracture repair have again been dependent upon the degree of venous stasis achieved. Fracture repair is a difficult entity to quantify, and the precise configuration achieved in a particular model is crucial to the outcome. The effects of venous *ligation* have been variable, some investigators finding no effect on fracture repair (Morton & Stabins 1927; Pearse & Morton 1928; Key & Walton 1933), while others have claimed enhanced healing in the presence of the impediment (Pearse & Morton 1930; McMaster & Roome 1934). Brookes & Helal (1968b) also found increased bone formation in a rat fibula osteotomy, following femoral vein ligation. The application of a venous tourniquet has more consistently produced accelerated fracture repair (Kruse & Kelly 1974), and Dale *et al.* (1989, 1993) also obtained significantly increased new bone formation in dogs in company with a sustained increase in venous and tissue pressure, following the use of the Aircast™ fracture fixation system.

Again, in reviewing the effects of a venous impediment on fracture repair, it is apparent that venous ligation may have a stimulatory function on osteogenesis, although the results are not always unequivocal. The sustained venous tissue pressure produced by a tourniquet may offer a more consistent model for investigation, although it must not be assumed that sustained elevation in venous pressure is a necessary condition for changes to occur. A discussion of potential mechanisms will be presented later. Another area of investigation concerns joint morphology changes, resulting from venous impediment; some of the reported effects are relevant to aetiological models of osteoarthrosis.

Effects of venous impediment on knee joint morphology

Brookes (1966b) and Brookes & Helal (1968b) sectioned the femoral vein between ligatures, as well as the internal iliac vein where it runs along the posterior border of the rat thigh. In addition, the saphenous vein was stripped from ankle to knee, care being taken to preserve the neighbouring arteries. Following ligation the limbs took full weight, and showed no sign of oedema, and upon sacrifice 8 weeks later it was verified that no regeneration of the resected veins had occurred; apart from the absence of these vessels the limb appeared normal. Microfocal radiography showed mild but obvious changes in the cancellous bone of the knee; trabeculation in femoral and tibial epiphyses was coarser in pattern in the ligated knee compared with the contralateral side, and individual trabeculae were thicker and more radiodense than in the control side (Fig. 21.4). Similar changes were noted in the patella. Histological examination of many anatomically matched pairs of sections tended to confirm the coarsening of trabeculae in the ligated knee; also, qualitatively, an impression was gained that the calcified zone of articular cartilage had thickened on the ligated side, compared with the non-ligated control, and that the femoral and tibial articular bone plates were thicker and denser in the ligated knee. It was also found that the articular cartilage in the ligated knee showed a diminished Schiff–periodic acid response, and it was concluded that there was a reduction in protein bound polysaccharide. These are mild changes, amounting to a thickening of the calcified zone of the articular cartilage and cancellous bone sclerosis. It was concluded that in the longer term the sclerotic articular cartilage, and the shift in balance of bone turnover towards

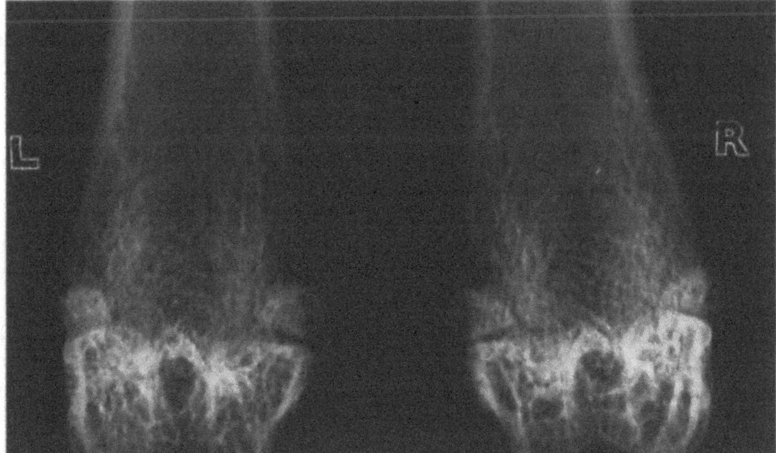

Fig. 21.4. Microradiographs of the inferior femoral epiphyses of a rat. The left is normal. The right shows coarsening of trabeculation and increased radiodensity 8 weeks after femoral vein ligation. (Original magnification ×3).

that of bone formation in the presence of venous obstruction, suggests that venous impediment may be a factor in the development of human osteoarthrosis.

Brookes (1990c) reported the results of a pilot study suggesting that simple femoral vein ligation *could* produce mild sclerotic changes in the rat knee joint, which possibly precede the effects of mechanical factors in osteoarthritis. A high unilateral femoral vein ligation was performed on 10-week-old Wistar rats. By 8 weeks, there were significant changes produced in the ligated bones; a frank sclerosis of cancellous bone, thickening and coarsening of epiphyseal trabeculae, accompanied by thinning and atrophy of the articular cartilage.

Venous impediment and clinical osteoarthrosis

The previous review has suggested an association between venous impediment and some alteration of bone metabolism, although not always, and also the production of some of the early features of clinical osteoarthrosis. Dieppe (1987) has defined osteoarthrosis (OA) as a group of diseases of synovial joints, characterized by loss of the articular cartilage with abnormal activity of the underlying bone. This concept is reflected in the typical radiological changes, which include joint space narrowing (due to cartilage loss), subarticular sclerosis, bone cysts and osteophytes (due to abnormal bone activity). Diagnosis is usually based upon some of these features, as well as pain and loss of mobility. An abnormality in joint mechanics, whatever its origins, is generally considered to be a major factor in the development of OA. However, in its primary form, it can be difficult in individual cases to define the nature of the mechanical disturbance. On the other hand, there is evidence that a deficiency in venous drainage of joint structures may be associated with OA, although whether causal or secondary remains contentious.

For many years it was commonly held that OA resulted from *ischaemia* (first postulated by Wollenberg 1909). Although osteoarthrotic lesions may be created experimentally by a prolonged ischaemic insult (Graf *et al.* 1992), Harrison *et al.* (1953) demonstrated that human sclerotic osteoarthrotic femoral heads showed subarticular *hypervascularity*; new vessels being superimposed on the normal arterial pattern. Angiographic studies of early osteoarthrotic femoral heads indicated that this vascular profusion and dilatation did not occur as a response to an ischaemic episode. A further constant feature was the presence of increased intercellular fluid in cancellous bone, suggestive of oedema.

Other investigators emphasize that the vascular pattern of the cancellous region beneath the pressure segment was dominated by venous engorgement, showing large numbers of dilated veins and sinusoids, although Trueta maintained that the hypervascularity was arterial, not venous. Rutishauser *et al.* (1952) and Rutishauser (1956) carefully studied the histology of osteoarthrotic bone. They consistently found numerous dilated and varicose-looking venous sinusoids in the intertrabecular spaces, and concluded that the essential vascular perturbation in osteoarthrosis was venous engorgement, caused by defective venous drainage. Intraosseous phlebography of lower limb bones involved in osteoarthrotic disease revealed venous dilatations in cancellous bone (Helal 1962; Wardle 1964). Delayed emptying of radiopaque media injected into cancellous bone of OA joints was demonstrated by Pistolesi (1962).

Furthermore, Brookes & Helal (1968a,b) reported their results of clinical intraosseous phlebography in 186 patients suffering from OA of the hip, knee or elbow. They found that wherever there was a normal control side for comparison, the articular sinusoids were distended. The injected fluid cleared more slowly from the affected side, suggesting a sluggish cancellous circulation. In 22 patients examined after treatment by osteotomy, relief of pain was concurrent with a return to normal size of the distended articular veins.

Similar reports have been published by Meriel *et al.* (1955), Phillips (1966), and Arnoldi *et al.* (1972). Interestingly, Phillips *et al.* (1967) showed that venous abnormalities can be reversed; a return to the normal pattern was observed in patients, 12–20 months following intertrochanteric osteotomy of osteoarthrotic femoral heads. Waisbrod & Tremain (1980) have described venous engorgement of the patella as a consistent feature in patients with chondromalacia patellae or patellofemoral OA, regardless of the severity of the pathological changes. A quantitative reduction of venous drainage rate in osteoarthrotic tibial metaphyses from knees of differing grades has been demonstrated by intraosseous phleboscintigraphy, which measures the clearance rate of ^{99m}Tc-labelled red blood cells. The clearance rate was significantly less in the affected bone, compared with the contralateral normal control, and decreased linearly with the severity of the pathology (Albuquerque & Isabel 1993).

Arnoldi *et al.* (1971, 1975) and Lemperg & Arnoldi (1978) determined the relationship between painful OA and a high resting intra-osseous venous pressure, and showed a reduction in pressure and pain following osteotomy. They suggested that the high intra-osseous venous pressure resulted from the blockage of outflow from periarticular veins, which was considered to be secondary to synovial effusion; there was a linear relationship between the two parameters (Arnoldi *et al.* 1979). This view was supported by Bunger (1987), who showed that simulated joint effusion resulted in intramedullary venous stasis and intra-osseous hypertension in the canine epiphysis and patella. In an acute experiment in puppies, Hansen *et al.* (1989) showed that knee joint tamponade, which increased intra-articular pressure in the knee to 75 mmHg, also resulted in decreased epiphyseal blood flow (see also Chapter 17; "Plasma shift and synovial water" in Chapter 17).

The various investigations cited above demonstrate the involvement of a venous impediment in OA, with associated intraosseous hypertension. He *et al.* (1990) examined the microvasculature of bone in an osteoarthrotic model of the rabbit knee, using SEM of intravascular casts. The pathological joint was produced by immobilizing the leg in extension for 5 weeks. Phlebography showed a dilated vascular bed, with prolonged clearance of contrast medium; intra-osseous pressures in the tibial metaphyses were elevated in the osteoarthrotic joint compared with the control (22.4 mmHg vs 11.2 mmHg). The morphology of the normal proximal tibiae showed clearly defined sinusoids with a few arteriovenous shunts, but in the osteoarthrotic bone substantial differences were found; large venous spaces, leakage of cast material through the sinusoid walls, and the presence of numerous arteriovenous shunts. Hansen *et al.* (1991) were not able to find haemodynamic evidence for arteriovenous shunts during acute knee tamponade experiments, but their presence could contribute to the elevation of intraossous pressure. The animal model used showed many similarities to clinical OA, including narrowing of the joint space, subchondral sclerosis and osteophyte formation. This study demonstrates that profound microanatomical changes may accompany the haemodynamic responses found in OA although whether these changes initiate the degenerative disease is open to question.

Chapter 22

Bone haemodynamics in venous impediment

The previous chapters have outlined evidence which, taken overall, suggests that venous impediment may stimulate increased production of bone, showing as bone sclerosis, increased weight, and in some cases length, or by accelerating the rate of fracture repair. There is some evidence that interference with venous return may also cause articular cartilage sclerosis. As these changes are produced by a vascular perturbation, it is not surprising that many studies have attempted to examine the haemodynamic sequelae produced in bone by vascular obstruction.

McPherson and co-workers (1961) used heat loss from a heated thermocouple to measure blood flow changes in the distal metaphysis of the femur, following femoral vein ligation in the cat. They noted a marked and instant *increase* in blood flow following occlusion of the ipsilateral femoral vein. Femoral diaphyseal marrow pressure also increased for the duration of the occlusion, thus supporting the previous findings of Stein *et al.* (1957, 1958), and confirmed later by Azuma (1964) and Shim *et al.* (1972). In contrast, occlusion of the femoral artery results in decreased blood flow. The application of a venous tourniquet above the site of the thermocouple also increased blood flow, and the authors concluded that blood is shunted from muscle through bone to circumvent the venous impediment. Similar flow changes were reported in bone marrow by Shaw (1963), who placed thermocouples in the femoral diaphysis of cats. Again, an increase in blood flow and marrow pressure followed femoral vein occlusion, and was put down to soft tissue shunting through bone.

Increased bone blood flow following venous ligation was not confirmed by White & Stein (1965), who employed a radioisotope technique to determine blood flow rate in the rabbit tibia. The authors, who were aware of reactive hyperaemia resulting from prolonged tourniquet use, recorded a 43% reduction in measured tibial blood flow following femoral vein ligation. In contrast to the previous studies using thermocouples, they concluded that in the acute phase, venous obstruction substantially *reduces* the rate of blood flow into the tibia. The two observations are perhaps not contradictory, but complementary observations; this is because venous diversion through the femoral marrow and its sinuses provides a readymade pathway, allowing blood from the limb to circumvent the obstructed femoral vein. It is a surprising omission that changes in tibial blood volume were not evaluated, which their methodology would have permitted.

Shim & Patterson (1966) used a qualitative method to determine circulatory changes in rabbit bone resulting from femoral vein occlusion. They cannulated the femoral nutrient vein and artery, and determined flow through the cannulae by drop counting of sampled blood. They showed that femoral vein ligation increased nutrient venous outflow from the rabbit femur, which was interpreted as venous congestion of bone rather than an increased blood supply; arterial supply to the bone was diminished, as measured by drop counting from the nutrient arterial anastomotic retrograde flow. This cannot be regarded as a method for measuring total rate of blood flow through a given bone, as measurement of blood flow through one or two vessels cannot be representative of the many complex inputs and drainage routes present in bone. These results were confirmed in a later investigation by Shim & co-workers (1972), when an increase in diaphyseal marrow pressure accompanied the venous congestion.

More recently Kiær *et al.* (1993) have examined acute blood flow changes in femoral condyles following femoral vein ligation in pigs, as part of a larger study comparing the use of inert gas (freon) washout and microsphere bone haemodynamic studies. Both methods, which showed a good correlation (r=0.53; P<0.013) for flow rates measured in normal bone, demonstrated a decrease in flow rate after femoral vein ligation, which was statistically significant (P<0.025; n=6) only when using microspheres.

Singh & Brookes (1971) measured femoral and tibial blood flow changes for periods up to 24 weeks following femoral vein ligation in groups of 10–14 rats. Blood flow was measured by arteriolar blockade (Brookes 1970), using ^{59}Fe radioferrous sulphate-labelled resin particles introduced into the left ventricle under direct vision. Blood flows in ligated femora and tibiae, relative to the contralateral non-ligated control, were significantly depressed only immediately postoperatively; from 1 day following ligation, up to 24 weeks, no further significant change in flow rate was observed (Table 22.1). It was concluded from this study that the medullary venous escape route was available.

This experiment was re-examined more recently by Revell & Brookes (1994), again examining the haemodynamic changes in blood flow and volume brought about by femoral vein ligation in the rat. However, in this case the authors were able to examine changes to the whole femora and tibia, together with localized regions of the distal femur and proximal tibia, particularly the diaphysis, metaphysis and epiphysis. Blood flow rates were measured by arteriolar blockade using resin particles; a validation for the use of this tracer material was given in Chapter 19. The experiment also examined concurrent changes in blood volume, using ^{51}Cr-labelled red blood cell dilution. Changes in blood flow rate and blood volume in whole femora and tibiae, and regions of the distal femur and proximal

Table 22.1 Arterial input to the femora of rats after ligation of the left femoral vein (Singh & Brookes 1971)

		Mean flow rate	
Number of animals	Postoperative period	Left	Right
10	Immediate	81.4	100
10	1 day	105.8	100
6	1 week	100	100
10	8 weeks	92.0	100
14	12 weeks	101.9	100
11	16 weeks	106.0	100
11	20 weeks	108.5	100
10	24 weeks	95.5	100

tibia of the rat, were obtained at 6 hours and 1, 3 and 7 days following unilateral femoral vein ligation, and at 8 and 16 weeks.

Results are shown in Figs 22.1–22.4 for whole bones and epiphyses. Diaphyseal and metaphyseal flow were largely unaltered as a result of the ligation. As already noted, there was a relative weight gain in the ligated femora and tibiae, increasing from 8 to 16 weeks; bone lengths also showed some increase. In particular, an initial postoperative depression in blood volume is followed by a relative increase in vascular volume during the first week post-ligation, clearly showing the presence of short-term venous congestion. Presumably later collateral circulatory changes act to reduce this. There is a tendency for relative vascular volume to be depressed when measured in whole bones on the ligated side by 16 weeks; in epiphyseal cancellous bone of the knee joint this reduction is also observed and, in this case, is statistically significant. A sustained relative reduction of arterial input on the ligated side to whole femora and tibia was present throughout the period of the investigation. This diminished blood flow to the bone could act as a compensatory mechanism to reduce congestion, and vasoconstrictive agents could be of importance here. The sustained reduction in blood flow eventually produces a slight ischaemic condition in the bones with respect to both flow and volume.

In the cancellous bone of the knee joint, a localized increase in flow was apparent in the first week, comparing ligated with non-ligated bone. It must be borne in mind that the rat knee joint epiphyses are compartmental isolates because of the persistence of growth cartilages. Vasoactive reflexes may act to produce vascular dilatation in the epiphysis in the short term, thereby adapting to the congestion; sympathetic vasodilator substances (Lundgaard *et al.* 1993) as well as

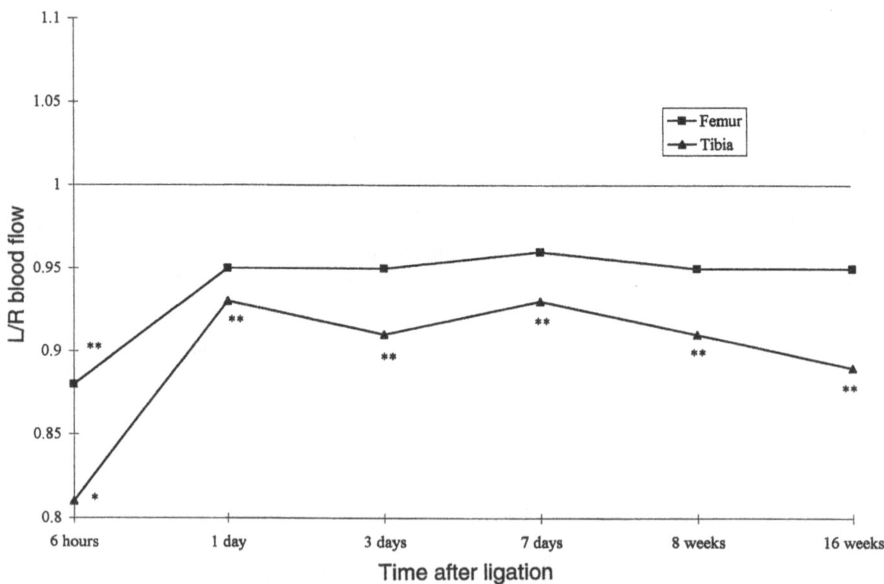

Fig. 22.1. Whole femora and tibiae: blood flow rates expressed as ratio L(ligated bone) / R(non-ligated control), at each time period. * $P<0.1$, ** $P<0.05$ for mean left and right difference at each time.

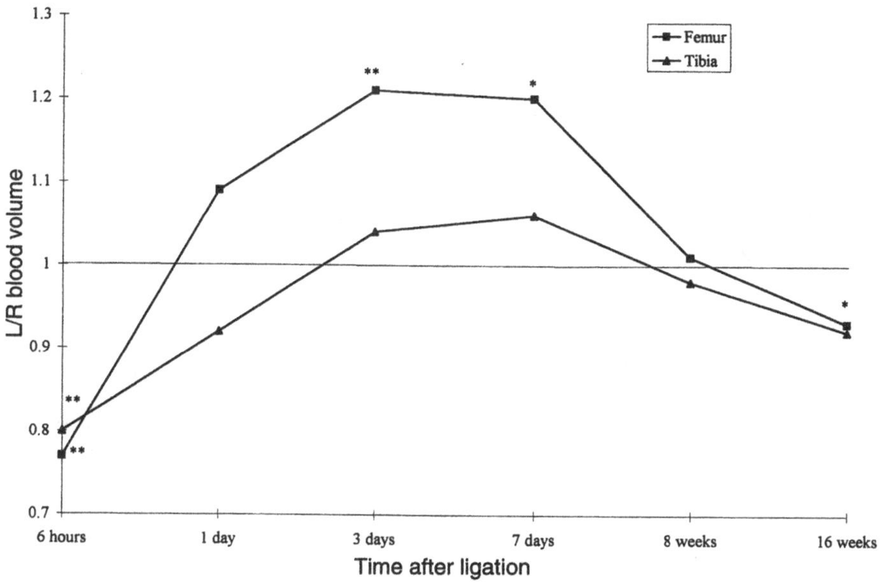

Fig. 22.2. Whole femora and tibiae: blood volumes, expressed as ratio L(ligated bone)/R(non-ligated control), at each time period. * $P<0.1$, ** $P<0.05$ for mean left and right difference at each time.

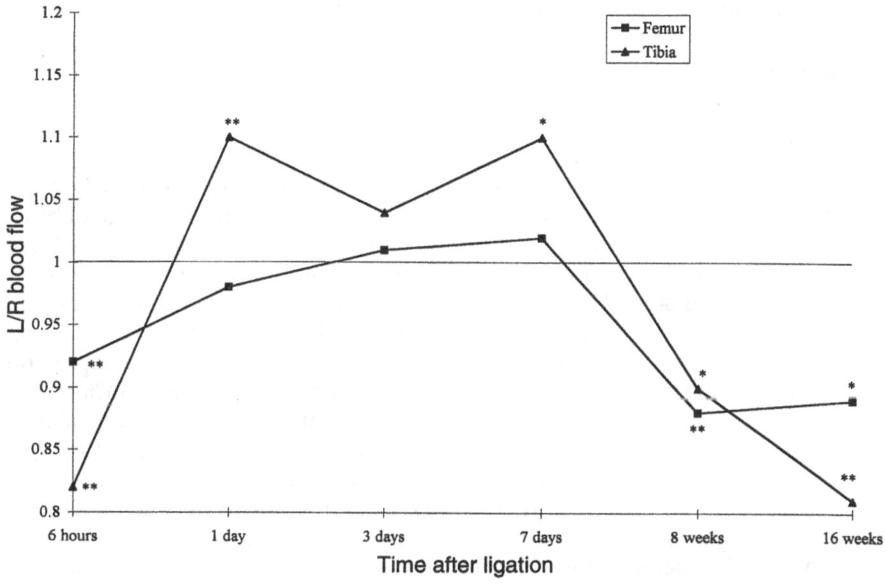

Fig. 22.3. Femoral and tibial epiphyses: blood flow rates expressed as ratio L(ligated bone)/R(non-ligated control), at each time period. * $P<0.1$; ** $P<0.05$ for mean left and right difference at each time.

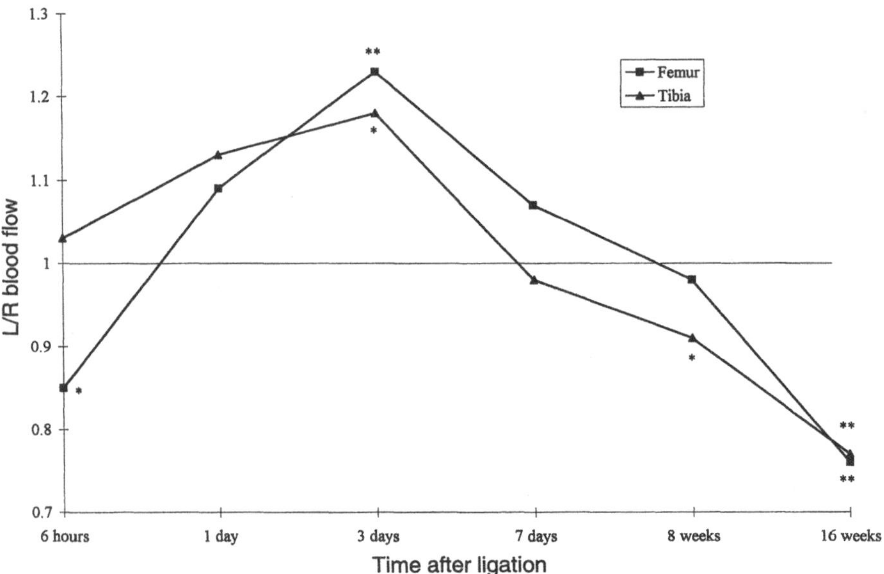

Fig. 22.4. Femoral and tibial epiphyses: blood volumes expressed as ratio L(ligated bone)/R(non-ligated control), at each time period. * $P<0.1$; ** $P<0.05$ for mean left and right difference at each time.

vasoconstrictor agents (Lindblad *et al.* 1993) are known to be active in bone. The metaphysis and diaphysis are in continuity, and venous escape routes are present to overcome vascular congestion and increased blood volume and flow, which would otherwise develop. These escape routes are via the medullary sinuses, linking with metaphyseal and periosteal veins. The presence of effective alternative venous drainage has been verified by perfusion studies (McPherson *et al.* 1961; Brookes & Singh 1972a)

Other studies have investigated bone blood volume changes resulting from venous obstruction. Blood volume describes the amount of blood contained in a unit amount of bone, whilst blood flow rate describes the rate of change of blood in that compartment. The measures, although often changing together in a linear relationship (Tøndevold & Eliasen 1982), are not necessarily linked in this way (Bunger 1987). Brookes (1966b) used a ^{51}Cr-labelled red blood cell haemodilution method to investigate blood volume changes following a severe venous stripping procedure in rats. Following occlusion of the femoral, iliac and saphenous veins, femoral and tibial knee joint epiphyseal bone showed a 36 and 43% relative increase in blood volume 8 weeks after ligation, compared with the contralateral unoperated controls. Tibial metaphyseal blood volume was increased by 20%; femoral metaphyseal volume was unaltered. In contrast, Brookes Singh (1972a) occluded the femoral vein in 80 rats, and examined blood volume changes, compared with unoperated contralateral controls, for periods up to 24 weeks. They reported that the mean value of the circulating red cell blood volume in whole femora and tibiae was relatively *lower* at all times on the operated side, although the fall only achieved statistical significance at 7 days post ligation. At 1 and 4 weeks they found a significant volume reduction ($P<0.05$) in isolated femoral and tibial diaphyses and epiphyses, but an increase in the metaphyses. Otherwise, no statistically significant changes were found in the regional determinations. These results do not agree with the substantial venous congestion found, following combined ligation of the iliac and femoral vein and saphenous stripping (Brookes 1966a); however, radical venous extirpation results in sustained bone venous engorgement, in contrast to the much milder effects of simple femoral vein ligation as observed by Brookes & Singh (1972a,b).

More recent studies have examined the effect of a venous tourniquet applied proximal to the knee joint in puppies (Annan *et al.* 1985). This experimental model showed an increased vascular space in the tourniquet-treated tibiae, compared with the contralateral control bone, 40 days after application of the tourniquet. These investigators measured a vascular space of 0.08 ml blood ml^{-1} bone in the tourniquet limb against a value of 0.05 ml ml^{-1} bone in the control side ($P<0.02$). Extracellular fluid space was also significantly increased in the tourniquet-treated limb. Kelly & Bronk (1990) obtained a similar result using a pressurized Aircast™ brace applied to the intact hind limb of dogs, finding a sustained (up to 42 days) elevation of saphenous vein pressure, vascular space, sucrose space and water of desiccation.

Welch *et al.* (1993) have examined the effect of increased intra-osseous pressure on new bone formation in the proximal metaphysis of the caprine tibia. Intra-osseous hypertension was achieved by popliteal ligation, followed by occlusion of the mid-diaphyseal medulla by insertion of a bone-cement plug; this raised the intramedullary pressure to a mean 28.7 mmHg, compared with 15.5 mmHg measured prior to the procedure, an 85% increase. In another group the previous venous blockage was accompanied by sustained intramedullary autoperfusion for a 5-day period, elevating the intramedullary pressure to between 30 and 45 mmHg. Histomorphometric analysis of the tibiae after a further 30 days showed substantial increases of periosteal, endosteal and cancellous new bone formation, correlated with the magnitude and duration of the induced hypertension.

There remains little doubt therefore that venous impediment elevates intramedullary venous pressure, the degree and duration of which varies with the particular model used and the investigator's ingenuity in sustaining it. Furthermore, the elevated hydrostatic pressure has been shown to increase blood congestion and transcapillary exudation of fluid into the extracellular space. Superimposed on these events are concomitant changes in the microenvironment – decreased pH and P_{O_2}, and increases in P_{CO_2} (Brookes & Helal 1968a,b; Arnoldi *et al.* 1972; Brookes & Singh 1972b; Lemberg & Arnoldi 1978; Grønlund *et al.* 1984; Kofoed 1986; Brinker *et al.* 1990; Liu & Ho 1991). Venous stasis *is* associated with osteogenesis; the question remains, how is this brought about?

Mechanisms of action of venous ligation

Haemodynamic changes

The investigations reviewed indicate that an altered haemodynamic status results from venous impediment, using only a mild venous obstruction (femoral vein ligation). If the impediment is severe and cannot be corrected (in the case of a permament tourniquet, or the Aircast™ brace, or by radical venous excision), then the bones are congested; if the venous impediment is mild, then bone venous congestion is evanescent and found only in the acute phase. The evidence also suggests that an altered haemodynamic state produces changes in bone turnover and joint morphology. Explanations for the mechanism of this interaction have been sought in the physicochemical changes produced by the changing relationships of venous and arterial blood. This paradigm was comprehensively developed and advocated by Brookes (1971), who has presented an elegant and detailed argument for the central position of the osseous circulation, and particularly vascular pH (related to blood flow rate, and Po_2/Pco_2) in the control of osteogenesis. In summary, he concluded that in the normal cortex, the bulk of blood which reaches the osteocytes has a reduced pH, a high Pco_2, and a reduced Po_2; i.e. the normal environment for osteocytes is characterized by a "drift to acidity". An acid environment alters the balance of bone formation and removal, leading to the production of hard cortical bone. Conversely, a shift to environmental alkalinity results in a light spongy bone being formed. Changes in pH/Pco_2/Po_2 are effected by changes in the vascular perfusion rate to the bone, and this argument facilitates a unifying explanation of many aspects of bone physiology, both normal and in pathological conditions, with reference to the haemodynamic status.

Brookes & Singh (1972b) examined bone blood pH and tissue gas tensions in rabbits, following femoral vein ligation, for periods up to 24 weeks. The results showed that pH and Po_2 fell in the diaphysis, compared with the non-ligated contralateral control, whilst Pco_2 increased. In the metaphysis, the pH was reduced, and both Po_2 and Pco_2 were elevated. It was suggested that these changes resulted from shunting of venous blood from the diaphysis into the metaphyseal sinusoids, and to abundant venous collateral branches which develop in the surrounding soft tissue. These were demonstrated by Thorotrast venography, performed 4 weeks after femoral vein ligation (Brookes & Singh 1972a). Also, contrast medium, injected simultaneously headward into both saphenous veins, reached the vena cava at the same time, showing that there was no delay in venous drainage in the ligated limb. In addition, no evidence of venous distension of the intraosseous vasculature was found. From the evidence of haemodynamic studies, showing an absence of long-term venous congestion following femoral vein ligation, it was argued that venous congestion, and hence venous hypertension, was not contributory to increased bone formation in the ligated limb. The cue to increased bone formation was therefore regarded as a reduced pH resulting from venous shunting.

Collateral drainage routes are able to circumvent venous obstructions. It is well known among those who practise perfusion techniques that an injection mass propelled into, say, the long saphenous vein at the ankle will bypass a ligature thrown around and completely obstructing the vessels of the soft tissues of the thigh. If the limb is now amputated above the level of the ligature, perfusate will be seen pouring out of the transected femoral marrow. Bearing in mind that the veins emerging from cancellous bone are without valves, it becomes apparent that an alternative venous drainage route for the leg from the level of the knee joint may be represented as:

> popliteal vein ⇒ femoral inferior metaphyseal veins ⇒ central venous sinus of femur ⇒ superior metaphyseal veins ⇒ medial and lateral circumflex femoral veins ⇒ gluteal veins ⇒ pelvis and inferior vena cava

In this schema, the profuse connections of the metaphyseal veins with the central venous sinus are given considerable importance in the provision of a venous escape mechanism. It is also possible that, with an obstructed femoral vein, venous blood from the thigh muscles joins that in the central venous sinus by flowing centripetally through the femoral cortex. The pathway for this flow lies in the connections that exist between cortical capillaries and the periosteal and interfascicular venules. The longitudinal periosteal veins presumably also contribute to the venous drainage of the obstructed limb, in view of the observed pooling of periosteal blood following experimental abolition of the muscle pump. These veins are in wide connection with the periarticular vascular plexus, and might equally provide a collateral venous drainage route for the whole limb in conditions of chronic venous obstruction. The ensuing engorgement of the periosteal and periarticular veins along the length of the appendicular skeleton may be expected to entrain disturbances in the circulation, metabolism and structure of joints as well as in the bones of the limb.

In human primary OA of the hip (Fig. 22.5), preliminary studies showed unusually low pH values (7.16) in samples of blood taken from the living femoral head prior to arthroplasty (Table 22.2). The mean Po_2 in seven unselected cases of coxarthrosis was 56 mmHg. In three cases of impacted subcapital fracture followed by the rapid development of a severe sclerosis of the head, pH depression was very marked (pH 6.87). The Pco_2 values for these cases was very high, 77 mmHg, providing evidence of venous obstruction of the circulation of the femoral head due to impaction. Presumably the arterial supply was intact, since the Po_2 was 59 mmHg. In primary OA the Pco_2 was 58 mmHg. On the other hand, in uncomplicated extracapsular fracture of the neck of femur seen 24 hours and

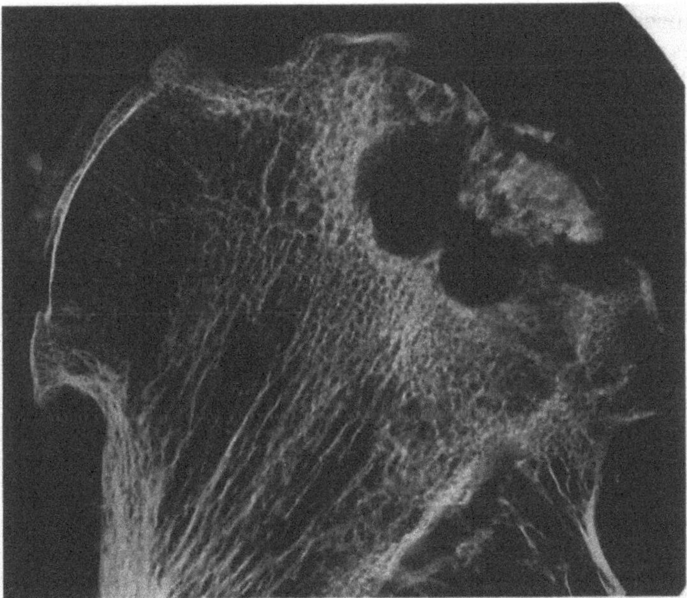

Fig. 22.5. Microradiograph of 2 mm thick coronal section through an osteoarthrotic femoral head, showing osteophytes, subarticular and cancellous bone sclerosis and the presence of "cysts". (Original magnification ×1.6)

Table 22.2 Intra-bone pH values measured on blood samples collected through bore holes during surgical anaesthesia

Cases (no.)	Source of blood sample	pH	P_{CO_2}	P_{O_2}
3	Impacted subcapital fracture	6.87	77	59
1	Non-union of tibial fracture	7.08		
7	Osteoarthrosis of the hip	7.16	58	56
2	Displaced cervical fracture (24 hours after injury)	7.22	47	73
1	Displaced cervical fracture (3 weeks after injury)	7.29	40	
1	Paget's disease of the hip	7.31	42	73
3	Femoral artery	7.36	38	85
24	Experimental osteotomies	7.36		

Table 22.3 Normal femoral and tibial pH values; data obtained from eight rabbits

Blood sampling site	pH
Femur	
Superior metaphysis ("non-growing end")	7.33
Marrow	7.40
Inferior metaphysis ("growing end")	7.30
Tibia	
Superior metaphysis ("growing end")	7.30
Inferior metaphysis ("non-growing end")	7.37

3 weeks after injury, pH elevation has been observed in the presence of bone rarefaction. The highest pH recorded (7.31) in human bone samples taken during surgical anaesthesia came from a pagetoid femoral head.

Brookes and Helal (1968a,b) measured the pH of blood samples taken from regions of normal rabbit tibiae and femora (Table 22.3). Their results indicate that normal bone blood is always on the alkaline side of neutrality; that marrow blood is more alkaline than metaphyseal; and that blood from a "growing" metaphysis is more acid than that from a "non-growing" metaphysis. They concluded that a mild acid drift occurs in those regions where net bone formation takes place at an increased rate. Such net bone formation is present in the sclerotic osteoarthrotic femoral heads mentioned above, where a reduced pH was also found.

Similarly, Pujol & Tran (1973) showed low pH and P_{O_2}, and raised P_{CO_2}, in trochanteric blood samples taken from cases of non-ischaemic coxarthrosis; i.e. OA of the hip. The results of these studies suggest that as a result of femoral vein ligation, a reduction in the pH and abnormal gas tensions of the blood to the knee joint is to be expected. As a result of such physicochemical changes, the micro-environment of the bone undergoes a mild acid drift, a complex tissue change brought about by changing haemodynamic conditions; acid drift forms a potent osteogenic stimulus.

Taken as a whole, then, the clinical and experimental evidence suggest that in OA a depressed pH of the micro-environment of bone cells, bought about by a local venous congestion, causes bone sclerosis by depressing the bone turnover rate and impeding preferentially the rate of bone removal. Total bone turnover is geared to the blood flow rate and P_{O_2} levels. The role of the P_{CO_2} is problematical, but possibly a high value increases the quantity of osteogenic blastemal cells available for the total turnover of bone in the area concerned and potentiates the calcification of both bone and cartilage. Depression of the pH in localized areas may be severe enough to abolish differentiation of blastemal tissue into bone. The removal of bone will then be followed by the substitution of fibrous tissue, as in the cyst formation of OA (Fig. 22.6).

Osteophyte production may be an expression of an attempt to improve the subchondral circulation by the reactive development of hypervascularity at the free border. This, by elevating local pH, may be the stimulus for spongy bone production (osteophytes) at the rim of the cartilage in non-weight-bearing areas, which is a characteristic sign of an osteoarthrotic joint pathology.

Intravascular pressure

Whilst this view offers a unifying paradigm, explaining many of the features associated with venous impediment, it is fair to admit that not all investigations have been able to find physicochemical changes of the type predicted by this hypothesis, and as in all branches of science, different opinions prevail. A reduced pH in blood samples from subchondral bone in osteoarthrotic human hips was not found by Kiær *et al.* (1988), or in sclerotic subchondral bone from a rabbit knee following production of an experimental OA (Kofoed 1986). Furthermore, acute measurements following venous tamponade in the canine knee, showed that $P\text{O}_2$, $P\text{CO}_2$ and pH were not altered in blood samples drawn from the distal femoral epiphyses, although epiphyseal intra-osseous pressure was significantly elevated (Holm *et al.*, 1990).

Kelly (1968, 1969) argued that changes in blood flow, pH, bone oxygen saturation, and partial pressures of oxygen and carbon dioxide, were the *consequences* of increased bone remodelling, and not factors that stimulated bone production following venous impediment. Yet, as Hansen (1993) has pointed out, "vascular

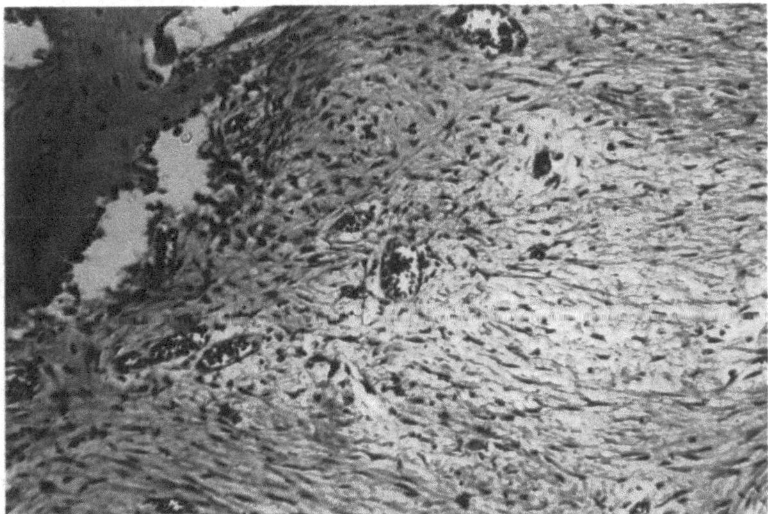

Fig. 22.6. Photomicrograph of a "cystic" area of the section shown in Fig. 22.5, showing vascular fibrous tissue. (Original magnification ×290)

invasion precedes osteogenesis in endochondral bones". In dogs, Kelly argues, there was always an increased saphenous vein pressure and intra-osseous pressure, following femoral vein ligation or a tourniquet (Keck & Kelly 1965; Kelly 1968); a hyperpressure which was sustained throughout the period of investigation in the case of tourniquet use, and from 6 to 9 weeks following venous ligation. They also showed microangiographic evidence of intra-osseous sinusoidal and capillary dilatation. It was argued that the prime cause of the increased bone remodelling was elevated intravascular pressure; and even the relatively transient increases following venous ligation (due to formation of collateral drainage routes) were adequate for metabolic stimulation.

More recent studies have shown that application of a proximal tourniquet to the canine hind limb stimulated new bone formation, in company with an increased intramedullary pressure (primarily determined by osseous venous resistance; Wilkes & Visscher 1975), vascular space, and an increased extracellular fluid compartment (Annan *et al.* 1985; Kelly & Bronk 1990; Bronk *et al.* 1993; Welch *et al.* 1994). They concluded that the elevated venous pressure increased fluid exudation from bone capillaries. Bone, being indistensible, cannot become oedematous and therefore increased centrifugal fluid flow will occur. Kelly & Bronk (1990) suggested, rather teleologically, that the long-term increase in vascular space resulted from increased blood flow to meet the metabolic demands of increased periosteal bone growth. Whether this is so remains debatable, but the results are consistent with a pressure-driven movement of fluid from the vascular space to the interstitium of bone.

Pressure transduction

In fact, this view accords with current hypotheses linking pressure with bone remodelling. Bone responds to mechanical stress by laying down more bone. This relationship between force and bone response was described by Julius Wolff (1892) in his classic exposition, *The Law of Bone Transformation.* Wolff's Law describes the piezotropic link (Treharne 1981) between stress and the shape and size of bone, and its internal structure. To achieve this dynamic response, some sort of a "pressure transducer" must be present in bone to detect local stresses and initiate a negative feedback loop to bone cells to counteract the increased load. Bone is exquisitely sensitive to dynamic loading; only four load reversal cycles per day have been shown to conserve bone mineral density in an avian disuse osteoporosis model (Rubin & Lanyon 1984, 1987). The same group, also using an avian model, showed a straight-line relationship between applied load and bone formation; below a threshold level (500 microstrains per day), bone resorption occurred.

Stress-generated streaming potentials

Anderson & Erickson (1970) suggested that electromechanical responses of bone in a normal physiological environment could be due to stress-generated streaming potentials (SGPs). Measurement of the dielectric properties of fluid saturated bone (Chakkalakal *et al.* 1980) demonstrated that the electromechanical effect observed in wet bone is several orders of magnitude higher than expected from a purely piezoelectrical effect (Johnson *et al.* 1980), and the view that streaming potentials are the dominant cause of stress-related electrical changes in *in vivo* bone is now widely accepted (Gross & Williams 1982; Johnson *et al.* 1982; Pollack *et al.* 1984). It has been known for many years that elastic deformation of dry bone produces a piezoelectric response (Gayda 1912, quoted in Cerquiglini *et al.* 1967; Yasuda 1953; Fukada & Yasuda 1957; Bassett & Becker 1962; Shamos *et al.* 1963). However, it is likely that a strictly piezoelectric stress-generated response is only found in dry bone; in physiologically wet bone piezoelectric signals, originating from charge separation in a deformed lattice, would attract mobile counter-ions, thus rapidly attenuating the amplitude and temporal survival of any signals.

Lanyon & Hartman (1977) demonstrated SGPs measured in sheep radii *in vivo* during walking and trotting. Other investigators have observed, however, that it is difficult to distinguish SGPs originating in bone, from interfering signals derived from muscle contraction and nerve action potentials. For instance, McDonald & Houston (1990) reported that maximum potentials of only 2.2 mV were recorded from rabbit tibias in response to sinusoidal loading, but found that this electrical activity was quite overwhelmed by muscle potentials following sciatic nerve stimulation. The authors argued that remodelling usually results from loading in relation to muscular activity, and that changes in electrical fields at the bone surface are predominantly influenced by muscle generated potentials. In fact, muscular activity *per se* may not be directly related to bone re-modelling; swimmers, for instance, can develop huge forearm muscles, but bone mineral density in the humerus, radius and ulna has been found to be less than sedentary controls. Furthermore, astronauts continue to lose bone mineral during weightlessness, in spite of having access to exercise bicycles. Dynamic vertical weight-bearing is a more important consideration in increasing bone mass.

Hydrostatic pressure

Streaming potentials develop between two points when an electrolyte flows past a charged solid surface. In bone, such potentials could arise in any of the fluid channels which facilitate interstitial fluid movement; junctional clefts between capillary endothelial cells, canaliculi, Haversian canals or Volkmann's canals (Kelly 1983). Montgomery *et al.* (1988), as mentioned in an earlier chapter, who convincingly described a pathway from capillary to matrix and thence into the general circulation, argued that the pattern of label movement suggested bulk interstitial fluid flow influenced by hydrostatic pressure. Current opinion holds that pressure applied to a bone may cause strain deformation leading to an increased exudation of fluid through the interstitium of the bone compactum. It is the hydrostatic pressure resulting from this increased flux through the non-distensible matrix that stimulates bone cells into an appropriate response. Thus it is found that both mechanical stress *and* increased intramedullary venous pressure resulting from venous impediment, may lead to increases in hydrostatic pressure in the linked environment of the osteocytes; this, in fact, raises the intriguing possibility of a common mechanism.

This possibility is not just of theoretical interest. McCarthy's group, working on just such a hypothesis, is currently investigating the potential of an intermittently applied proximal venous tourniquet to ameliorate bone mineral loss in astronauts' lower limbs (McCarthy & Hughes 1996). It should be noted that Goodship's group are also concerned with amelioration of bone loss in the skeleton of astronauts, but their approach has been to intermittently strike the heel of the orbiting subject with a pneumatic "mallet" (Goodship *et al.* 1997), thus again drawing attention to the possibility of a common pathway between external and internal pressure transduction. It should be borne in mind, however, that pathways of bone loss through disuse, and the pathway of mineral gain via weight-bearing activity, are almost certainly different. There is a clear discrepancy between the greater bone loss following disuse, perhaps through weightlessness or immobilization, and the amount gained by physical loading. A 1–2% increase in bone mass may occur within 12 months of increased activity (shown by longitudinal studies), but 3–4% of regional bone mass may be lost within a single month of immobilization, for instance as a result of prolonged bed rest.

The above discussion implicates streaming potentials as intermediary between pressure and osteocyte response, thus reflecting the current vogue. Annan *et al.* (1985) used a computer simulation which predicted small voltage changes resulting from increased transudation following tourniquet application. Others have criticized the concept on the grounds that the magnitude of SGPs are simply too small to be significant when placed amongst the electrical "noise" generated during normal musculoskeletal function. Fluid *pressure* may directly stimulate cells, and Jendrucko *et al.* (1976) have argued on theoretical grounds that osteocytes experience high hydrostatic pressures in response to stress. Several studies have also shown that bone cells can respond to pressure without electrical signals acting as an intermediary (Rodan *et al.* 1975; Somjen *et al.* 1980; Binderman *et al.* 1984; Yeh & Rodan 1984). It should be noted, however, that transcortical streaming potentials have been associated with pulse pressure in the canine tibia (Otter *et al.* 1990), *in the absence of movement*. Furthermore, both pressure oscillations and electrical potentials disappeared following occlusion of the femoral artery. Occlusion of the femoral vein caused a reduction in amplitudes of streaming potentials and pulse pressure.

In this section attention has been drawn to current ideas of the link between venous impediment and bone formation, implicating both physicochemical changes in the micro-environment of bone-forming cells, and elevated hydrostatic pressures resulting from increased capillary transudation. The latter consideration has led to the suggestion of a common mode of action between the bone adaptations effecting Wolff's law phenomena and increased bone formation following venous obstruction. It must be noted, however, that whilst bone formation is increased in the presence of a constant impediment to venous drainage, *static* loads applied to the skeleton are not recognized as osteogenic stimuli (Lanyon & Rubin 1984). Venous impediment, of course, alters the physicochemical environment of the bone-producing cells, lowering pH and Po_2, and increasing Pco_2; external loading of bone does not produce these effects. To be taken as a valid consideration, then, the suggestion of a common mechanism for venous impediment effects, and external load transduction, must take account of these clear *differences* in biological circumstance, as well as the similarities.

Chapter 23
Vascular control of osteogenesis

Mechanical influences on bone formation

The factors of stress and immobilization (Table 23.1) are clearly important stimuli affecting the operation of Wolff's law. Rubin & Lanyon (1987) are of the opinion that bone remodelling is regulated by an equilibrium between a systemic tendency towards bone resorption and mechanically derived stimuli driving bone formation. This allows them to explain such phenomena as disuse osteoporosis resulting from immobilization or weightlessness. At a mechanical equilibrium the amount of bone production is determined by the relative activities of osteolytic and osteogenic processes. Many hypotheses have been promoted to explain Wolff's law phenomena, but whilst most can explain bone formation in response to load, they often fail to explain bone resorption in absence of load.

Bone, when stressed with either a tensile or compressive force, will lay down more bone. The amount of extra bone formed reaches a maximum as load increases, the peak-magnitude of which varies with any particular bone. Thereafter bone mass decreases in response to a continuing increase in load. Treherne (1981) has termed this effect excess load resorption, but it is sometimes known as pressure necrosis. It is well known that bone decreases in mass if the compressive load is reduced. If a reduction in tensile force also reduces bone mass, then a minimum amount of bone must exist where the effective load

Table 23.1 Factors affecting bone formation and resorption (Arnett 1991)

Systemic hormones	Local factors	Miscellaneous agents
PTH/PTH related peptide	Prostaglandins	Immobilization/weightlessness
1,25 $(OH)_2D_3$	Interleukin-1	Stress/exercise
Calcitonin	Colony stimulating factors	Protons
Sex steroids	Tumour necrosis factors α, β	Calcium
Glucocorticoids	Interferon-γ	Phosphate
Growth hormone	Insulin-like growth factors 1,11	Fluoride
Thyroid hormone	Transforming growth factor α	Biphosphonates
	Epidermal growth factor	Alcohol/tobacco
	Transforming growth factor β	
	Bone morphogenic proteins	
	Platelet-derived growth factor	
	Fibroblast growth factor	
	Vasoactive intestinal peptide	
	Calcitonin gene-related protein	

approaches zero (Treherne 1981). If this is true, it offers a strictly biomechanical explanation for why tubular bones are hollow. The bone medulla is in a region termed by engineers, the neutral axis, which experiences little if any load and hence will show minimal stress-induced bone formation. Prolonged space flight experiments have shown that bone mineral density decreases. There are large regional differences in loss of bone mineral, perhaps related to the unequal distribution of venous pressure (McCarthy & Hughes 1996). Bed rest experiments have also shown rapid bone mineral loss and similar effects have been seen using a rat tail-suspension model; here, the mineral loss is in the suspended hind limb skeleton (see review in Dillaman & Roer 1993).

An adequate explanation of the transduction mechanisms affecting Wolff's law must therefore explain both sides of the force equation. Early theories were concerned with bone mineral solubility, and its alterations in response to pressure. If the applied load changes, then the solubility of hydroxyapatite is changed, altering the calcium concentration in the extracellular fluid. Alteration in calcium concentration would stimulate differential osteoblast or osteoclast activity to adjust the amount of bone according to the load experienced (Justus & Luft 1970). Eriksson (1974) developed this further, equating changes in calcium levels with generation of streaming potentials. Another ingenious theory on the bone mineral theme was proposed by Radin (1974), and was concerned with microfracture formation. It was proposed that increasing compressive loads cause strain or internal bending of bone trabeculae, resulting in microfractures. Each microfracture causes callus to form reparatively, which in turn stiffens the trabecula,eventually preventing further strain and fracture deformation. Yet, for some experimentalists, trabecular microfractures are a great rarity. Anyway, these theories do not explain disuse osteoporosis or excess load resorption.

Strain generated streaming potentials

As discussed in the preceding chapter the majority opinion relating mechanical forces to bone remodelling, holds that streaming potentials are the intermediary stimulus, resulting from deformation-induced changes in interstitial fluid flow. Piezoelectric phenomena as formerly believed are not relevant to physiological wet-bone conditions. Streaming potentials are the predominant electrogenic mechanism for stress-generated signals in physiological conditions, and can arise from the flow of any electrolyte past a charged surface; they are not related to piezoelectricity, and can be recorded from plants by bending their stems, and from plants and bone as a result of "sucking-through" electrolytes by application of a vacuum (Cerquiglini *et al.* 1967).

Pressure hypothesis

Stress-generated electrical activity, whilst an attractive hypothesis, is by no means essential to what is in essence a pressure hypothesis for bone formation (see Chapter 22). Bone cells may respond directly to extracellular fluid shear-pressures resulting from bone deformation, or from the increased intravascular pressures resulting, for instance, from venous impediment. The osteocyte, which represents the final stage in the osteoblast lineage, is the most popular candidate for a transduction cell. The cells are ideally placed in the lacunae of the bone matrix, their communicating processes extending everywhere through the fluid-filled canaliculi. Much biochemical evidence suggests that osteocyte deformation brought about by hydrostatic pressure, is responsible for signals promoting differentiation and matrix remodelling in the Haversian systems of bone cortex. However this ignores many studies which have produced evidence against the simple hypothesis presented here; it may well be that many of the diverse cell types within bone (mast cells, macrophages, fibroblasts, precursor cells, as well as endothelial cells, osteoblasts, osteoclasts and osteocytes) are able to respond to compressive/tensile pressure deformation of their membranes and cyto-architecture. It would be surprising if it were not so (El Haj 1990).

Vascular control of osteogenesis

Irrespective of the cell type and biochemical cascades involved in transduction between applied load and bone cell response, it is clear that many of the processes affecting both normal bone and the changes observed in pathology, entrain changes in the physicochemical environment of the cells. The ways in which mechanical forces may affect bone formation is fully comprehended in the wider concept of the vascular control of osteogenesis, which has the advantage of offering an explanation for the control of bone removal as well as bone formation, the two sides of the osteogenic coin. No offence is intended when we emphasize our subject; the living bone. Applied loads have little effect on dead and dry bone cortex, except a weak piezoelectric one. In wet dead bone, even that is obliterated by streaming potentials of a much greater magnitude generated in the deformed microchannels of bone substance.

The osseous circulation subserves many functions, for example blood formation and the continual remodelling of bone cortex, involving simultaneous bone formation and bone removal in response to applied forces, and the nutritional requirements of the skeleton and, in pregnant women, that of the fetus. Of the most immediate importance to the economy of the body, the blood supply of bone makes possible the rapid exchange of ions, particularly calcium, phosphate, sodium and hydrions, between bone crystal and the circulating blood, thus ensuring the homeostasis of body fluids. For example, a single tracer dose of ^{45}Ca radio-calcium gluconate injected into the living subject vanishes from the blood in less than 30 seconds, lost in the vast quantity of skeletal bone crystal, and thereby conserving the constancy of calcium concentration in blood plasma. At the same time it is also responsible for the proliferation of bone cells, and for the growth and renewal of bone substance, and thus for the provision and maintenance of a system of mechanical levers for locomotion, respiration and mastication.

There are many factors, hormones, peptides, vitamins, amino acids and salts,which participate in bone growth in general, and in the constant renewal of bone substance by virtue of their being carried by the osseous circulation to the skeleton as a whole. Local variations, however, in bone turnover are almost certainly linked with changes in the local vascular conditions and in particular, from one autonomous microregion to the next (Pfeiffer *et al.* 1995).

Brookes (1971) built up an hypothesis that a *diminished pH and raised* Pco_2 brings about *bone accumulation*, on physicochemical evidence derived from: normal bones possessing growing and non-growing ends, as well as in experimental venous engorgement; clinical osteoarthrosis of the hip; impacted fractures of the femoral neck; experimental osteotomies and arteriovenous anastomoses present either by accident or design; heterotopic bone formation in scar tissue; tuberculous foci and in the lungs in mitral stenosis; and in the dactylitis associated with tertiary syphilitic end-arteritis. All of the above lend support to the concept that a *local acidosis* in the microenvironment of cells possessing an osteogenic potency, provides a stimulus for bone accumulation. Furthermore, he also showed that the contrary applied (a difficulty for pure mechanists) in that a *raised pH and reduced* Pco_2 brings about *bone softening*. The physicochemical evidence was found in the alkalotic environment of normal cancellous bone; soft callus formation and bone remodelling in experimental fracture repair; extracapsular fractures of the femoral neck prior to internal fixation; cortical bone softening in occlusive vascular disease following periosteal arterialization; and also following experimental generation of a periosteal arterial inflow; from the facts of senescence; the relief of osteoarthritis by osteotomy; and in Paget's disease of bone. In all the above circumstances, a *local alkalosis* was associated with bone loss. Davis & Wood (1993) in their canine *ex vivo* perfusion model, further confirm that osteogenesis is under vascular control. Essentially, they have found that alkalosis increases the vascular resistance by more than 50%, severely depressing the blood flow, whereas acidosis reduces it by 18%, i.e. elevating the blood flow.

Sufficient evidence has been put forward in the preceding pages to indicate the importance to be attached to haemodynamic factors in the control of osteogenesis. More still needs to be known concerning the variability in the osseous circulation of the pH, the Pco_2 and Po_2, the rate of blood flow, and intravascular pressures and mural shear forces generated in blood vessels during normal usage and locomotion.

Envoi

It is clear that the major haemodynamic characteristics of the osseous circulation command a central position in the control of bone growth and renewal, and also make possible the transduction of applied forces. Against the vascular background a plethora of factors operate, variously modulating bone formation and resorption. Table 23.1 shows a list of substances and conditions drawn up by Arnett (1991), to which many more may now be added including the ubiquitous nitric oxide. A full discussion of these factors is outside the scope of this book, but see Chapters 8 ("Regulators and mediators") and Chapter 9 ("Factors acting on blood flow in cortex). It is plain that time is needed before the molecular factors controlling bone micrometabolism, have been salted out and verified.

The evidence to date indicates that the dynamics of the living osseous circulation are variable, and new equilibria can be set up between bone cells and their environment. More data from a variety of experimental situations, and not only those confined to a Petri dish, are clearly needed before a precise, quantitative and molecular description of the vascular control of osteogenesis can be given.

The evidence available, however, does point to the importance of the pH and the respiratory gas tensions in bone blood vessels for maintaining the life of bone, and making possible the production and release of cell-to-cell messengers. These chemical factors and electrical signals provide precision and accuracy to the control of normal bone formation and renewal, and determining whether excess bone accumulates, or bone softening and excavation occurs in bone disease.

Bibliography

Aalto K, Slätis P (1984) Blood flow in rabbit osteotomies studied with radioactive microspheres. *Acta Orthop Scand* **55:** 637–639.
Abramson DI (1962) In: *Blood Vessels and Lymphatics* (ed DI Abramson), London: Academic.
Acheson RM (1960) In: *Human Growth* (ed JM Tanner), Oxford: Pergamon.
Adkins EWO, Davies DV (1940) Absorption from the joint cavity. *QJ Exp Physiol* **30:** 147–154.
Ahlqvist J, Harlilainen A, Aalto K, Sama S, Lalia M, Osterlund K (1994) High hydrostatic pressures in traumatic joints require elevated synovial capillary pressure probably associated with arteriolar vasodilation. *Clin Physiol* **14:** 671–679.
Akeson WH, Eichelberger L, Roma M (1958) Biochemical studies of articular cartilage. II. Values following the denervation of an extremity. *J. Bone Joint Surg* **40A:** 153–162.
Albinus BS (1754) *Academicarum Annotationum Liber III*, Leidae: J & H Verbeek.
Albuquerque M, Isabel A (1993) Phleboscintigraphy of the superior tibial metaphysis in the osteoarthritic knee. *ARCO News Letter* **5:** 6–12.
Altmann K (1950) Untersuchungen über Frakturheilung unter besonderen experimentallen Bedingungen. Ein Beitrag zur Biomechanik der Frakturheilung. *Z Anat EntwGesch* **115:** 52–81.
Amato VP, Bombelli R (1959) The normal vascular supply of the vertebral column in the growing rabbit. *J Bone Joint Surg* **41B:** 782–795.
Amprino R (1953) La croissance et la remaniement des os étudiées par l'emploi du radiocalcium. *C R Assoc Anat* **74:** 493–498.
Amprino R (1955) Struttura microscopica e rinnovamente delle ossa. *Atti Soc Ital Patol* **4:** 9–68.
Amprino R (1968) Bone histophysiology. *Guy's Hosp Rep* **116:** 51–69.
Amprino R, Bairatti A (1936) Processi di ricostruzione e di riassorbimento nella sostanza compatta delle ossa dell'uomo. *Z Zellforsch Mikrosk Anat* **24:** 439–511.
Amprino R, Marotti G (1964) A topographic quantitative study of the bone formation and reconstruction. In: *Proceedings of the First European Bone and Tooth Symposium*, Oxford: Pergamon.
Amprino R, Sisto L (1946) Analogies et différences de structure dans les différentes régions d'un même os. *Acta Anat* **2:** 202–214.
Anderson CE, Parker J (1966) Invasion and resorption in endochondral ossification. An electron microscopic study. *J Bone Joint Surg* **48A:** 899–914.
Anderson DW (1960) Studies of the lymphatic pathways of bone and bone marrow. *J Bone Joint Surg* **42A:** 716–717.
Anderson JC, Eriksson C (1970) Piezoelectric properties of dry and wet bone. *Nature* **227:** 491–492.
Anderson R (1951) Diodrast studies of the vertebral and cranial venous systems. *J Neurosurg* **8:** 411–422.
Annan I, Bronk J, An K-N, Kelly PJ (1985) Stimulation of bone growth and remodelling by raised venous pressure: a proposed explanation. *Fed Proc* **44:** 1760.
Anseroff NJ (1934) Die Arterien der langen Knochen des Menschen. *Z Anat EntwGesch* **103:** 793–812.
Archie JP, Fixler DE, Ullyot DJ, Hoffman JI, Utley JR, Carlson (1973) Measurement of cardiac output with end organ trapping of radioactive microspheres. *J Appl Physiol* **35:** 148–154.
Ardan NI, Janes JM, Herrick JF (1957) Ultrasonic energy and surgically produced defects in bone. *J Bone Joint Surg* **39A:** 394–402.
Aries LJ (1941) Experimental analysis of the growth pattern and rates of appositional and longitudinal growth in the rat femur. *Surg Gynecol Obstet* **72:** 679–689.
Arkin AM, Katz JF (1956) The effects of pressure on epiphyseal growth. The mechanism of plasticity of growing bone. *J Bone Joint Surg* **38A:** 1056–1076.

Arlet J, Ficat P, Sebag D (1968) Intéret de la mesure de la pression intra-médullaire dans le massif trochantérien chez l'homme, en particulier pour le diagnostic de l'ostéonécrose fémoro-capitale. *Rev Rhum* **35:** 250–256.

Arnett TR (1991) Physiology of the skeleton. In: *Osteoporosis* (ed Stevenson), Update Postgraduate Centre Series, Guildford: Reed Healthcare Communications, 10–13.

Arnett TR, Dempster DW (1990) Perspectives, protons and osteoclasts. *J Bone Min Res* **5:** 1099–1103.

Arnett TR, Boyde A, Jones SJ, Taylor ML (1994) Effects of medium acidification by alteration of carbon dioxide or bicarbonate concentrations on the resorptive activity of rat osteoclasts. *J Bone Min Res* **9:** 375–379.

Arnoldi CC, Lemperg RK, Linderholm H (1971) Immediate effect of osteotomy on the intramedullary pressure of the femoral head and neck in patients with degenerative osteoarthritis. *Acta Orthop Scand* **42:** 357–365.

Arnoldi CC, Linderholm H, Müssbichler H (1972) Venous engorgement and intraosseous hypertension in osteoarthritis of the hip. *J Bone Joint Surg* **54B:** 409–421.

Arnoldi CC, Lemperg RK, Linderholm H (1975) Intra-osseous hypertension and pain in the knee. *J Bone Joint Surg* **57B:** 360–363.

Arnoldi CC, Reinmann I, Christenson S, Mortensen S (1979) The effect of increased intra-articular pressure on juxtachondral bone marrow pressure. *IRCS Med Sci* **7:** 471.

Asbø-Hansen G (1950) The origin of synovial mucin; Ehrlich's mast cell, secretory element of connective tissue. *Ann Rheum Dis* **9:** 149–157.

Aschoff KAL (1906) Zur Frage der Cholesterinbildung in der Gallenblase. *Münch Med Wschr* **3:** 1847–1848.

Aschoff KAL (1922) Das retikulo-endotheliale System und seine Beziehungen zur Gellenfarbstoffbindung. *Münch Med Wschr* **69:** 1352–1356.

Aschoff KAL (1924) Das retikulo-endotheliale System. *Ergebn Inn Med Kinderheilkd* **3:** 1–118.

Aschroft GP, Evans NT, Roeda D, Dodd M, Mallard J, Porter W, Smith F (1992) *In vivo* bone blood flow measurement with positron emission tomography (a study of patients with tibial fractures). *J Bone Joint Surg* **74B:** 673–677.

Asling CW, Evans HM (1956) In: *The Biochemistry and Physiology of Bone* (ed GH Bourne), New York: Academic.

Aubin ML, Leriche H, Aboulker J, Ernest C, Ecoiffier J, Metzger J (1976) Cavo-spinal phlebography in myelopathies of venous origin. Application of the method in 115 cases *Acta Radiol Suppl* **347:** 403–413.

Aukland K, Bower BF, Berlinger RW (1964) Measurement of local blood flow with hydrogen gas. *Circ Res* **14:** 10–22.

Axhausen G (1926) Die aseptische Knochennecrose und ihre Bedeutung für die Knochen und Gelenkchirugie. *Acta Chir Scand* **60:** 369–396.

Azuma H (1964) Intraosseous pressure as a measure of haemodynamic changes in bone marrow. *Angiology* **15:** 396–406.

Bachmann G, Pfeifer T, Spies H, Katthagen BD (1993) 3D-CT and angiography of cast preparations of pelvic vessels: demonstration of arterial blood supply of the acetabulum. *ROFO* **158:** 214–220.

Baldes EJ, Herrick JF, Essex HE (1933) Modification in thermostromuhr method of measuring flow of blood. *Proc Soc Exp Biol Med* **30:** 1109–1111.

Balthasar A (1952) Die Bedeutung der Aufsplitterung nach Kirschner für die Behandlung der verzörten Callusbildung. *Mschr Unfallheilk Invalidenw* **55:** 308–314.

Barcroft J (1946) *Researches on Prenatal Life*; Oxford: Blackwell.

Barkow JCL (1868) *Comparative Morphologie des Menschen und der Thiere*, Theil 6, Breslau: Hirt.

Barland P, Novikoff AB, Hamerman D (1962) Electron microscopy of human synovial membrane. *J Cell Biol* **14:** 207–220.

Barnett CH, Harrison, RJ, Tomlinson JDW (1958) Variations in the venous systems of mammals. *Biol Rev* **33:** 442–487.

Barnett CH, Davies DV, MacConaill MA (1960) *Synovial Joints, their structure and mechanics*, London: Longmans.

Bassett CAL (1965a) Electro-mechanical factors regulating bone architecture. In: *Calcified Tissues* (ed. H Fleisch *et al.*), Berlin: Springer.

Bassett CAL (1965b) Electrical effects in bone. *Sci Am* **213:** 18–25.

Bassett CAL, Becker RO (1962) Generation of electrical potentials in bone in response to mechanical stress. *Science* **137:** 1063–1064.

Batson OV (1940) Function of vertebral veins and their role in the spread of metastases. *Ann Surg* **112:** 138–149.

Bauer W, Short CL, Bennett GA (1933) The manner of removal of proteins from normal joints. *J Exp Med* **57:** 419–433.
Bauer W, Ropes MW, Waine H (1940) The physiology of articular structures. *Physiol Rev* **20:** 272–312.
Bazett HC, McGlone B (1928) Notes on pain sensations which accompany deep punctures. *Brain* **51:** 18–23.
Bednar MS, Arnoczky SP, Weiland AJ (1991) The microvasculature of the triangular fibrocartilage complex: its clinical significance. *J Hand Surg* **16A:** 1101–1105.
Bélanger EF (1954) Autoradiographic visualization of the entry and transit of S^{35} in cartilage, bone and dentine of young rats and the effects of hyaluronidase *in vitro*. *Can J Biochem Physiol* **32:** 161–169.
Bélanger EF, Migicovsky BB, Copp DH, Vincent J (1963) Resorption without osteoclasts (osteolysis). In: *Mechanisms of Hard Tissue Destruction* (ed RF Sognnaes), Washington: American Association for the Advancement of Science.
Belchier J (1736) An account of the bones of animals being changed to a red colour by aliment only. *Phil Trans R Soc* **39:** 287–288.
Bell J (1823) *The Anatomy and Physiology of the Human Body*, 5th edn, London: Longman, Hurst, Rees, Orme & Brown.
Benassi E (1931) Lo sviluppo e trofismo dello scheletro degli arti in rapporto alla allacciatura dei vasi principali. *Archo Ital Chir* **28:** 49–68.
Bennett GA, Shaffer MF (1939) The passage of proteins from the vascular system into joints and certain other body cavities. *J Exp Med* **70:** 277–291.
Bérard A (1835) Mémoirs sur le rapport qui existe entre la direction des conduits nourriciers des os longs, et l'ordre suivant lequel les épiphyses se soudent au corps de l'os. *Arch Gén Méd Series 2* **7:** 176–183.
Bergmann E (1927) Theoretisches, Klinisches und Experimentelles zur Frage der aseptischen Knochennekrosen. *Dt Z Chir* **206:** 12–87.
Bernstein MA (1933) Experimental production of arthritis by artificially produced pasive congestion *J Bone Joint Surg* **15:** 661–673.
Berry JL, Thaeler-Oberdoerster DA, Greenwald AS (1986) Subchondral pathways to the superior surface of the human talus. *Foot Ankle* **7(1):** 2–9.
Bhaskar SN, Weinmann JP, Schour I, Greep RO (1950) The growth pattern of the tibia in normals and in rats. *Am J Anat* **86:** 439–477.
Bichat X (1801) *Anatomie Générale*, vol. 3, Paris: Brosson, Gabon.
Bick EM (1948a) Criteria of healing in fractures following internal fixation. *NY State J Med* **48:** 277–279.
Bick EM (1948b) Structural patterns of callus in fractures of long bones; with special reference to healing after internal fixation. *J Bone Joint Surg* **30A:** 141–150.
Bick EM (1951) The ring apophysis of the human vertebra. *J Bone Joint Surg* **33A:** 783–787.
Bick EM, Copel JW (1950) Longitudinal growth of the human vertebra. A contribution to human osteogenesis. *J Bone Joint Surg* **32A:** 803–814.
Bidder A (1906) Osteobiologie. *Arch Mikrosk Anat* **68:** 137–213.
Bier AKG (1905) *Hyperaemia as a Therapeutic Agent* (translated edition by GM Blech), Chicago.
Bier AKG (1918) Beobachtungen über Regeneration beim Menschen. Regeneration der Knochen. *Dtsch Med Wschr* **44:** 281–284.
Bikle DD, Stesin A, Halloran B, Steinbach L, Recker R (1993) Alcohol-induced bone disease: relationship of age and parathyroid hormone levels. *Alcoholism Clin Exp Res* **17:** 690–695.
Bill A (1962) Studies of the heated thermocouple principle for determinations of blood flow in tissues *Acta Physiol Scand* **84:** 111–126.
Binderman I, Shimshoni Z, Sonjen D (1984) Biochemical pathways involved in the translation of physical stimulus into biological message. *Calcif Tiss Int* **36:** S82–S85.
Bing RJ, Hammond M, Handelsman J, Powers S, Spencer F (1949) Coronary blood flow, cardiac oxygen consumption and cardiac efficiency in man. *Bull Johns Hopkins Hosp* **84:** 396–400.
Bing RJ, Maraist FM, Dammann JF, Draper A, Heimbecker R, Daley R, Gerard R, Calazel P (1950) Effect of strophanthus on coronary blood flow and cardiac oxygen consumption of normal and failing human hearts. *Circulation* **2:** 513–516.
Bisgard JD (1931) Effect of sympathetic ganglionectomy upon bone growth *Proc Soc Exp Biol Med* **29:** 229–230.
Bisgard JD (1933) Longitudinal bone growth. Influence of sympathetic deinnervation. *Ann Surg* **97:** 374–380.
Bisgard JD, Bisgard ME (1935) Longitudinal growth of bones *Arch Surg* **31:** 568–578.
Bizzozero G (1868) Sulla funzione ematopoietica del midollo delle ossa *Zentbl Med Wiss* **6:** 885.

Bizzozero G (1869) Sul midollo dell ossa. *Il Morgagni, Naples* **11:** 617.
Bizzozero G (1872) Sul midollo dell ossa. *Il Morgagni, Naples* **14:** 23.
Bloom W, Fawcett DW (1962) *Textbook of Histology*, 8th edn, Philadelphia: Saunders.
Bloom W, Bloom MA, McLean FC (1941) Calcification and ossification. Medullary bone changes in the reproductive cycle of female pigeons *Surg Gynecol Obstet* **94:** 215–222.
Bloomenthal ED, Olsen WH, Necheles H (1952) Studies on bone marrow cavity of the dog. Fat embolism and marrow pressure. *Surg Gynecol Obstet* **94:** 215–222.
Blount WP (1937) Blount's disease; osteochondrosis of medial aspect of upper tibial epiphysis causing tibia vara.
Bourliére F (1950) Senescence et vitesse de cicatrisation chez le rat. *Rev Méd Liège* **5:** 669–671.
Bove AA, Famiand FC, Levin LL, Carey RA, Pierce AL, Lynch PR (1977) Alteration in long bone regional blood flow associated with inadequate decompression in dogs. *Undersea Biomed Res* **4:** 169–182.
Bowsher D (1954) Comparative study of azygos venous system in man, monkey, dog, cat and rabbit. *J Anat* **88:** 400–406.
Bragdon JH, Foster L, Sosman MC (1949) Experimental infarction in bone and marrow. *Am J Pathol* **25:** 709–723.
Brånemark P-I (1958) A method for vital microscopy of mammalian bone marrow *in situ. Univ Arsska Lund* **54:** 5–41.
Brånemark P-I (1959) Vital microscopy of bone marrow in the rabbit. *Scand J Clin Lab Invest* **11:** Suppl 38.
Brash JC (1924) The growth of the jaws and palate. In: *The Growth of the Jaws, Normal and Abnormal, in health and disease*, London: Dental Board of the United Kingdom.
Bray RC, Butterwick DJ, Doschak MR, Tyberg JV (1996) Coloured microsphere assessment of blood flow to knee ligaments in adult rabbits; effects of injury. *J Orthop Res* **14:** 618–625.
Breschet G (1820) *Recherches anatomiques, physiologiques et pathologiques sur le Système veineux, et specialement sur les canaux des os*, Thèse. Paris.
Briant TD, Dale GG, Harris WR (1961) Referred to in: *Histology*, 4th edn, by AW Ham & TS Leeson, Philadelphia: Lippincott.
Bridgeman G, Brookes M (1990) The blood supply of the patella in the aged. In: *Bone Circulation and Bone Necrosis*, (ed. J Arlet, B Mazières), Berlin: Springer, 20–25.
Bridgeman G, Brookes M (1996) Blood supply to the human femoral diaphysis in youth and senescence. *J Anat* **188:** 611–621.
Bridgeman G, Brookes M (1997) Unpublished data.
Brinker MR, Lipton HL, Cook SD (1990) Pharmacological regulation of the circulation of bone. *J Bone Joint Surg* **72A:** 964–975.
Broca PP (1856) *Des anévrysmes et de leur traitement*, Paris: Labé.
Brodin H (1955) Paths of nutrition in articular cartilage and intervertebral discs. *Acta Orthop Scand* **24:** 177–183.
Bronk JT, Meadows TH, Kelly P (1993) The relationship of increased capillary filtration and bone formation. *Clin Orthop Rel Res* **293:** 338–345.
Brookes CH, Revell WJ, Heatley FW (1993) Vascularity of the humeral head after proximal humeral fractures; an anatomical cadaver study. *J Bone Joint Surg* **75B:** 132–136.
Brookes M (1957) Femoral growth after occlusion of the principal nutrient canal in day-old rabbits. *J Bone Joint Surg* **39B:** 563–571.
Brookes M (1958a) The vascularization of long bones in the human fetus. *J Anat* **92:** 261–267.
Brookes M (1958b) The vascular architecture of tubular bone in the rat. *Anat Rec* **132:** 25–47.
Brookes M (1960a) The vascular reaction of tubular bones to ischaemia in peripheral occlusive vascular disease. *J Bone Joint Surg* **42B:** 110–125.
Brookes M (1960b) Sequelae of experimental partial ischaemia in long bones of the rabbit. *J Anat* **94:** 552–561.
Brookes M (1963) Cortical vascularization and growth in fetal tubular bones. *J Anat* **97:** 597–609.
Brookes M (1964) The blood supply of bones. In: *Modern Trends in Orthopaedics - 4: Science of Fractures* (ed JMP Clark), London: Butterworths.
Brookes M (1965) Red cell volumes and vascular patterns in long bones. *Acta Anat* **62:** 35–52.
Brookes M (1966a) The vascular factor in osteoarthritis. *Surg Gynecol Obstet* **123:** 1255–1260.
Brookes M (1966b) Haemodynamic data on the osseous circulation. In: *Calcified Tissue* (eds H Fleisch, HJJ Blackwood, M Owen), Berlin: Springer, 101–104.
Brookes M (1967a) The osseous circulation. *Biomed Eng* **2:** 294–299.
Brookes M (1967b) Blood flow rates in compact and cancellous bone and bone marrow. *J Anat* **101:** 533–541.

Brookes M (1968) A measurement of the rates of blood flow, circulating red cell volume and velocity in bone marrow and cortex. *Acta Anat* **69:** 201–209.
Brookes M (1970) Arteriolar blockade: a method of measuring blood flow rates in the skeleton. *J Anat* **106:** 557–563.
Brookes M (1971) *The Blood Supply of Bone: an approach to bone biology*, London: Butterworth.
Brookes M (1972) Restoration of blood flow to ischaemic knee joints by vitallium implants. *Guy's Hosp Rep* **121:** 31–35.
Brookes M (1974a) La circulation osseuse normal et pathologique. In: *La Circulation Osseuse* (eds J Ficat, J Arlet), Paris: INSERM, 5–13.
Brookes M (1974b) Approaches to non-invasive blood flow measurements in bone. *Biomed Eng* **9:** 342–347.
Brookes M (1978) Blood flow measurements by fractional distribution compared with ^{18}F uptake in the skeleton. In: *Circulation Osseuse (2nd SICO)* (eds J Arlet, P Ficat), Toulouse: Université Paul Sabatier, 141–147.
Brookes M (1986) An anatomy of the osseous circulation. *Bone* **3:** 32–34.
Brookes M (1987a) Blood flow measurement in bone, Part I. *Bone* **4:** No 2, 22–24.
Brookes M (1987b) Blood flow measurement in bone, Part II. *Bone* **4:** No 3, 33–36.
Brookes M (1988) *Blood Flow in the Diaphysis of Long Bones*, Strasbourg: AIOD.
Brookes M (1990a) Arteriosclerosis in the arteries of bone. A translation from the German, of a "lost" paper by the late Erich Ramseier. *ARCO Bull* **2:** No 2, 104–112.
Brookes M (1990b) Blood flow in the diaphysis of long bones. *ARCO Bull*, **2:** No 2, 75–85.
Brookes M (1990c) The effect of a pulsed electromagnetic field on sclerosing bone. In: *Proceedings of Symposium on the Response of Bone to Electrical Stimulation*, University of Bristol.
Brookes M (1993) Morphology and distribution of blood vessels and blood flow in bone. In: *Bone Circulation and Vascularization in Normal and Pathological Conditions* (eds A Schoutens, SPF Hughes, J Gardenières, J Arlet), New York: Plenum, 19–28.
Brookes M, Gallanaugh SC (1975) Circulatory depression in bone after acrylic implantation. *Clin Orthop Rel Res* **107:** 274–276.
Brookes M, Harrison RG (1957) The vascularization of the rabbit femur and tibiofibula. *J Anat* **91:** 61–72.
Brookes M, Helal B (1968a) Vascular factors in osteogenesis. In: *Proceedings of the Symposium Ossium, London, Edinburgh: Livingstone*, 129–132.
Brookes M, Helal B (1968b) Primary arthritis, venous engorgement and osteogenesis. *J Bone Joint Surg* **50B:** 493–504.
Brookes M, Irving M (1962) Neural factors in the genesis of bone atrophy. *J Anat* **96:** 413–414.
Brookes M, Landon DN (1963) The juxta-epiphyseal vessels in the long bones of fetal rats. *J Bone Joint Surg* **46B:** 336–345.
Brookes M, May KU (1972) The influence of temperature on bone growth in the chick. *J Anat* **111:** 351–363.
Brookes M, Richards DJ (1968) Osteogenesis and the pH of the osseous circulation. *Calcif Tissue Res* **2:** Suppl 93–93A.
Brookes M, Richards DJ (1969) Physico-chemical sequelae of experimental osteotomy. *Proc R Soc Med* **62:** 435–438.
Brookes M, Singh M (1972a) Venous shunt in bone after ligation of the femoral vein. *Surg Gynecol Obstet* **135:** 85–88.
Brookes M, Singh M (1972b) Bone blood pH and gas tensions after femoral vein ligation. *Surg Gynecol Obstet* **135:** 873–876.
Brookes M, Wardle EN (1962) Muscle action and the shape of the femur. *J Bone Joint Surg* **44B:** 398–411.
Brookes M, Richards DJ, Singh M (1970) Vascular sequelae of experiment osteotomy. *Angiology* **21:** 355–367.
Brookes M, Elkin AC, Harrison RG, Heald CB (1961) A new concept of capillary circulation in bone cortex. Some clinical applications. *Lancet* **i:** 1078–1081.
Bruch CWL (1852) Beiträge zur Entwicklungsgeschichte des Knochensystems. *Denkschr schweiz Naturf Ges* **12:** 1–76.
Brueton RN, Brookes M (1995) Intramedullary reaming and callus formation. In: *Dynamische Osteosynthese* (eds RH Gahr, W Hein, H Seidel), Berlin Heidelberg: Springer, 7–17.
Brueton RN, Hughes SW, Revell WJ (1996) Bone volume changes following reaming and nailing of the rabbit tibia. *ARCO Newslett* **8:** 106.
Brueton RN, Revell WJ, Brookes M (1993a) Haemodynamics of bone healing in a model stable fracture. In: *Bone Circulation and Vascularization in Normal and Pathological Conditions* (eds, A Schoutens, SPF Hughes, J Gardenières, J Arlet), New York; Plenum, 121–128.

Brueton RN, Revell WJ, Brookes M (1993b) Surgical interventions on unfractured bones: vascular and histological sequelae. *ARCO Bulletin, Toulouse*, **5:** 88–89.

Buckberg GD, Luck JC, Payne DG, Hoffman LIE, Archie JP, Fixler DE (1971) Some sources of error in measuring regional blood flow with radioactive microspheres. *J Appl Physiol* **31:** 598–604.

Buckland-Wright JC, MacFarlane DG, Lynch J, Clark B (1990) Quantitative microfocal radiographic assessment of progression in generalized osteoarthritis of the hands. *Arth Rheum* **33:** 57.

Buerger L, Oppenheimer A (1908) Bone formation in sclerotic arteries. *J Exp Med* **10:** 354–367.

Bullough WS, Laurence EB (1961) The control of mitotic activity in the skin. In: *Wound Healing* (ed D Slome), London: Pergamon.

Bullough WS, Laurence EB, Iversen OH, Elgjo K (1967) The vertebrate chalone *Nature, Lond* **214:** 578–580.

Bunger C (1987) Haemodynamics of the juvenile knee. Joint effusion and synovial inflammation studied in dogs. *Acta Orthop Scand Suppl* **222:** 1–104.

Bunger C, Harving S, Hjermind J, Bunger EH (1983) Relationship between intra-osseous pressures and intra-articular pressures in arthritis of the knee. *Acta Orthop Scand* **54:** 188–193.

Bunting CH (1919) The regulation of the red blood-cell supply. *Contr Med Biol Res NY* **2:** 824–828.

Burger RE, Estavillo JA (1977) Pulmonary circulation-vertebral venous interconnections in the chickens. *Anat Rec* **188:** 39–43.

Burrows HJ (1941) Coxa plana, with special reference to its pathology and kinship. *Br J Surg* **29:** 23–36.

Bywaters EGL (1937) The metabolism of joint tissues. *J Path Bact* **44:** 247–268.

Caeiro JC, Mainetti H (1932) La circulatión diafisiara en los huesos largos. Su importancia en la etiologia de las seudo-artrosis. *Prensa Méd Argent* **18:** 1156–1167.

Caesar J, Shaldon S, Chiandussi L, Guevara L, Sherlock S (1961) The use of indocyanine green in the measurement of hepatic blood flow and as a test of hepatic function. *Clin Sci* **21:** 43–57.

Cajori FA, Crouter CY, Pemberton R (1926) The physiology of synovial fluid. *Arch Intern Med* **37:** 92–101.

Calvo W (1968) The innervation of bone marrow in laboratory animals. *Am J Anat* **123:** 315–328.

Camera U (1953) A proposito delle arthroplastiche dell'anca ed un proposito di un nuovo indovizzo nel trattamento del artrosi. *Minerva Orthop* **4:** 1.

Cameron DA (1961) Erosion of the epiphysis of the rat tibia by capillaries. *J Bone Joint Surg* **43B:** 590–594.

Carey EJ (1929) Studies in the dynamics of histogenesis. Experimental, surgical and roentgenological studies in the architecture of human cancellous bone, the resultant of back pressure vectors of muscle action. *Radiol* **13:** 127–168.

Carlson CS, Meuten DJ, Richardson DC (1991) Ischemic necrosis of cartilage in spontaneous and experimental lesions of osteochondroses. *J Orthop Res* **9:** 317–329.

Carlson CS, Cullins LD, Meuten DJ (1995) Osteochondrosis of the articular-epiphyseal cartilage complex in young horses: evidence for a defect in cartilage canal blood supply. *Vet Pathol* **32:** 641–647.

Carlson H (1957) Reaction of rabbit patellar cartilage following operative defects. *Acta Orthop Scand Suppl* **28:** 1–104.

Carrel A, Ebeling AH (1921) Age and multiplication of fibroblasts. *J Exp Med* **34:** 599–623.

Castor CW (1957) Production of mucopolysaccharides by synovial cells in a simplified tissue culture medium. *Proc Soc Exp Biol Med* **94:** 51–56.

Castor CW (1960) The microscopic structure of normal human synovial tissue. *Arthritis Rheum* **3:** 140–151.

Castor CW, Fries FF (1961) Composition and function of human synovial connective tissue cells measured *in vitro*. *J Lab Clin Med* **57:** 394–407.

Castor CW, Muirden KD (1964) Collagen formation in monolayer cultures of human fibroblasts. The effects of hydrocortisone *Lab Invest* **13:** 560–574.

Cerquiglini S, Cignitti M, Marchetti M, Salleo (1967) On the origins of electrical effects produced by stress in the hard tissues of living organisms. *Life Sci* **6:** 2651–2660.

Chakkalakal DA, Johnson MW, Harper RA, Katz JL (1980) Dielectric properties of fluid saturated bone. *IEE Trans Biomed Eng* **BM27:** 95–100.

Charkes ND, Brookes M (1976) Unpublished: A private discussion resulting in the design of a 5-compartmental model for blood flow measurement: the Claude Bernard model.

Charkes ND, Makler PT, Philips C (1978) Studies of skeletal tracer kinetics I: Digital computer solution of a five compartment model of [^{18}F] in humans. *J Nucl Med* **19:** 1302–1309.

Charkes ND, Brookes M, Makler PT (1979a) Radiofluoride kinetics. In: *Principles of Radiopharmacology, III* (ed. LG Colombetti), Boca Raton, Florida: CRC Press, 225–242.

Charkes ND, Brookes M, Makler PT (1979b) Studies of skeletal tracer kinetics: evaluation of a five compartmental model of ^{18}F fluoride. *J Nucl Med Technol* **20:** 1150–1157.

Charnley J (1959) The lubrication of animal joints. In: *Proceedings of a Symposium on Biomechanics*. London: Institute of Mechanical Engineers.
Cheselden W (1741) *The Anatomy of the Human Body*, 6th edn, London: W Bowyer.
Chidgey LK (1991) Histologic anatomy of the triangular fibrocartilage. *Hand Clin* **7:** No 2, 249–262.
Cho MH, Neuhaus OW (1960) Absence of blood clotting substances from synovial fluid. *Thromb Diath Haemorh* **5:** 108–111.
Christ B (1975) *Die Entwicklung der Körperwandmetamerie: experimentelle Untersuchungen an Hühnerembryonen*. Bochum: *Habilitationsschrift* Ruhruniversität.
Clark WE, Le Gros (1928) An experimental study of the nature of the synovial membrane in joints. *J Anat* **63:** 152–154.
Clark ER, Clark EL (1942) Microscopic observations on new formation of cartilage and bone in the living animal. *Am J Anat* **70:** 167–200.
Clarke JM (1990) The structure of vascular channels in the subchondral plate. *J Anat* **171:** 105–115.
Cochran GV, Pawluk RJ, Bassett CA (1968) Electromechanical characteristics of bone under physiologic moisture conditions. *Clin Orthop* **58:** 249–270.
Cockett FB (1955) The pathology and treatment of venous ulcers of the leg. *Br J Surg* **43:** 260–278.
Coessens BC, Adams ML, Wood MB (1995) Evaluation of influence of 24-hour cold preservation in endothelin production, and on endothelin receptors in the bone vasculature. *J Orthop Res* **13:** No 5, 725–732.
Coessens BC, Miller VM, Wood MB (1996) Endothelin induces vasoconstriction in the bone vasculature *in vitro*: an effect mediated by a single receptor population. *J Orthop Res* **14:** No 4, 611–617.
Cofield RH, Bassingthwaite JB, Kelly P (1975) Strontium-85 extraction during transcapillary passage in tibial bone. *J Appl Physiol* **39:** 596–602.
Cohen J, Harris WH (1958) The three dimensional anatomy of Haversian systems. *J Bone Joint Surg* **40A:** 419–434.
Caollin-Osdoby P (1994) Role of vascular endothelial cells in bone biology. *J Cell Biochem* **55:** No 3, 304–309.
Colt JD, Iger M (1963) An attempt to stimulate bone growth by creating a venous stenosis. *Angiology* **14:** 584–587.
Compère EL, Adams CO (1937) Studies of longitudinal growth in long bones: influence of trauma to the disphysis. *J Bone Joint Surg* **19:** 922–936.
Cooper, Sir Astley Paston (1822) *A Treatise on Dislocations and Fractures of the Joints*. London: Longman, Hurst, Rees, Orme & Brown.
Cooper, Sir Bransby (1837) An experimental enquiry respecting the process of reparation after simple fracture. *Guy's Hosp Rep* **11:** 179–198.
Cooper RR, Milgram JW, Robinson RA (1966) Morphology of the osteon: an electron microscopy study. *J Bone Joint Surg* **48A:** 1239–1271.
Copp DH, Shim SS (1963) The homeostatic function of bone as a mineral reservoir. *Oral Surg* **16:** 738–744.
Copp DH, Shim SS (1965) Extraction ratio and bone clearance of ^{85}SR as a measure of effective bone blood supply. *Circulation Res* **16:** 461–467.
Copp DH, Mensen ED, McPherson GD (1960) Regulation of blood calcium. *Clin Orthop* **17:** 288–296.
Courbil JL (1954) *Recherches sur les artères périostées des os du membre inférieur*, Thèse. Marseille: Schneider.
Cretin A (1952) Paralèlle entre les éléments anatomiques normaux et pathologiques de la maladie rhumatismale. *CR Acad Sci Paris* **235:** 1447–1448.
Crock HV (1967) *The Blood Supply to the Lower Limb Bones in Man*, London: Livingstone.
Crock HV (1996) *An Atlas of the Vascular Anatomy of the Skeleton and Spinal Cord*, London: Martin Dunitz.
Cumming JD (1962) A study of blood flow through bone marrow by a method of venous effluent collection. *J Physiol Lond* **162:** 13–20.
Cumming JD, Nutt ME (1962) Bone marrow blood flow and cardiac output in the rabbit. *J Physiol Lond* **162:** 30–34.
Cunningham GJ (1960) Microradiography. In: *Tools of Biological Research* vol 2 (ed. Sir Hedley JB Atkins), Oxford: Blackwell.
Cunningham RS (1922) On the origin of the free cells of serous exudates. *Am J Physiol* **59:** 1–36.
Curtain CC (1960) Photoelectric comparator for Rayleigh fringe electrophoresis patterns. *J Scient Instrum* **37:** 190–193.
Cuthbertson EM, Siris E, Gilfillan RS (1964) The effect of ligation of the canine nutrient artery on intramedullary pressure. *J Bone Joint Surg* **46A:** 116–122.

Daftari TK, Whitesides TE Jr, Heller JG, Goodrich AC, McCarey BE (1994) Nicotine in the revascularization of bone graft. An experimental study in rabbits. *Spine* **19:** 904–911.

Dahl B (1934) Effets des rayons X sur les os longs en développement: étude radiographique et anatomique. *J Radiol Electrol* **18:** 131–140.

Dale GG, Harris WR (1958) Prognosis of epiphyseal separation an experimental study. *J Bone Joint Surg* **40B:** 116–122.

Dale PA, Bronk JT, Kelly PJ (1989) Fracture healing with elevated venous pressure. *Proc Am Orth Res Soc (Las Vegas)* **35:** 590.

Dale PA, Bronk JT, O'Sullivan ME, Chao EY, Kelly PJ (1993) A new concept in fracture immobilization: the application of a pressurized brace. *Clin Orthop Rel Res* **295:** 264–269.

Damsin JP, Lazennec JY, Gonzales M, Guerin-Surville H, Hannoun L (1992) Arterial supply of the acetabulum in the fetus: application to periarticular surgery in childhood. *Surg Radiol Anat* **14:** No 3, 215–221.

Daniels (1952) Personal communication from the late Professor RG Harrison of Liverpool University. Harrison knew Daniels in Oxford University as the one who devised the first usable continual soft Xray apparatus.

Davies DR, Bassingthwaite JB, Kelly PJ (1979) Blood flow and ion exchange in bone. In: *Skeletal research: an experimental approach (ed. DJ Simmons, AS Kunin)*, New York: Academic Press, 397–420.

Davies DV (1942) The staining reactions of normal synovial membrane with special reference to the origin of synovial mucin. *J Anat* **77:** 160–169.

Davies DV (1950) The structure and functions of the synovial membrane. *Br Med J* **1:** 92–95.

Davies DV (1967) Properties of synovial fluid. In: *Proceedings of a Symposium on Lubrication and Wear in Living and Artificial Human Joints*, London: Institution of Mechanical Engineers.

Davies DV, Edwards DAW (1948) Blood supply of synovial membrane and intra-articular structure. *Ann R Coll Surg* **2:** 142–156.

Davies DV, Young L (1954) The distribution of radioactive (^{35}S) in the fibrous tissues, cartilages and bones of the rat following its administration in the form of inorganic sulphate. *J Anat* **88:** 174–183.

Davies R, Tothill P, Hooper G, Fleming RH, McCarthy ID, Hughes SP (1984) The early effects of sympathectomy on bone blood flow. *Calcif Tissue* **36:** No. 5, 622–624.

Davis TR, Wood MB (1992) Endothelial control of long bone vascular resistance. *J Orthop Res* **10:** No 3, 344–349.

Davis TR, Wood MB (1993) The effects of acidosis and alkalosis on long bone vascular resistance. *J Orthop Res* **11:** 834–839.

Davis TR, Holloway I, Pooley J (1990) The effect of anaesthesia on the bone blood flow of the rabbit. *J Orthop Res* **8:** 479–484.

Davson H, Eggleton G (1968) *Starling and Lovatt Evans Principles of Human Physiology*, 14th edn, London: Churchill

Dean MT, Wood MB, Vanhoutte PM (1992) Antagonist drugs and bone vascular smooth muscle. *J Orthop Res* **10:** No. 1, 104–111.

de Bruyn PPH, Breen PC, Thomas TB (1970) The microcirculation of the bone marrow. *Anat Rec* **168:** 55–68.

Decker B, McGuckin WF, Slocumb CH (1959) Concentration of hyaluronic acid in synovial fluid. *Clin Chem* **5:** 465–469.

Delesse A (1848) In: *Annls Mines* 13: 378. Cited by Dunnill, Anderson & Whitehead (1967) *J Path Bact* **94:** 271–291.

Delesse A (1887) Procédé méchanique pour déterminer la composition des roches (extrait). *CR Acad Sci, Paris* **25:** 544.

de Marneffe R (1951) *Recherches morphologiques et expérimentales sur la vascularisation osseuse*, Brussels: Acta medica Belgica.

de Saint-Georges L, Miller SC (1992) The microcirculation of bone and marrow in the diaphysis of the rat hemopoietic long bones. *Anat Rec* **233:** 169–177.

DeSimone DP, Reddi AH (1992) Vascularization and endochondral bone development: changes in plasminogen activator activity. *J Orthop Res* **10:** 320–324.

Deutsch SD, Gandsman EJ, Spraragen SG (1981) Quantitative regional blood flow analysis and its clinical application during routine bone scanning. *J Bone Joint Surg* **63A:** 295–305.

Dewardener HE (1967) *The Kidney*, 3rd edn, London: Churchill.

Dickinson PH (1953) Venous stasis and bone growth. *Exp Med Surg* **11:** 49–53.

Dieppe P (1987) Clinical aspects of osteoarthritis. In: *Studies in Osteoarthritis; Pathogenesis. intervention, assessment* (ed DJ Lott, MK Jasani, GFB Birdwood), London: Wiley and Sons, 17–20.

Dietz JR, Zucker IH, Bie P, Gilmore JP (1979) Haematocrit as an index of changes of plasma volume in conscious dogs. *Experimentia* **35:** 1064–1065.
Digby KH (1916) The measurement of diaphyseal growth in proximal and distal directions. *J Anat* **50:** 187–188.
Dillaman RM (1984) Movement of ferritin in the 2-day-old chick femur. *Anat Rec* **209:** 445–453.
Dillaman RM, Roer RD (1993) Bone blood flow and space flight osteopaenia. In: *Bone Circulation and Vascularization in Normal and Pathological Conditions.* (Ed. Schoutens A, Arlet J, Gardeniers JWM & Hughes SFF) pp. 185–194. New York: Plenum Press.
Dillaman RM, Roer RD, Gay DM (1991) Fluid movement in bone: theoretical and empirical. *J Biomechan* **24:** Suppl 12, 163–177.
Dintenfass L (1963) Lubrication in synovial joints: a theoretical analysis. *J Bone Joint Surg* **45A:** 1241–1256
Doan CA (1922a) The capillaries of the bone marrow of the adult pigeon. *Bull Johns Hopkins Hosp* **33:** 222–226.
Doan CA (1922b) The circulation of the bone marrow. *Contrib Embryol Carnegie Inst* **13:** 29.
Doan CA (1931) Clinical implications of experimental hematology. *Medicine, Baltimore* **10:** 323–371.
Dodds GS (1930) Row formation and other types of arrangement of cartilage cells in endochondral ossification. *Anat Rec* **46:** 385–399.
Dohler JR, Hennig FF, Hughes SP (1995) Reactivity of cortical bone capillaries. Functional TEM analysis with adrenaline, ATP and insulin. *Langenbecks Arch Chirurg* **380:** 176–183.
Dole WP, Jackson DL, Rosenblatt JI, Thompson WL (1982) Relative error and variability in blood flow measurements with radio-labelled microspheres. *Am J Physiol* **243:** H371–H378.
Dowson D, Higginson GR (1966) *Elasto-hydrodynamic Lubrication*, Oxford: Pergamon.
Draenart K, Draenart Y (1980) The vascular system of bone marrow. *Scan Electron Microsc* **4:** 113–122.
Drinker CK, Drinker KR (1916) A method for maintaining an artificial circulation through the tibia of the dog, with a demonstration of the vasomotor control of the marrow vessels. *Am J Physiol* **40:** 514.
Drinker CK, Drinker KR, Lund CC (1922). Circulation in the mammalian bone marrow. *Am J Physiol* **62:** 1–92.
Dubreuil G (1929) *Leçons d'embryologie humaine*, Paris: Vigot.
Duhamel HL (1739) Sur une racine qui a la faculté de teindre en rouge les os des animaux vivants. *Mém Acad r Sci* **52:** 1–13.
Duhamel HL (1743) Quatrième mémoire sur les os. *Mém Acad r Sci* **56:** 87–111.
Duncan CP, Shim SS (1977) The autonomic nerve supply of bone. *J Bone Joint Surg* **59B:** 323–330.
Dunnhill MS, Anderson JA, Whitehead R (1967) Quantitative histological studies on age changes in bone. *J Path Bact* **94:** 271–291.
du Noüy PL (1932) Une mesure de l'activité physiologique. *Cr Séanc Soc Biol* **109:** 1227–1230.
du Noüy PL (1936) *Biological Time* London: Methuen.
Eckert-Möbius A (1924) Über die Rolle der gefässhaltigen Dtsch Knorpelkanäle bei der enchondralen Verknöcherung. *Dtsch Med Wochenschr* **50:** 1798–1799.
Edholm OG, Howarth S, McMichael J (1945) Heart failure and blood flow in osteitis deformans. *Clin Sci* **5:** 249–260.
Edlund T (1949) Studies in absorption of colloids and fluid from rabbit knee joint. *Acta Physiol Scand* **18:** Suppl 62, 1–108.
Eichelberger L (1960) Hyaline cartilage: the histochemical characterization of the extracellular and intracellular compartments. *Clin Orthop* **17:** 77–91. (See also Akeson *et al.* 1958)
Ekholm R (1951) Articular cartilage nutrition: how radioactive gold reaches the cartilage in rabbit knee joints. *Acta Anat* **11:** suppl 15, 1–76.
Ekholm R (1953) Nutrition of articular cartilage. A radioautographic study. *Acta Anat* **24:** 329–338.
Ekholm R (1956) Osteoarthritis in the knee joint with special reference to the weight-bearing in the joint. *Acta Neerl Morphol* **1:** 1–39.
Ekholm R, Ingelmark BE (1952) Functional thickness variations of human articular cartilage. *Acta Soc Med Upsal* **57:** 39–59.
Eletto L (1933) Ricerche topografiche e radiografiche sulla circolazione arteriosa delle grandi ossa lunghe degli arti, nell' uomo. I Arto superior. *Archo ital Anat Embriol* **31:** 569–581.
El Haj A (1990) Biomechanical bone cell signalling: is there a grapevine? *J Zool Lond* **220:** 689–693.
Enlow DH (1962) A study of the postnatal growth and remodelling of bone. *Am J Anat* **110:** 269–305.
Enneking WF (1948) The repair of complete fractures of rat tibias. *Anat Rec* **101:** 515–537.
Eriksson C (1974) Streaming potentials and other water dependent effects in mineralised tissues. *Ann NY Acad Sci* **238:** 321–338.

Evans EB, Eggers GWN, Butler JK, Blumel J (1960) Experimental immobilization and remobilization of rat knee joints. *J Bone Joint Surg* **42A:** 737–738.
Fahey JJ (1936) Effect of lumbar sympathetic ganglionectomy on longitudinal bone growth as determined by the teleroentgenographic method. *J Bone Joint Surg* **23:** 1042–1046.
Fahraeus R (1929) The suspension stability of the blood. *Phys Rev* **9:** 241.
Failla G (1960) The ageing process and somatic mutations. In: *The Biology of Ageing. AIBS Symposium 6: Washington*, 170–175.
Failla JM (1993) Hook of hamate vascularity: vulnerability to osteonecrosis and nonunion. *J Hand Surg* **18A:** No 6, 1075–1079.
Fan FC, Schuessler GB, Chen RY, Chien S (1979). Determinations of blood flow and shunting of 9 and 15 μm spheres in regional beds. *Am J Physiol* **237:**H25–H33.
Farquhar MG, Palade GE (1963) Junctional complexes in various epithelia. *J Cell Biol* **17:** 375–412.
Fawcett DW (1942) The amedullary bone of the Florida manatee (*Trichechus latirostris*). *Am J Anat* **71:** 271–309.
Fein RS (1967) Are synovial joints squeeze film lubrication? In: *Proceedings of a Symposium on Lubrication and Wear in Living and Artificial Human Joints*, London: Institution of Mechanical Engineers.
Felts WJL (1954) The prenatal development of the human femur. *Am J Anat* **94:** 1–44.
Ferguson WR (1950) Some observations on the circulation in fetal and infant spines. *J Bone Joint Surg* **32A:** 640–648.
Fischer A (1946) Regeneration. In: *Biology of Tissue Cells*, Cambridge: University Press, Chap 7.
Fischer AGT (1923) Physiological principles underlying the treatment of injuries and disease of the articulations. *Lancet* **ii:** 541–548.
Fischer AGT (1929) *Chronic (Non-tuberculous) Arthritis*, London: HK Lewis.
Fischer LP, Noyer D, Gonon GP, Carret JP, Morin A, Clermont A (1977) Arterial vascularization of the os coxae. *Bull Assoc Anatomistes* **61:** 343–356.
Fitzgerald TC (1961) Blood supply of the head of the canine femur. *Vet Med* **56:** 389–394.
Flaim SF, Morris ZQ, Kennedy TJ (1978) Dextran as a radioactive microsphere suspending agent: severe hypotensive effect in the rat. *Am J Physiol* **235:** H587–H591.
Flavell G (1956) Reversal of pulmonary hypertrophic osteoarthropy by vagotomy. *Lancet* **i:** 260–262.
Folkman J (1985) Toward an understanding of osteogenesis: search and discovery. *Perspect Biol Med* **29:** 10–36.
Forsyth RP, Hoffbrand BI (1970) Redistribution of cardiac output after sodium pentobarbitone anaesthetic in the monkey. *Am J Physiol* **218:** 214–217.
Foster LN, Kelly RP, Watts WM (1951) Experimental infarction of bone and bone marrow. *J Bone Joint Surg* **33A:** 396–406.
Foxon GEH (1961) The radiography of small animals in biological research. *Guy's Hosp Rep* **110:** 345–355.
Francis JRD (1958) *A Textbook of Fluid Mechanics for Engineering Students*, London: Edward Arnold.
Frazer EF (1940) *The Anatomy of the Human Skeleton*, London: Churchill.
Frazer JRE, McCall JF (1965) Culture of synovial cells *in vitro*. Notes on isolation and propagation. *Ann Rheum Dis* **24:** 351–359.
Frederickson JM, Honour AJ, Copp DH (1955) Measurement of initial bone clearance of Ca^{45} from blood in the rat. *Fed Proc* **14:** 49.
Frost HM (1960) *In vivo* osteocyte death. *J Bone Joint Surg* **42A:** 138–143.
Fukada E, Yasuda I (1957) On the piezoelectric effect of bone. *J Phys Soc Japan* **12:** 1158–1162.
Fyfe FW (1964) Predominance of epiphyseal over metaphyseal blood supply in nourishment of epiphyseal cartilage. *J Anat* **98:** 471–427.
Gahr RH, Hein W, Seidel H (eds) (1995) *Dynamische Osteosynthese*, Berlin: Springer, xi, 289.
Gardner E (1950) Physiology of movable joints. *Physiol Rev* **30:** 127–176.
Gardner E, Gray DJ (1950) Prenatal development of the human hip joint. *Am J Anat* **87:** 219–260.
Gebhardt W (1901) Über funktionell wichtige Anordnungsweisen der grösseren und feineren Bauelemente des Wirbeltierknochens. *Arch Entw-Mech Org* **11:** 383–498.
Gebhardt W (1905) Über funktionell wichtige Anordnungsweisen der grösseren und feineren Bauelemente des Wirbeltierknochens. *Arch Entw-Mech Org* **20:** 187–334.
Geigy (1962) *Documenta Geigy Scientific Tables*, 6th edn (ed K Diem), Manchester: Geigy Pharmaceutical Company.
Gelberman RH, Gross MS (1986) The vascularity of the wrist. Identification of arterial patterns at risk. *Clin Orthop Rel Res* **202:** 40–49.
Gelberman RH, Menon J (1980) The vascularity of the scaphoid bone. *J Hand Surg* **5A:** No 5, 508–513.

Gelberman RH, Bauman TD, Menon J, Akeson WH (1980) The vascularity of the lunate bone and Kienbock's disease. *J Hand Surg* **5A:** No 3, 272–278.
Gelberman RH, Panagis JS, Taleisnik J, Baumgaertner M (1983) The arterial anatomy of the human carpus. Part I: The extraosseous vascularity. *J Hand Surg* **8A:** No 4, 367–375.
Gelbke (1950) The influence of pressure and tension on growing bone in experiments with animals. *J Bone Joint Surg* **33A:** 947–954.
Girgis FG, Pritchard JJ (1958) Experimental production of cartilage during the repair of fractures of the skull vault in rats. *J Bone Joint Surg* **40B:** 274–281.
Gleaton HE, Alexander SC, Wollman H (1968) Effects of sympathetic blockade and epidural anaesthesia on resting blood flow in the anterior tibial muscle of man. In: *Blood Flow Through Organs and Tissues* (eds WH Bain, AM Harper), London: Livingstone.
Godman GC, Porter KR (1960) Chondrogenesis studied with the electron microscope. *J Biophys Biochem Cytol* **8:** 719–760.
Goldhaber B (1958) The effect of hyperoxia on bone resorption in tissue culture. *Arch Pathol* **66:** 635–641.
Goodship AE, Cunningham JL, Walker P, Organov V, Darling J, Miles AW, Owen G (1997) The application of an impulsive mechanical stimulus prevents bone loss during long term space flight. *J Bone Joint Surg* **79B (suppl III):** 369.
Gowin W (1983) Significance of the venous system of the spine in the formation of metastases *Strahlentherapie* **159:** 682–689.
Graf J, Neusel E, Freese U, Simank H-G, Niethard FU (1992) Subchondral vascularisation and osteoarthritis. *Int Orthop (SICOT)* **16:** 113–117.
Grant WC, Root WS (1947) The relation of O_2 in bone marrow blood to post-hemorrhagic erythropoiesis. *Am J Physiol* **150:** 618–627.
Gray H (1989) *Grays Anatomy*, 37th edn (ed PL Williams *et al.*), London: Churchill Livingstone.
Gray DJ, Gardner E (1950) The prenatal development of the human knee and superior tibiofibular joints. *Am J Anat* **86:** 235–287.
Gray DJ, O'Rahilly R (1957) Prenatal development of the skeleton and joints of the human hand. *Am J Anat* **101:** 169–224.
Gray SJ, Sterling K (1950) The tagging of red cells and plasma proteins with radioactive chromium. *J Clin Invest* **29:** 818.
Greene EC (1935) *The Anatomy of the Rat*, Philadelphia: American Philosophical Society.
Greger R, Winhorst U. (1996) *Comprehensive Human Physiology* (2 volumes), Berlin: Springer.
Gregg PJ, Walder DN (1980) Regional distribution of circulating microspheres in the femur of the rabbit. *J Bone Joint Surg* **62B:** 222–226.
Grégoire R, Carrière C (1921) Circulation arterielle intra-osseuse du fémur et du tibia. *C R Assoc Anat* **16:** 179–185.
Greulich RC, Leblond CP (1953) Radioautographic visualization of radiocarbon in the organs and tissues of new born rats following administration of ^{14}C labelled bicarbonate. *Anat Rec* **115:** 559–585.
Grey EG, Carr GL (1915) An experimental study of the factors responsible for non-infectious bone atrophy. *Bull Johns Hopkins Hosp* **26:** 381–385.
Grey SJ, Sterling K (1950a) The tagging of red cells and plasma proteins with radioactive chromium. *J Clin Invest* **29:** 1604–1613.
Grey SJ, Sterling K (1950b) Determination of circulating red cell volume by radioactive chromium. *Science* **112:** 179.
Grønlund J, Koefod H, Svalastoga E (1984) Effect of increased knee joint pressure on oxygen tension and blood flow in subchondrial bone. *Acta Physiol Scand* **121:** 127–131.
Gross D, Williams (1982) Streaming potentials and the electromechanical response of physiologically wet bone. *J Biomech* **15:** 277–295.
Gross PM, Heistad D, Marcus ML (1979) Neurohumoral regulation of blood flow to bones and marrow: *Am J Physiol* **237:** H440–H448.
Grossfield H, Meyer K, Godman G (1955) Differentiation of fibroblasts in tissue culture as determined by mucopolysaccharide production. *Proc Soc Exp Biol Med* **88:** 31–35.
Gunst MA (1980) Interference with bone blood supply through plating of intact bone. In: *Current Concepts of Internal Fixation of Fractures* (ed HK Uhthoff), Berlin: Springer, 268–276.
Gunter GS (1949) The determination of "Spinnbarkeit" of synovial fluid and its destruction by enzymic action. *Aust J Exp Biol Med Sci* **27:** 265–274.
Guyton AC (1963) Concept of negative interstitial pressure based on pressures in implanted perforated capsules. *Circ Res* **12:** 399–414.
Guyton AC, Hall JE (1996) *Textbook of Medical Physiology* 9th edition. Philadelphia: Saunders & Co.

Haas SL (1939) Growth in length of the vertebrae. *Arch Surg* **38:** 245–249.
Hadhazy C, Varga S (1976) Studies on cartilage formation XIX. Oxygen and glucose supply of the regenerating articular surface. *Acta Biol Sci Hung* **27:** No 4, 215–230.
Haines RW (1933) Cartilage canals. *J Anat* **68:** 45–64.
Haines RW (1947) The development of joints. *J Anat* **81:** 33–55.
Hales JRS (1974) Radioactive microsphere technique for studies of the circulation. *Clin Exp Pharmacol Physiol* suppl 1: 31–46.
Hales Rev Stephen (1727) *Static Essays, vol I: Vegetable Staticks*, London: W. Innys & Woodward.
Haliburton RA, Sullivan CR, Kelly PJ, Peterson LFA (1958) The extra-osseous and intra-osseous blood supply of the talus. *J Bone Joint Surg* **40A:** 1115–1120.
Hall MC (1965) *The Locomotor System: Functional Histology*, Springfield, Illinois: Thomas.
Hally AD (1964) A counting method for measuring the volumes of tissue components in microscopical sections. *Q J Microsc Sci* **105:** 503–517.
Ham AW (1930) A histological study of the early phase of bone repairs. *J Bone Joint Surg* **12:** 827–844.
Ham AW (1932) In: *Cowdry's Special Cytology*, 2nd edn, New York: Hoeber.
Ham AW (1953) *Histology*, 2nd edn, New York: Lippincott.
Ham AW, Leeson TS (1964) In: *Ham's Histology*, 4th edn, New York: Lippincott.
Hamerman D, Ruskin J (1959) Histologic studies on human synovial membrane. I. Metachromatic staining and the effects of streptococcal hyaluronidase. *Arthritis Rheum* **2:** 546–552.
Hamerman D, Schubert M (1962) Diarthrodial joints: an essay. *Am J Med* **33:** 555–590.
Hamerman D, Rojkind M, Sandson J (1966) Protein bound to hyaluronate: chemical and immunological studies. *Fed Proc* **25:** 1040–1045.
Handley RC, Pooley J (1991) The venous anatomy of the scaphoid. *J Anat* **178:** 115–118.
Hansen EB, Hjortdal VE, Kjolseth D, He SZ, Hoy K, Soballe K Bunger C (1991) Arteriovenous shunting is not associated with venous congestion in bone: knee tamponade studied with 15 μm and 50 μm microspheres in immature dogs. *Acta Orthop Scand* **62:** 268–275.
Hansen ES (1993) Microvascularization, osteogenesis and myelopoiesis in normal and pathological conditions. In: *Bone Circulation and Vascularization in Normal and Pathological Conditions* (eds A Schoutens, J Arlet, JWM Gardeniers, SPF Hughes), London: Plenum, 229–242.
Hansen ES, Henriksen TB, Noer I, Bunger C (1989) Haemodynamic effects of knee joint tamponade: ^{99m}Tc-diphosphonate scintimetry in growing dogs. *Acta Orthop Scand* **60:** 549–553.
Harpunder K (1926) Physikalisch-chemische Untersuchungen am normalen Knorpel. *Biochem Z* **169:** 308–319.
Harris HA (1929) Vascular supply of bone, with special reference to epiphyseal cartilage. *J Anat* **64:** 3–4.
Harris HA (1933) *Bone Growth in Health and Disease*, London: Oxford University Press.
Harris RI, MacDonald JL (1936) The effect of lumbar sympathectomy upon the growth of legs paralysed by anterior poliomyelitis. *J Bone Joint Surg* **18:** 35–45.
Harris WH, Haywood EA, Lavorgna J, Hamblen DA (1968) Spatial and temporal variations in cortical bone formation in dogs. *J Bone Joint Surg* **50A:** 1118–1128.
Harrison MHM, Trueta J, Scajowicz F (1953) Osteoarthritis of the hip: a study of the nature and evolution of the disease. *J Bone Joint Surg* **35B:** 598–626.
Harrison RG, Gossman HH (1955) Fate of radiopaque media injected into the cancellous bone of the extremities. *J Bone Joint Surg* **37B:** 150–156.
Harrison RJ (1961) In: *Recent Advances in Anatomy*, 2nd series (eds F Goldby, RJ Harrison), London: Churchill.
Hartles RL, Leaver AG (1961) Citrate in mineralized tissues. III. The effect of purified diets low in calcium and vitamin D on the citrate content of the rat femur. *Arch Oral Biol* **5:** 38–44.
Hasán A, Brookes M (1990) Angiogenesis in early fracture repair. In: *Bone Circulation and Bone Necrosis* (eds J Arlet, B Mazières, D Hungerford), Berlin: Springer, 169–175.
Hashimoto M (1936) Über das kapilläre Blutgefässsystem des Kaninchenknochenmarks. *Trans Soc Path Jap* **26:** 300–307.
Havers C (1691) *Osteologia Nova, or some New Observations of the Bones etc*, London: Samuel Smith.
He S-Z, Zhenhua X, Hansen EB, Bunger C (1990) Microvascular morphology of bone in arthrosis: scanning electron microscopy in rabbits. *Acta Orthop Scand* **61:** 195–200.
Heister L (1732) *Compendium Anatomicum*, 4th edn, Norimbergi et Altorfi: GC Weber.
Helal B (1962) *Osteoarthritis of the Knee Joint*, Thesis, Liverpool.
Helal B (1965) The pain in primary osteoarthritis of the knee: its causes and treatment by osteotomy. *Postgrad Med J* **41:** 172–181.
Helferich H (1887) Über künstliche Vermehrung der Knochenneubildung. *Arch Klin Chir* **2:** 142.

Hellstadius A (1947) An investigation by experiments on animals of the role played by the epiphyseal cartilage in longitudinal growth. *Acta Chir Scand* **95:** 156–166.
Hendel PM, Hattner RS, Rodrigo J, Buncke HJ (1982) The functional anatomy of the rib. *Plast Reconstr Surg* **70:** No 5, 578–587.
Hensel H, Ruef J (1954) Fortlaufende Registrierung der Muskeldurchblutung am Menschen mit einer Calorimetersonde. *Arch Physiol* **259:** 267–280.
Heřt J (1960) Primary vascular architechtonics in the diaphyseal cortex of growing bones. *Čská Morf* **8:** 89–102.
Heřt J, Hladiková J (1961) Die Gefässversorgung des Haversschen Knochens. *Acta Anat* **45:** 344–361.
Herzig E, Root WS (1959) Relation of sympathetic nervous system to blood pressure of bone marrow. *Am J Physiol* **196:** 1053–1056.
Heymann MA, Payne BD, Hoffman JI, Rudolph AM (1977) Blood flow measurements with radionuclide labelled particles. *Proc Cardiovasc Dis* **20:** 55–79.
Hickey DS, Hukins DWL (1981) Collagen fibril diameter and elastic fibres in the annulus fibrosus of the human fetal intervertebral disc. *J Anat* **133:** 351–357.
Hildebrand O (1896) Experimenteller Beitrag zur Lehre von den freien Gelenkörpern. *Dtsch Z Chir* **42:** 292–308.
Hintzche E (1928) Über die Beitrag der Gefässkanäle im Knorpel nach Befunden am distalen Ende des menschlichen Schenkelbeines. *Z Mikrosk Anat Forsch* **12:** 61–126.
Hintzche E (1931) Über Umbildungen im jungen menschlichen Hyalinknorpel. *Z Mikrosk Anat Forsch* **25:** 320–361.
Hirsch C (1944) A contribution to pathogenesis of chondromalacia of patella: physical, histologic and chemical study. *Acta Chir Scand* **90:** suppl 83, 10–106.
Ho SS, Coel MN, Kagawa R, Richardson AB (1994) The effects of ice on blood flow and bone metabolism in knees. *Am J Sports Med* **22(4):** 537–540.
Hoffbrand B, Forsyth R (1969) Validity studies of the radioactive microsphere method for the study of the distribution of cardiac output, organ blood flow, and resistance in the conscious rhesus monkey. *Cardiovasc Res* **3:** 426–432.
Holdsworth FW (1966) Epiphyseal growth: speculations on the nature of Perthes' disease. *Ann R Coll Surg* **39:** 1–16.
Holm IE, Ewald H, Bulow J, Bunger C (1990) Vasoactive substances in subchondral bone of the dog knee. *J Orthop Res* **8:** 205–212.
Holmdahl DE, Ingelmark BE (1948) Der Bau des Gelenkknorpels unter verschiedenen funktionellen Verhältnissen. *Acta Anat* **6:** 309–375.
Holmdahl DE, Ingelmark BE (1950) The contact between the articular cartilage and the medullary cavities of the bone. *Acta Orthop Scand* **20:** 156–165.
Holthofer H, Virtanen I, Kariniemi AL, Hormia H, Linder E, Miettinen A (1982) *Ulex europeus* I lectin as a marker for vascular endothelium in human tissues. *Lab Invest* **47:** 60–66.
Holtrop ME (1965) The origin of bone cells in endochondral ossification. In: *Calcified Tissues, 1965* (ed H Fleisch, HJJ Blackwood, M Owen, MP Fleisch-Ronchetti), Berlin: Springer.
Horton BT (1932) Hemihypertrophy of extremities associated with congenital arterio-venous fistula. *J Am Med Assoc* **98:** 373–379.
Horváth L (1959) Analysis of mast cells by means of polarization microscopy. *Nature, Lond* **183:** 1067–1068.
Howe WW, Lacey T, Schwartz RP (1950) A study of the gross anatomy of the arteries supplying the proximal portion of the femur and the acetabulum. *J Bone Joint Surg* **32A:** 856–866.
Hoyer H (1869) Zur Histologie des Knochenmarkes. *Zentralbl Med Wiss* **7:** 257.
Hoyer H (1882) *Biol Centralbl* **ii:** 19–22.
Hudlicka O, Tyler KR (1986) *Angiogenesis: the growth of the vascular system*, London: Academic.
Hueter C (1866) Zur Histologie der Gelenkflächen und Gelenkkapseln mit einem kritischen Vorwort über dem Knochenmark. *Virchows Arch Path Anat Physiol* **36:** 25–80.
Huggins C (1939) A quantitative study of the activity of the reticulo-endothelial structures in bone marrow in normal and ischaemic limbs as indicated by India ink and titanium dioxide. *Anat Rec* **74:** 231–256.
Huggins C, Wiege E (1939) The effect on the bone marrow of disruption of the nutrient artery and vein. *Ann Surg* **110:** 940–947.
Hughes H (1952) The factors determining the direction of the canal for the nutrient artery in the long bones of mammals and birds. *Acta Anat* **15:** 261–280.
Hughes S, Blount M (1979) The structure of capillaries in cortical bone. *Ann R Coll Surg Engl* **61:** 312.
Hughes SPF, Davies DR, Bassingthwaighte JB, Knox FG, Kelly PJ (1977) Bone extraction and blood clearance of diphosphonate in the dog. *Am J Physiol* **23:** H341–H347.

Hughes SPF, Lemon GJ, Davies DR, Bassingthwaite JB, Kelly PJ (1979) Extraction of minerals after experimental fractures of the tibia in dogs. *J Bone Joint Surg* **61A:** 857–866.

Hughes-Jones NC, Mollison PL, Veall N (1957) Removal of incompatible red cells by the spleen. *Br J Haematol* **3:** 125–133.

Humphry GM (1858) *A Treatise on the Human Skeleton including the Joints*, Cambridge: Macmillan.

Humphry GM (1861) Observations on the growth of long bones. *Med-Chir Trans* **44:** 117–122.

Hunter J (1772) Experiments and observations on the growth of bones. In: *The Works of J Hunter FRS* (1837), vol 4 (ed JF Palmer), London: Longman.

Hunter J (1790) Some observations on the loose cartilages found in joints and most commonly met with in that of the knee. In: *The Works of J Hunter FRS (1837)* vol 3 (ed JF Palmer), London: Longman.

Hunter W (1743) Of the structure and diseases of articulating cartilages. *Phil Trans R Coll* **42:** 514–521.

Hunter WL, Arsenault AL (1990) Endothelial cell division in metaphyseal capillaries during endochondral bone formation in rats. *Anat Rec* **227:** 351–358.

Hunter WL, Arsenault AL, Hodsman AB (1991) Rearrangement of the metaphyseal vasculature of the rat growth plate in rickets and rachitic reversal: a model of vascular arrest and angiogenesis renewed. *Anat Rec* **229:** 453–461.

Hurrell DJ (1934) The vascularisation of cartilage. *J Anat* **69:** 47–61.

Hutchison WJ, Burdeaux BD (1959) The influence of stasis on bone growth. *Surg Gynecol Obstet* **99:** 413–420.

Hyman H (1961) Linear system for quantitating hydrogen at a platinum electrode. *Circ Res* **9:** 1093–1097.

Hyrtl J (1864) Normale und abnorme Verhältnisse der Schlagadern des Unterschenkels. *Denkschr Akad Wiss, Wien* **23:** 245–288.

Ida R, Lee A, Huang J, Brandi ML, Yamaguchi DT (1994) Prostaglandin-stimulated second messenger signalling in bone-derived endothelial cells is dependent on confluency in culture. *J Cell Physiol* **160:** no 3, 585–595.

Ingebrigsten R, Krog J, Lerand S (1963) Circulation distal to experimental arterio-venous fistulas of the extremities. A polarographic study. *Acta Chir Scand* **125:** 308–317.

Ingelmark BE, Ekholm R (1948) A study on variations in the thickness of articular cartilage in association with rest and periodical load. *Ups LäkFör Förh* **53:** 61–74.

Ingelmark BE, Sääf J (1948) Über die Ernährung des Gelenkknorpels und die Bildung der Gelenkflüssigkeit unter verschiedenen funktionellen Verhältnissen. *Acta Orthop Scand* **17:** 303–357.

Irino, S, Ono T, Watanabe K, Toyota K, Uno J, Takasugi N, Murakami T (1975) SEM studies on microvascular architecture, sinus wall, and transmural passage of blood cells in the bone marrow by a new method of injection replica and noncoated specimens. *Scan Electron Microsc* **1:** 267–274.

Irving MH (1965) The blood supply of the growth cartilage and metaphysis in rachitic rats. *J Pathol Bacteriol* **89:** 461–471.

Ishido B (1923) Gelenkuntersuchungen. *Virchows Arch Path Anat Physiol* **244:** 424–428.

Israel J (1877) Angiectasie im Stromgebiete der Arteria tibialis antica. *Arch Klin Chir* **21:** 109–131.

Iversen PO, Nicolaysen G, Benestad HB (1994) Endogenous nitric oxide causes vasodilation in rat bone marrow, bone and spleen during accelerated hematopoiesis. *Exp Hematol* **22:** 1297–1302.

Jackson RW, MacNab (1959) Fractures of the shaft of the tibia: a clinical and experimental study. *Am J Surg* **97:** 543–557.

Jaffe HL (1929) The vessel canals in normal and pathological bone. *Am J Pathol* **5:** 323–333.

Jaffe HL, Pomeranz MM (1934) Changes in the bones of extremities amputated because of arterio-vascular disease. *Arch Surg* **29:** 566–588.

Jamieson RA, Kay AW (1965) *A Textbook of Surgical Physiology*, 2nd edn, London: Livingstone.

Jarry L, Uhthoff HK (1960) Activation of osteogenesis by the petal technique. An experimental study. *J Bone Joint Surg* **42B:** 126–136.

Jaya Y (1958) Contralateral vasoconstriction in the hind limb of the rat and rabbit. *Clin Sci* **17:** 55–61.

Jendrucko RJ, Hyman WA, Newell PH, Chakraborty BK (1976) Theoretical evidence for the generation of high pressure in bone cells. *J Biomech* **9:** 87–91.

Jodal M, Lundgren O (1970) Plasma skimming in the intestinal tract. *Acta Physiol Scand* **80:** 50–60.

Johnson EF, Berryman H, Mitchell R, Wood WB (1985) Elastic fibres in anulus fibrosus of the adult human intervertebral disc. A preliminary report. *J Anat* **143:** 57–63.

Johnson MW, Chakkalakal DA, Harper RA, Katz JL (1980) Comparison of the electromechanical effects in wet and dry bone. *J Biomech* **13:** 437–442.

Johnson MW, Chakkalakal DA, Harper RA, Katz JL, Rouhana SW (1982) Fluid flow in bone *in vitro*. *J Biomech* **15:** 881–885.

Johnson PC (1974) The microcirculation, local and humoral control of the circulation. In: *Cardiovascular Physiology* Physiology Series 1. (eds AC Guyton, CE Jones), London: Butterworths & Baltimore: University Park Press, 163.
Johnson RW (1927) A physiological study of the blood supply of the diaphysis. *J Bone Joint Surg* **9:** 153–184.
Johnston TB, Davies DV, Davies F (1958) In: *Grays Anatomy* 32nd edn (TB Johnston, DV Davies, F Davies), London: Longmans.
Jones ES (1936) Joint lubrication. *Lancet* **i:** 1043–1045.
Jones LC, Niv AI, Davis RF, Hungerford DS (1982) Bone blood flow in the femora of anaesthetised and conscious dogs in a chronic preparation, using the radioactive tracer microsphere method. *Clin Orthop* **170:** 286–295.
Jost A (1947) Expériences de décapitation de l'embryon du lapin. *C R hebd Séanc Acad Sci, Paris* **225:** 322–324.
Jost A (1961) The role of fetal hormones in prenatal development. *Harvey Lect* **55:** 201–226.
Jowsey J (1960) Age changes in human bone. *Clin Orthop* **17:** 210–218.
Judet J, Judet R, Lagrange J, Dunoyer J (1955) A study of the arterial vascularization of the femoral neck in the adult. *J Bone Joint Surg* **37A:** 663–680.
Justus R, Luft JH (1970) A mechanomechanical hypothesis for bone remodelling induced by mechanical stress. *Calcif Tissue Res* **5:** 222–235.
Just-Viera JO, Yeager GH (1965) Venous stasis I: Effects of venous resection on bone growth. *Surgery* **58:** 694–702.
Kahn D, Weiner GJ, Ben-Haim S, Ponto LL, Madsen MT, Bushnell DL, Watkins GL, Argenyi EA, Hichwa RD (1994) Positron emission tomographic measurement of bone marrow blood flow to the pelvis and lumbar vertebrae in young normal adults *Blood* **83:** 958–63.
Kaihara S, Van Heerden PD, Migita T, Wagner HN (1968) Measurement of distribution of cardiac output. *J Appl Physiol* **25:** 696–700.
Kajava Y (1919) Beitrag zur Kenntnis der Entwicklung des Gelenknorpels. *Acta Soc Sci Fenn* **48:** 1–128.
Kalser MH, Ivy HK, Prevsner L, Marbarger JP, Evy AC (1951) Changes in bone marrow pressure during exposure to simulated altitude. *J Aviat Med* **22:** 286–294.
Kane WJ, Grim E (1969) Blood flow to canine hindlimb bone, muscle and skin. *J Bone Joint Surg* **51A:** 309–322.
Kapitola J, Andrie J, Kubickova J (1993) Local blood circulation and bone mineral content in the bones of rats: the effect of castration, estradiol and testosterone in male and female rats. *Sbornik Lekarsky* **94:** 219–227.
Kapitola J, Andrie J, Kubickova J (1994) Possible participation of prostoglandins in the increase in the bone blood flow in oophorectomized female rats. *Exp Clin Endocrinol* **102:** 414–416.
Kassowitz M (1881) *Die Normale Ossification, etc*, I Teil Vienna: W Braunmüller.
Katthagen BD, Spies H, Bachmann G (1995) Arterial vascularization of the bony acetabulum. *Z Orthop* **133:** no 1, 7–13.
Katz MA, Blantz RC, Floyd DR, Seldin DW (1971) Measurement of intrarenal blood flow. I; analysis of microspheres method. *Am J Physiol* **220:** 1903–1921.
Keck SW, Kelly PJ (1965) The effect of venous stasis on intra-osseous pressure and longitudinal bone growth in the dog. *J Bone Joint Surg* **47A:** 539–544.
Keith Sir Arthur (1919) Bone growth and bone repair. *Br J Surg* **6:** 160–165.
Keith Sir Arthur (1927) Concerning the origin and nature of the osteoblasts. *Proc R Soc Med* **21:** 1–8.
Kelly PJ (1968) Effect of unilateral increased venous pressure on bone remodelling in canine tibia. *J Lab Clin Med* **72:** 410–418.
Kelly PJ (1969) Oxygen saturation, PO_2 and pH in the tibial bone distal to a femoral arteriovenous fistula in puppies. *J Lab Clin Med* **73:** 418–424.
Kelly PJ (1973) Comparison of marrow and cortical bone blood flow by ^{125}I-labelled 4-iodoantipyrine (I-Ap) washout. *J Lab Clin Med* **81:** 497–505.
Kelly PJ (1983) Pathways of transport in bone. In: *Handbook of Physiology*; section 2, vol. 3, part 1 (eds JT Sheppard, FM Abboud), Baltimore: Williams & Wilkins, 371–396.
Kelly PJ, Bronk JT (1990) Venous pressure and bone formation. *Microvasc Res* **39:** 364–375.
Kelly PJ, Janes JM, Peterson LFA (1959) The effect of arterio-venous fistulae on the vascular pattern of the femora of immature dogs: a micro-angiographic study. *J Bone Joint Surg* **41A:** 1101–1108.
Kelly PJ, Yipintsoi T, Bassingthwaite JB (1971) Blood flow from the canine tibial diaphysis estimated by iodo-antipyrene-125I washout. *J Appl Physiol* **31:** 38–47.
Kety SS (1949) Measurement of regional circulation by local clearance of radioactive sodium. *Am Heart J* **38:** 321–328.

Kety SS, Schmidt CF (1945) The determination of cerebral blood flow in man by use of nitrous oxide in low concentrations. *Am J Physiol* **143:** 53–56.

Kety SS, Schmidt CF (1946) Effects of active and passive hyperventilation on cerebral blood flow, cerebral oxygen consumption, cardiac output and blood pressure of normal young men. *J Clin Invest* **25:** 107–119.

Key JA, Walton F (1933) Healing of fractures and bone defects after venous stasis. *Arch Surg* **27:** 935–940.

Kiær T, Dahl B, Lausten GS (1993) The relationship between inert gas-washout and radioactive tracer microspheres in measurement of bone blood flow: effect of decreased arterial supply and venous congestion on bone blood flow in an animal model. *J Orthop Res* **11:** 28–35.

Kiær T, Gronlund J, Sorenson KH (1988) Subchondral PO_2, PCO_2, pressure, pH, and lactate in human osteoarthritis of the hip. *Clin Orthop Rel Res* **229:** 149–155.

Kienböck R (1910) *Avascular Necrosis of the Lunate*, described in Vienna.

Kirkby OJ, Berg-Larsen T (1991) Regional blood flow and strontium-85 incorporation rate in the rat hindlimb skeleton. *J Orthop Res* **9:** 862–868.

Kirkpatrick JS, Callaghan JJ, Vandemark RM, Goldner RD (1990) The relationship of the intrapelvic vasculature to the acetabulum. Implications in screw-fixation acetabular components. *Clin Orthop Rel Res* **258:** 183–190.

Kishikawa E (1936) Studien über einige lokale Reize, welche das Langenwachstum des Langrohrenknochens steigern (abstract). *Acta Med (Fukuoka)* **29:** 4.

Kissoon N, Peterson R, Murphy S, Gayle M, Ceithami E, Harwood-Nuss A (1994) Comparison of pH and carbon dioxide tension values of central venous and intraosseous blood during changes in cardiac output. *Crit Care Med* **22:** 1010–1015.

Kistler GH (1934) Sequences of experimental bacterial infarction of the femur in rabbits. *Arch Surg* **29:** 589–611.

Kistler GH (1935) Sequences of experimental bacterial infarction of the femur in rabbits. *Surg Gynecol Obstet* **60:** 913–925.

Kita K, Kawai K, Hirohata K (1987) Changes in bone marrow blood flow with aging (sic). *J Orthop Res* **5:** 569–575.

Klein A (1864) Zur Geschichte der Entstehung der Gelenkmaüse. *Virchows Arch Path Anat Physiol* **29:** 190–197.

Kling DH, Levine MG, Wise S (1955) Mucopolysaccharides in tissue cultures of human and mammalian synovial membrane. *Proc Soc Exp Biol Med* **89:** 261–263.

Kobrin I, Kardon MB, Oigman W, Pegram BL, Frohlich ED (1984) Role of site of microsphere injection and catheter position on systemic and regional haemodynamics in rat. *Am J Physiol* H35–H39.

Kofoed H (1986) Haemodynamics and metabolism in arthrosis: studies in the rabbit knee. *Acta Orthop Scand* **57:** 119–122.

Kofoed H (1993) Intraosseous pressure, gas tension and bone blood flow in normal and pathological situations: a survey of methods and results. In: *Bone Circulation and Vascularization in Normal and Pathological Conditions* (eds A Schoutens, SPF Hughes, J Gardenieres, J Arlet), Boca Raton: Plenum, 121–128.

Köhler A (1908) *Köhler's First Disease: osteochondritis of the tarsal navicular*, Wiesbaden, Germany.

Koken EW (1975) Anatomical investigation of the blood supply of the lunate zone. *Z Orthop* **113:** no 6, 1022–6.

Kölliker A (1873) *Die normale Resorption des Knochengewebes und ihre Bedeutung für die Entstehung der Knochenformen*, Leipzig: FCW Vogel.

Koltze H (1951) Studie zur äusseren Form in den Gelenken. *Z Anat Entw-Gesch* **115:** 584–591.

Konerding MA, Blank M (1987) The vascularization of the vertebral column of rats. *Scan Microsc* **1:** no 4, 1727–1732.

König F (1887) Ueber freie Körper in den Gelenken. *Dt Z Chir* **27:** 90–109.

Koskinen EVS (1959) The repair of experimental fractures. *Ann Chir Gynaecol Fenn* **48:** suppl 90.

Kowallik P, Schulz R, Guth B, Schade A, Paffhausen W, Gross R, Heusch G (1991) Measurement of regional myocardial blood flow with multiple coloured microspheres. *Circulation* **83:** 974–982.

Krompecher S (1937) *Die Knochenbildung*, Jena: Fischer.

Kruse RL, Kelly PJ (1974) Acceleration of fracture healing distal to a venous tourniquet. *J Bone Joint Surg* **56A:** 730–739.

Kuhlmann JN, Guerin-Surville H (1981) Extrinsic and intrinsic vascularization of the scaphoid and lunate bones. *Bull Assoc Anat* **65:** 433–446.

Kuhlmann JN, Guerin-Surville H, Chrétien Y (1982) Vascularization of the pyramidal and pisiform bones. *Bull Assoc Anat* **66:** 79–88.

Kuhns JG, Weatherford HL (1936) Role of the reticulo-endothelial system in the deposition of colloidal and particulate matter in articular cavities. *Arch Surg* **33:** 68–82.
Kuntz A, Richins CA (1945) Innervation of bone marrow. *J Comp Neurol* **83:** 213–222.
Kunze (1933) Cited by M Burger (1954) In: *Altern und Krankeit*, Leipzig: Georg Thieme.
Kushkhabiev VI (1993) The topographical characteristics of the blood vessels of the human spine. *Morfologia* **104:** 103–111.
Lacroix P (1947) Excitation de la croissance en longueur du tibia par décollement de son périoste diaphysaire. *Revue Orthop Chir Appar Mot* **33:** 3–6.
Lacroix P (1948) La disposition du canal de l'artère nourricière dans les os longs. *Arch Biol Paris* **59:** 391–403.
Lacroix P (1951) *The Organization of Bones*, London: Churchill.
Ladanyi J, Hidvegi E (1954) Blood supply of experimental callus formation. *Acta Morph Hung* **4:** 35–44.
Lahtinen R, Lahtinen T, Romppanen (1982) Bone and bone marrow blood flow in chronic granulocytic leukaemia and primary myelofibrosis. *J Nucl Med* **23:** 218–224.
Lamas A, Amado D, Da Costa JC (1946) La circulation du sang dans l'os. *Presse Méd* **54:** 862–863.
Landauer W (1927) Untersuchungen über Chondrodystrophie. I Embryonen. *Arch EntwMech Org* **110:** 195–278.
Landauer W (1929) Funktionelle Strukturen von Knorpel und Knochen und ihre Entstehung. *Arch EntwMech Org* **115:** 911–915.
Landauer W (1931) Untersuchungen über das Krüperhuhn. II. Morphologie und Histologie des Skelets, insbesondere des Skelets der langen Extremitätenknochen. *Z Mikrosk Anat Forsch* **25:** 115–180.
Lane LB, Villacin A, Bullough PG (1977) The vascularity and remodelling of subchondral bone and calcified cartilage in adult human femoral and humeral heads. An age- and stress related phenomenon. *J Bone Joint Surg* **59B:** no 3, 272–278.
Langer K (1876) Über das Gefässystem der Röhrenknochen, mit Beiträgen zur Kenntnis des Baues und der Entwicklung des Knochengewebes. *Denkschr K K Akad Wiss Wien* **36:** 1–40
Langer K (1877) Über die Blutgefässe der Knochen des Schädeldaches und der harten Hirnhaut. *Denkschr K K Akad Wiss Wien* **37:** 217–240.
Lanyon LE, Hartman W (1977) Strain related electrical potentials recorded *in vitro* and *in vivo*. *Calcif Tissue Res* **22:** 315–327.
Lanyon L, Rubin CT (1984) Static versus dynamic loads as an influence on bone remodelling. *J Biomech* **17:** 897–905.
Larson B, Light TR, Ogden JA (1987) Fracture and ischemic necrosis of the immature scaphoid. *J Hand Surg* **12A:** no 1, 122–127.
Laughlin MH, Armstrong RB (1982) Muscular blood flow distribution patterns as a function of running speed in rats. *Am J Physiol* **243:** H296–H306.
Laughlin MH, Armstrong RB, White J, Rouk K (1982) A method of using microspheres to measure muscle blood flow in exercising rats. *J Appl Physiol: Resp Environ Exercise Physiol* **52:** 1629–1635.
Laugier S (1952) Saignée des os. *Union Méd* **6:** 587.
Launder WJ, Hungerford DS, Jones LH (1981) Haemodynamics of the femoral head. *J Bone Joint Surg* **63A:** 442–448.
Lavender JP, Khan RA, Hughes SPF (1979) Blood flow and tracer uptake in normal and abnormal canine bone: comparison with Sr-85 microspheres, Kr-81m, and Tc99m MDP. *J Nucl Med* **20:** 413–418.
Leblond CP, Wilkinson GW, Bélanger LF, Robichon J (1950) Radioautographic visualization of bone formation in the rat. *Am J Anat* **86:** 289–341.
Lee AB (1924) *The Microtomist's Vade-Mecum*, 8th edn (ed. JB Gatenby *et al.*), London: Churchill.
Leger L, Frileux C (1950) La phlébographie par injection intramedullo-osseuse du produit de contraste. *Presse Méd* **58:** 29.
Lemon GJ, Davies DR, Hughes SPF, Bassingthwaite JB, Kelly PJ (1980) Transcapillary exchange and retention of fluoride, strontium, EDTA, sucrose and iodoantipyrene in bone. *Calcif Tissue Int* **31:** 173–181.
Lemperg RK, Arnoldi CC (1978) The significance of intraosseous pressure in normal and diseased states with special reference to the intraosseous engorgement-pain syndrome. *Clin Orthop Rel Res* **136:** 143–156.
Leonhardt H (1967) *Histologie und Zytologie des Menschen*, Stuttgart: Thieme.
Leotta N (1907) Sulla legatura delle grandi vene del corpo: ricerche sperementali. *Atti R Acad med Roma* **34:** 80–83.
Leriche R, Policard A (1926) *Les problèmes de la physiologie normale et pathologique de l'os*, Paris: Masson.

Levander G (1929) Über die Behandlung von Brüchen des Oberschenkelschaftes, nebst Beitrag zur Kenntnis des gesteigerten Langenwachstums der Röhrenknochen der unteren Extremitäten nach Bruch derselben. *Acta Chir Scand* **65:** suppl 12, 5–237.

Lever JD, Ford EHR (1959) Histological, histochemical and electron microscope observations on synovial membrane. *Anat Rec* **132:** 525–539.

Levick JR (1995) Microvascular architecture and exchange in synovial joints. *Microcirculation* **2:** no 3, 217–233.

Lewis OJ (1956) The blood supply of developing long bones with special reference to the metaphyses. *J Bone Joint Surg* **38B:** 928–933.

Lewis PR, McCutchen CW (1959) Experimental evidence for weeping lubrication in animal joints. *Nature, Lond* **184:** 1285.

Lexer E (1922) Über die Entstehung von Pseudarthrosen nach Frakturen und nach Knochentransplantationen. *Arch Klin Chir* **119:** 520–607.

Lexer E, Kuliga, Turk W (1904) *Untersuchungen über Knochenarterien*, Berlin: Hirschwald.

Li G, Bronk JT, Kelly PJ (1989) Canine bone blood flow estimated with microspheres. *J Orthop Res* **7:** 61–67.

Lilly AD, Kelly PJ (1970) Effects of venous ligation on bone remodelling in the canine tibia. *J Bone Joint Surg* **52A:** 515–520.

Lindblad BE, Nielsen LB, Bjurholm A, Bunger C, Hensen ES (1993) Vasoconstrictive action of neuropeptide Y and norepinephrine in bone: a comparative study in the *in situ* perfused porcine tibia. *Trans Eur Orthop Res Soc* **3:** 31.

Liu SL, Ho TC (1991) The role of venous hypertension in the pathogenesis of Legge-Perthes disease. A clinical and experimental study. *J Bone Joint Surg* **73A:** 194–200.

Lloyd-Roberts GC (1953) Role of capsular changes in osteoarthritis of hip joint. *J Bone Joint Surg* **35B:** 627–642.

Lockhart RD, Hamilton GF, Fyfe FW (1959) *Anatomy of the Human Body*, London: Faber & Faber.

Longmore D (1969) Personal communication.

Loomis WF (1961) Cell differentiation: a problem in selective gene activation through self-produced micro-environmental differences of carbon dioxide tension. In: *Biological Structure and Function* (ed. TW Goodwin, O Lindberg), London: Academic.

Lopez-Curto JA, Bassingthwaighte JB, Kelly PJ (1980) Anatomy of the microvasculature of the tibial diaphysis of the adult dog. *J Bone Joint Surg* **62:** 1362–1369.

Lorenz M, Plenk H (1977) A perfusion method of incubation to demonstrate horseradish peroxidase in bone. *Histochemistry* **53:** 257–263.

Loud AV, Barany WC, Pack BA (1965) Quantitative evaluation of cytoplasmic structures in electron micrographs. *Lab Invest* **14:** 996–1008.

Lovén OC (1863) *Studier och undersökninger öfver benäfuaden, fönämigast med afseende på dess utveckling*, Stockholm: Hërberg.

Lowenstein JM, Pauporte J, Richards V, Davison R (1958) Effects of sympathectomy on blood turnover rates in muscle and bone. *Surgery* **43:** 768–773.

Lunde PKM, Michelson K (1970) Determination of cortical blood flow in rabbit femur by radioactive microspheres. *Acta Physiol Scand* **80:** 39–44.

Lundgaard A, Aalkjaer C, Mulvaney MJ, Bjurholm A, Hensen ES (1993) Calcitonin gene-related peptide, vasoactive intestinal peptide, and substance P induce relaxation of resistance arteries isolated from cancellous bone. *Trans Eur Res Soc* **3:** 30.

Lutken P (1950) Investigations into the position of the nutrient foramina and the direction of the vessel canals in the shafts of the humerus and femur in man. *Acta Anat* **9:** 57–68.

McAuley GO (1958) The blood supply of the rat's femur in relation to the repair of cortical defects. *J Anat* **92:** 665.

McCarthy ID, Hughes SPF (1983) The role of skeletal blood flow in determining the uptake of 99mTc methylene diphosphonate. *Calcif Tissue Int* **35:** 508–511.

McCarthy ID, Hughes SPF (1990) Is there a blood bone barrier? In: *Bone Circulation and Bone Necrosis* (eds J Arlet, B Mazieres), Berlin: Springer, 30–33.

McCarthy ID, Hughes SPF (1996) The role of bone circulation in changes of bone mass during prolonged exposure to microgravity. *ARCO Newslett* **8:** 106–107.

McCarthy ID, Orr JS, Hughes SPF (1980) An experimental model to study the relationship between blood flow and uptake for bone seeking radionuclides in normal bone. *Clin Phys Physiol Meas* **1:** 135–143.

MacConaill MA (1932) The function of the intra-articular fibrocartilages, with special reference to the knee and inferior radio-ulnar joints. *J Anat* **66:** 210–227.

MacConaill MA (1967) Basic anatomy of weight-bearing joints. In: *Proceedings of a Symposium on Lubrication and Wear in Living and Artificial Human Joints*, London: Institution of Mechanical Engineers.
McCutchen CW (1962) The frictional properties of animal joints. *Wear* **5:** 1.
McCutchen CW (1967) Physiological lubrication. In: *Proceedings of a Symposium on Lubrication and Wear in Living and Artificial Human Joints*, London: Institution of Mechanical Engineers.
McDonald F, Houston WJB (1990) An *in vivo* assessment of muscular activity and the importance of electrical phenomena in bone remodelling. *J Anat* **172:** 165–175.
McElfrish EC, Kelly PJ (1974) Simultaneous determination of blood flow in cortical bone, marrow and muscle in canine hind limb by femoral artery catheterization. *Calcif Tissue Res* **14:** 301–307.
Macewen W (1912) *The Growth of Bone: observations on osteogenesis*, Glasgow: James Maclehose.
McGrory BJ, Moran CG, Bronk J, Weaver AL, Wood MB (1994) Canine blood flow measurements using serial microsphere injections. *Clin Orthop Rel Res* **303:** 264–279.
Macklin CC (1920) Cited by Keith A (1927) *Proc R Soc Med* **21:** 1–8.
Macklin CC, Macklin MT (1920) A study of brain repair in the rat by use of trypan blue, with special reference to the vital staining of macrophages. *Arch Neurol Psychiat Lond* **3:** 353–394.
McLean FC (1958) The ultrastructure and function of bone. *Science, NY* **127:** 451–456.
McLean FC, Urist MR (1961) *Bone: an introduction to the physiology of skeletal tissue*, 2nd edn, London: University of Chicago Press.
McMaster P, Roome N (1934) The effect of sympathectomy and of venous stasis on bone repair; an experimental study. *J Bone Joint Surg* **16:** 365–371.
McMaster PD (1941) An inquiry into the structural conditions affecting fluid transport in the interstitial tissue of the skin. *J Exp Med* **74:** 9–28.
McMurray TP (1935) Osteoarthritis of hip joints. *Br J Surg* **22:** 716–727.
MacNab I (1957) Blood supply of the tibia (Abstract). *J Bone Joint Surg* **39B:** 799.
McPherson A, Scales J, Gordon L (1961) A method of estimating qualitative changes of blood flow in bone. *J Bone Joint Surg* **43B:** 791–799.
Major P, Resnick D, Greenway G (1980) Heterotopic ossification in paraplegia: a possible disturbance of the paravertebral venous plexus. *Radiology* **136:** no 3, 797–799.
Maki Y, Breidenbach WC, Firrell JC (1993) Evaluation of a local microsphere injection method for measurement of blood flow in the rabbit lower extremity. *J Orthop Res* **11:** 20–27.
Malik AB, Kaplan JE, Saba TM (1976) Reference sample method for cardiac output and regional blood flow determinations in the rat. *J Appl Physiol* **40:** 472–475.
Malkin SAS (1936) Femoral osteotomy in treatment of osteoarthritis of the hip. *Br Med J* **1:** 304–305.
Marnell P (1967) A theoretical analysis of hip joint lubrication. In: *Proceedings of a Symposium on Lubrication and Wear in Living and Artificial Human Joints*, London: Institution of Mechanical Engineers.
Maroudas A (1967) Hyaluronic acid films. In: *Proceedings of a Symposium on Lubrication and Wear in Living and Artificial Human Joints*, London: Institution of Mechanical Engineers.
Maroudas A, Stockwell R, Nachemson A, Urban J (1975) Factors involved in the nutrition of human lumbar intervertebral disc, cellularity and diffusion of glucose *in vitro*. *J Anat* **120:** 113–130.
Mascagni P (1819) *Prodromo della grande Anatomia*, Florence: Giovanni Marenghi.
Matthews BF (1953) Composition of articular cartilage in osteoarthritis. *Br Med J* **2:** 660–661.
Maximov AA, Bloom W (1952) *Textbook of Histology*, London: Saunders.
Menck J, Lierse W (1990) The arterial supply of the thoracic and lumbar spine in newborns. *Acta Anat* **137:** no 2, 170–174.
Mendel PL, Hollenberg NK (1971) Cardiac output distribution in the rat; comparison of rubidium and microsphere methods. *Am J Physiol* **221:** 1617–1620.
Meriel P, Ruffie R, Fournie A (1955) La phlébographie de la hanche dans les coxarthoses. *Rev Rhum Mal Osteoartic* **22:** 238–241.
Mestdagh H, Bailleul JP, Chambon JP, Laraki A (1979) The dorsal arterial network of the wrist with reference to the blood supply of the carpal bones. *Acta Morphol Neerl Scand* **17:** no 1.
Mestdagh H, Houcke M, Mairesse JL, Vilette B, Depreux R (1984) Vascular anatomy of the pisiform bone. *Ann Chir Main* **3:** no 2, 145–148.
Meyer K (1957) The chemistry of the mesodermal ground substances. *Harvey Lect* **51:** 88–112.
Michel (1872) Quoted by Langer (1876) from *Ber K Sächs Ges Wiss* 331.
Michelson K (1967) Pressure relationships in the bone marrow. *Acta Physiol Scand* **71:** 16–29.
Mikic ZD (1992) Blood supply of the articular disc of the antebrachiocarpal joint in dogs. *J Anat* **181 (Pt 3):** 447–453.
Miller ME, Christenson GC, Evans HE (1964) *Anatomy of the Dog*, Philadelphia, Saunders and Co.

Miodoński AJ, Kus J, Tyrankiewicz R (1981) SEM blood vessel casts analysis. In: *Three-dimensional Anatomy of Cells and Tissue Surfaces* (eds JA Didio, PM Motta, DJ Allen), Amsterdam: Elsevier, 71–87.

Misrahy GA, Hardwick DF, Brooks CJ, Garwood VP, Hall WP (1962) Bone, bone marrow and brain oxygen. *Am J Physiol* **202:** 225–231.

Mody BS, Belliappa PP, Dias JJ, Barton NJ (1993) Non-union of fractures of the scaphoid tuberosity. *J Bone Joint Surg* **75B:** 423–425.

Montgomery RJ, Sutker BD, Bronk JT, Kelly PJ (1988) Interstitial fluid flow in cortical bone. *Microvasc Res* **35:** 295–307.

Montis S, Ridola C (1959a) Vascolarizzazione dell' astragolo. *Quad Anat Prat* **15:** 574–580.

Montis S, Ridola C (1959b) Vascolarizzasione del calcagno. *Quad Anat Prat* **15:** 565–573.

Moore CD, Gewertz BL, Wheeler HT, Fry WJ (1981) An additional source of error in microsphere measurement of regional blood flow. *Microvasc Res* **21:** 377–383.

Moran CG, Wood MB (1992) Failure of perfusion with oxygenated Krebs-Ringer solution to preserve the eccrine function of the vascular endothelium in bone. *J Orthop Res* **10:** 813–817.

Morgan JD (1959) Blood supply of the growing rabbit's tibia. *J Bone Joint Surg* **41B:** 185–203.

Mørkrid L, Ofstad J, Willassen Y (1976) Effect of steric restriction on the intracortical distribution of microspheres in dog kidney. *Circ Res* **39:** 608–615.

Morris MA, Kelly PJ (1980) Use of tracer microspheres to measure bone blood flow in conscious dogs. *Calcif Tissue Int* **32:** 69–76.

Morton JJ, Stabins SJ (1927) An experimental study of certain factors influencing osteogenesis. *NY State J Med* **27:** 1197–1198.

Moschcowitz E (1916) The relation of angiogenesis to ossification: based upon the study of five cases of calcification and ossification of the ovary. *Bull Johns Hopkins Hosp* **27:** 71–78.

Moses MA, Sudhalter J, Langer R (1990) Identification of an inhibitor of neovascularization from cartilage. *Science* **248:** 1408–1410.

Müller H (1858) Über die Entwicklung der Knochensubstanz nebst Bemerkungen über den Bau rachitischer Knochen. *Z Wiss Zool* **9:** 147–233.

Mueller W (1926) Über das Verhalten des Knochengewebes bei herabgesetzter Zirkulation und das Bild von Nekrose der Zwischenlamellen. *Beitr Klin Chir* **138:** 614–624.

Murray PDF, Kodiček E (1949) Bones, muscles and vitamin C. II. Partial deficiencies of vitamin C and mid-diaphyseal thickenings of the tibia and fibula in guinea-pigs. *J Anat* **83:** 205–223.

Murray PDF, Selby D (1930) Intrinsic and extrinsic factors in the primary development of the skeleton. *Arch EntwMech Org* **122:** 629–662.

Nagel A (1993) The clinical significance of the nutrient artery. *Orthop Rev* **22:** 557–561.

Nakano T, Thompson JR, Christopherson RJ, Aherne FX (1986) Blood flow distribution in hind limb bones and joint cartilage from young growing pigs. *Can J Vet Res* **50:** 96–100.

Needham J (1931) *Chemical Embryology*, vol 3, Cambridge: University Press.

Nelson GG, Kelly PJ, Lowell FA, Peterson LFA, Janes JM (1960) Blood supply of the human tibia. *J Bone Joint Surg* **42A:** 625–635.

Nesbitt R (1736) *Human Osteogeny Explained in Two Lectures, etc.*, London: T Wood.

Neuman WF, Neuman MW (1958) *The Chemical Dynamics of Bone Mineral*, Chicago: Chicago University Press.

Neutze JM, Wyler F, Rudolph AM (1968) Use of radioactive microspheres to assess distribution of cardiac output in rabbits. *Am J Physiol* **315:** 486–495.

Nicoladoni K (1875) Von Dumreicher's Methode zur Behandlung drohender Pseudarthrosen. *Wien Med Wochenschr* **25:** 124.

Nicholas JS (1950) Development of contractility. *Proc Am Phil Soc* **94:** 175–183.

Nilsonne U (1959) Biophysical investigations of the mineral phase in healing fractures. *Acta Orthop Scand Suppl* **37:** 1–81.

Nilsson GE, Tenland T, Oberg PA (1980) A new instrument for continuous measurement of tissue blood flow by light spectroscopy. *IEEE Trans Biomed Eng* **27:** 12–19.

Nissen KI (1963) The arrest of early primary osteoarthritis of the hip by osteotomy. *Proc R Soc Med* **56:** 1051–1060.

Niv AI, Hungerford DS (1979) Bone blood flow in anaesthetized and conscious dogs. *Proc 25th Meet Orthop Res Soc* **4:** 17.

Noback CR, Robertson GG (1951) Sequences of appearance of ossification centers in the human skeleton during the first five prenatal months. *Am J Anat* **89:** 1–28.

Noden DM (1990) Origins and assembly of avian embryonic blood vessels. *Ann NY Acad Sci* **588:** 236–249.

Nomina Anatomica (1989) 6th edn. Authorized by the 12th International Congress of Anatomists. Edinburgh: Churchill Livingstone.

Notzli HP, Swiontowski MF, Thaxter ST, Carpenter GK, Wyatt JR (1989) Laser Doppler flowmetry for bone blood flow measurement: He-Ne laser light attenuation and depth of perfusion assessment. *J Orthop Res* 7: 413–424.

Novack P, Goluboff B, Bortin L, Soffe A, Shenkin HA (1953) Studies of the cerebral circulation and metabolism in congestive heart failure. *Circulation* 7: 724–731.

Novak V (1959) Arrangements of vessels in the periosteum of long bones in the newborn. *Čslká Morf* 7: 353–362.

Nussbaum A (1923) Anatomie der Knochenarterien und Knochencapillaren, ihre Beziehuing zur Entstehung der Gelenkmaüse, der Tuberkulose und der Osteomyelitis. *Arch Klin Chir* **126:** 40–42.

Nutton RW, Fitzgerald RH, Brown ML, Kelly PJ (1984) Dynamic radioisotope bone imaging as a non-invasive indicator of canine tibial blood flow. *J Orthop Res* **2:** 67–74.

Oberdahlhoff H (1946) Zur Frage der Knochenneubildung. *Chirurg* **17:** 123–129.

Oberlin C, Salon A, Pigeau I, Sarcy JJ, Guidici P, Treil N (1992) Three-dimensional reconstruction of the carpus and its vasculature: an anatomic study. *J Hand Surg* **17A:** 67–72.

Obletz BE, Halbstein BM (1938) Non-union of fractures of carpal navicular. *J Bone Joint Surg* **20:** 424–428.

Oehmke HJ (1987) Blood supply and function of the scaphoid bone. *Unfallchirurgie* **13:** 174–177.

Ohtani O, Gannon B, Ohtsuka A, Murakami T (1982) The microvasculature of bone and especially of bone marrow as studied by scanning electron microscopy of vascular casts, a review. *Scan Electron Microsc* **1:** 427–434.

Oki S, Matsuda Y, Itoh T, Shibata T, Okumura H, Desaki J (1994) Scanning electron microscopic observations of the vascular structure of vertebral end-plates in rabbits. *J Orthop Res* **12:** 447–449.

Okubo M, Kinoshita M, Yukimura T, Abe Y, Shimazu A (1979) Experimental study of measurement of regional blood flow in the adult mongrel dog using radioactive microspheres. *Clin Orthop Rel Res* **138:** 263–270.

Oliveira H de (1932) Contribution à la connaissance de la mécano-structure du tibia humain. *Folia Anat Univ Conimbr* **7:** 1–10.

Ollier L (1867) *Traité expérimentale et clinique de la régénération des os et de la production artificielle du tissu osseux*, Paris: Masson.

O'Malley AG, Law WA (1963) The influence of the flexor and adductor muscles in osteoarthritis of the hip joint. *Proc R Soc Med* **56:** 122–125.

Omura K, Osogoe B (1951) Saponin-induced colonization of the bone marrow elements in foreign organs in rabbits. *Anat Rec* **110:** 289–312.

Oni OA, Dearing S, Pringle S (1993) Endothelial cells and bone cells. In: *Bone Circulation and Vascularization in Normal and Pathological Conditions* (eds A Schoutens, J Arlet, JWM Gardeniers, SPF Hughes), London: Plenum Press, 43–48.

Orr JW, Strickland LH (1938) The metabolism of bone marrow. *Biochemistry* **32:** 567–571.

Osgood RB (1903) Lesions of the tibial tubercle occurring during adolescence. *Boston Med Surg J* **148:** 114 (see also Schlatter C).

Ostrup LT, Stromberg B, Alm A (1976) The vascular anatomy of the dorsal part of the caudal ribs in the dogs. A microangiographic study with special reference to the microvascular free transfer of living rib grafts. *Scand J Plast Reconstr Surg* **10:** no 2, 1129–1134.

Otter MW, Palmieri VR, Cochran GVB (1990) Transcortical streaming potentials are generated by circulatory pressure gradients in living canine tibia. *J Orthop Res* **8:** 119–126.

Ottolenghi D (1902) Sur les nerfs de la moelle des os. *Arch Ital Biol* **37:** 73–80.

Paff GH (1948) Influence of pH on growth of bone in tissue culture. *Proc Soc Exp Biol Med* **68:** 288–293.

Paget Sir James (1867) In: *Lectures on Surgical Pathology* (ed. William Turner), London: Longman.

Panagis JS, Gelberman RH, Taleisnik J, Baumgaertner M (1983) The arterial anatomy of the human carpus *Part II:* The intra vascularity. *J Hand Surg* **8A:** 375–382.

Pappenheimer JR (1953) Passage of molecules through capillary walls. *Physiol Rev* **33:** 387–423.

Park EA (1939) Observations on the pathology of rickets with particular reference to the changes at the cartilage shaft junctions of the growing bones. *Bull NY Acad Med* **15:** 495–543.

Park EA (1954) Bone growth in health and disease. *Arch Dis Child* **29:** 269–281.

Parke WW, Whalen JL, Van Demark RE, Kambin P (1994) The infra-aortic arteries of the spine: their variability and clinical significance. *Spine* **19:** 1–5.

Parouti JP (1962) *Contribution à l'étude de la vascularization interne du fémur du chien*, Thèse, Toulouse: Imprimerie Moderne.

Parsons FG (1905) On pressure epiphyses. *J Anat Physiol Lond* **39:** 402–412.

Payton CG (1934) The position of the nutrient foramen and direction of the nutrient canal in the long bones of the madder-fed pig. *J Anat* **68:** 500–510.
Pearse HE Jr (1928) An experimental study of arterial collateral circulation. *Ann Surg* **88:** 227–232.
Pearse HE Jr, Morton JJ (1928) The stimulation of bone growth by venous stasis. *J Bone Joint Surg* **12:** 97–111.
Pearse HE, Morton JJ (1930) The influence of alterations in the circulation and repair of bone. *J Bone Joint Surg* **13:** 68–74.
Peck ME (1957) Obstructive anomalies of the iliac vein associated with growth shortening in the ipsilateral extremity. *Ann Surg* **146:** 619–629.
Perthes GC (1910) Über Arthritis deformans juvenilis. *Dtsch Z Chir* **101:** 779.
Petersen H (1930) Die Organs des Skeletsystems. In: *Handbuch der mikroskopischen Anatomie des Menschen* (ed W von Möllendorf), Berlin: Springer.
Peterson LFA, Neher M, Janes JM, Kelly PJ (1959) A stereoscopic microradiographic camera with vacuum filmholder and a steromicroscope. *Proc Staff Meet Mayo Clin* **34:** 283.
Petrakis NL (1952) Temperature of human bone marrow. *J Appl Physiol* **4:** 549–553.
Pfeiffer S, Lazenby R, Chiang J (1995) Brief communication: cortical remodelling data are affected by sampling location. *Am J Phys Anthrop* **96:** 89–92.
Phemister DB (1940) Changes in bones and joints resulting from interruption of circulation. *Arch Surg* **41:** 1455–1482.
Phibbs RH, Dong L (1970) Nonuniform distribution of microspheres in blood flowing through a medium sized artery. *Can J Physiol Pharmacol* **48:** 415–421.
Phillips RS (1966) Phlebography in osteoarthritis of the hip. *J Bone Joint Surg* **48B:** 280–288.
Phillips RS, Bulmer JH, Hoyle G, Davis W (1967) Venous drainage in osteoarthritis of the hip. *J Bone Joint Surg* **49B:** 301–309.
Pinard A (1952) *Structure et vaisseaux de la diaphyse des os longs chez le fetus humain*, Thèse, Bâle: S Karger.
Piney A (1922) Anatomy of the bone marrow with special reference to the distribution of red marrow. *Br Med J* **2:** 792–795.
Piollet P (1905) Sur la direction des artères nourricières des os longs. *J Anat Physiol Paris* **41:** 50–57.
Pistolesi GF (1962) *Il circolo venoso profondo dell'anca nell'artrosi*, film produced by Istituto di Ortopedia e Traumatologia, Universitá di Padova, Italy.
Platt D, Pigman W, Holley HL, Patton FM (1956) An electrophoretic study of normal and post mortem human and bovine synovial fluids. *Arch Biochem* **64:** 152–163.
Pollack S, Petrov N, Salzstein R, Brankov G, Blagoeva R (1984) An anatomical model for streaming potentials in osteons. *J Biomech* **17:** 627–636.
Polster J (1970) *Zur Hæmodynamik des Knochens*, Stuttgart: Ferdinande Enke.
Pommer G (1927) Über Begriff und Bedeutung der durchbohrenden Knochenkanäle. *Z Mikrosk Anat Forsch* **9:** 540–584.
Post M, Shoemaker WC (1962) Bone electrolyte response to intravenous acid loads. *Surg Gynecol Obstet* **115:** 749–756.
Pratt CMW (1957) Observations of osteogenesis in the femur of the fetal rat. *J Anat* **91:** 533–544.
Pratt CMW (1959) Postnatal changes in the shaft of the rat's femur. *J Anat* **93:** 309–322.
Preston BN, Davies DV, Ogston AG (1965) The composition and physico-chemical properties of hyaluronic acids prepared from ox synovial fluid and from a case of mesothelioma. *Biochemistry* **96:** 449–474.
Pridie KH (1952) The development of osteoarthritis of the hip joint. *J Bone Joint Surg* **34B:** 153.
Pringle S, De Bono DP (1988) Monoclonal antibodies to damaged and regenerating vascular endothelium. *J Clin Lab Immunol* **26:** 159–162.
Pritchard JJ (1961) Hard tissues – bone and bones. In: *Recent Advances in Anatomy* (eds F Goldby, RJ Harrison), London: Churchill.
Pritchard JJ (1963) Bone healing. *Scient Basis Med Annual Rev* (eds I Gilliland, J Francis), London: Athlone Press, 288–301.
Pritchard JJ, Ruzicka AJ (1950) A comparison of fracture repair in the frog, lizard and rat. *J Anat* **84:** 236–261.
Prives MG, Funstein LV, Scherban EI, Shishova VG (1959) Method of labelled atoms in *in vivo* investigations of arterial system of bone. *Arkh Anat Gistol Embriol* **37:** 56–64.
Pujol M, Tran M (1973) Étude gazométrique sur sang osseux trochanterien dans les coxopathies. In: *Proc Symp International sur la Circulation Osseuse*, pp. 259–265, (eds J Arlet, P Ficat), Toulouse: University Paul Sabatier.
Quain Jones (1894) *Elements of Anatomy* (eds Shäfer, GD Thane), London: Longmans, Green.

Radin EL (1974) Trabecular microfractures in response to stress: the possible mechanism of Wolff's law. In: *Proc 12th Int Soc Orthop Surg Traum*, Excerpta Medica: Amsterdam.

Ramseier E (1962) Untersuchungen über arteriosklerotische Veränderungen der Knochenarterien. *Virchows Arch Pathol Anat* **336:** 77–86.

Ranvier L (1875) *Traité technique d'histologie*, Paris: Savy.

Ray RD, Aouad R, Galante J (1963) Isotope studies of the circulatory dynamics of bone. *Symp Soc Int Chir Orthop Traumat* **1:** 6–9.

Reddi AH, Kuettner KE (1981) Vascular invasion of cartilage: correlation of morphology with lysosome, glycosaminoglycans, protease, and protease inhibitor activity during endochondral bone development. *Dev Biol* **82:** 217–223.

Reeve J, Arlot M, Wootton R, Edouard C, Tellez M, Hesp R, Green J, Meunier P (1988) Skeletal blood flow, iliac histomorphometry, and strontium kinetics in osteoporosis: a relationship between blood flow and corrected apposition rate. *J Clin Endocrinol Metab* **66:** 1124–1131.

Reichel SM (1947) Vascular system of the long bones of the rat. *Surgery, St Louis* **22:** 146–157.

Reichert ILH, McCarthy ID, Hughes SPF (1994) Acute haemodynamic effects of intramedullary reaming in the intact ovine tiba. In: *Association Internationale pour la Recherche sur la Circulation Osseuse (Toulouse), ARCO News Letter* **6:** no 2, 95.

Rehn E (1923) Fraktur und Muskel. *Arch Klin Chir* **128:** 640–666.

Remak R (1855) *Untersuchungen über die Entwicklung der Wirbeltiere*. Berlin: Reimer.

Revell WJ, Brookes M (1991) The effect of a pulsed electromagnetic field on bone sclerosis. *Proc Bioelec Repair Growth Soc* **11:** 8.

Revell WJ, Brookes M (1993a) Bone blood flow in the rat using arteriolar blockade; comparisons between labelled resin particles and microspheres. *J Anat* **182:** 305–312.

Revell WJ, Brookes M (1993b) Arteriolar blockade revisited. In: *Bone Circulation and Vascularization in Normal and Pathological Conditions* (eds A Schoutens, SPF Hughes, JWM Gardeniers, J Arlet), New York: Plenum, 73–84.

Revell WJ, Brookes M (1994) Haemodynamic changes in the rat femur and tibia following femoral vein ligation. *J Anat* **184:** 625–633.

Revell WJ, Heatley FW (1990) Long term sequential measurements of bone blood flow within a single animal by the hydrogen washout method. In: *Bone Circulation and Bone Necrosis* (eds J Arlet, B Mazières), Berlin: Springer, 124–128.

Revell WJ, Heatley FW, Brookes M (1991) The vascular response of the intact rabbit femur to simulated plating. Proceedings of the Anatomical Society. *J Anat* **179:** 220.

Reynolds O (1883) An experimental investigation of the circumstances which determine whether the motion of water shall be direct or sinuous and of the law of resistance in parallel channels. *Phil Trans R Soc* **174:** 935–982.

Reynolds SRM (1948) Morphological determinants of the flow characteristics between an artery and its branch, with special reference to the ovarian spiral artery in the rabbit. *Acta Anat* **5:** 1–6.

Rhinelander FW (1965) Some aspects of the microcirculation of healing bone. *Clin Orthop* **40:** 12–16.

Rhinelander FW (1968) The normal microcirculation of diaphyseal cortex and its response to fracture. *J Bone Joint Surg* **50A:** 784–800.

Rhinelander FW (1980) Vascular proliferation and blood supply during fracture healing. In: *Current Concepts of Internal Fixation of Fractures.* (Ed Uhthoff HK, Stahl E), Berlin: Springer-Verlag.

Rhinelander FW, Baragry RA (1962) Microangiography in bone healing. I. Undisplaced closed fractures. *J Bone Joint Surg* **44A:** 1273–1298.

Rhinelander FW, Bennett GA, Bauer W (1939) Exchange of substances in aqueous solution between joints and the vascular system. *J Clin Invest* **18:** 1–13.

Richards DJ, Brookes M (1968) Osteogenesis and the pH of the osseous circulation. *Calcif Tissue Res* **2:** suppl 93.

Richards DJ, Brookes M (1969) Physico-chemical sequelae of experimental osteotomy. *Calcif Tissue Res* **2:** suppl 93.

RICRP (1955) Recommendations of the International Commission on Radiological Protection. *Br J Radiol* suppl 6.

Riggi K, Wood MB, Ilstrup DM (1990) Dose-dependent variations in blood flow evaluation of canine nerve, nerve grafts, tendon, and ligament tissue by the radiolabelled microsphere technique. *J Orthop Res* **8:** 909–916.

Riggs SA, Wood MB, Cooney WP, Kelly PJ (1984) Blood flow and bone uptake of ^{99m}Tc labelled methylene diphosphonate. *J Orthop Res* **1:** 236–243.

Rindfleisch GE (1879) Über Knochenmark und Blutbildung. *Arch Mikrosk Anat* **17:** 1, 21.

Robertson DE (1927) Acute haematogenous osteomyelitis. *J Bone Joint Surg* **9:** 8–23.

Rodan GA, Bourret LA, Harvey BA, Mensi T (1975) Cyclic AMP and cyclic GMP: mediators of mechanical effects on bone remodelling. *Science* **189:** 467–469.

Rogers WM, Gladstone H (1950) Vascular foramina and arterial supply of the distal end of the femur. *J Bone Joint Surg* **32A:** 867–874.

Rojos LS (1961) La estimulación del crecimiento de los huesos largos en niños por bloqueo quirurgico del canal medular. *Gaz Med Mexico* **91:** 145–158.

Roome NW, McMaster PE (1934) Influence of venous stasis on heterotopic formation of bone. *Arch Surg Chicago* **29:** 54–58.

Rosen V, Theis RS (1995) *The Cellular and Molecular Basis of Bone Formation and Repair*, Heidelberg: RG Landes Co. Springer.

Rosenthal G, Bowie MA, Wagoner G (1941) Studies in the metabolism of articular cartilage. I. Respiration and glycolysis in cartilage in relation to its age. *J Cell Comp Physiol* **17:** 221–233.

Ross JD, Treadwell PE, Syverton JT (1962) Cultural characterization of animal cells. *Ann Rev Microbiol* **16:** 141–188.

Rowbotham GF, Little E (1962) The circulations and reservoir of the brain. *Br J Surg* **50:** 244–250.

Rowbotham GF, Little E (1965) New concepts on the aetiology and vascularization of meningiomata, etc. *Br J Surg* **52:** 21–24.

Rubascheva A, Prives MG (1932) Blutversorgung der langen Röhrenknochen des Hundes. *Z Anat Entwgesch* **98:** 361–374.

Rubin CT, Lanyon L (1984) Regulation of bone formation by applied dynamic load. *J Bone Joint Surg* **66A:** 397–402.

Rubin CT, Lanyon L (1987) Osteoregulatory nature of mechanical stimuli: function as a determinant for adaptive remodelling in bone. *J Orthop Res* **5:** 300–310.

Ruch TC, Fulton JF (1962) *Medical Physiology and Biophysics*, 18th edn, Philadelphia: Saunders.

Rutishauser E (1956) Vascularity of bone in relation to pathological studies. In: *CIBA Symposium, Bone Structure and Metabolism* (ed. GEW Wolstenholme), London: Churchill.

Rutishauser E, Forestier J, Herbert JJ, Rabinowicz T, Grasset E (1952) Aspects anatomo-cliniques des arthropathies de la hanche. *Rev Rhum Mal Ostéoartic* **19:** 869.

Sabin FR (1932) Bone marrow. In: *Cowdry's Special Cytology*, 2nd edn, New York: Hoeber.

Sakul BU, Guzel MB, Islam C (1994) The location and the nutrient foramina on the shafts of the limb bones. *Keibogaku Zasshi J Anat* **69:** 410–411.

Salter RB, Field P (1960) The effects of continuous compression on living articular cartilage. *J Bone Joint Surg* **42A:** 31–49.

Saperstein LA (1958) Regional blood flow by fractional distribution of indicators. *Am J Physiol* **193:** 161–168.

Sapia FS de (1953) Scollamento del periostio ed allungamento degli arti. *Ortop Traumat Appar Mot* **21:** 339–345.

Sappey Ph C (1867) *Traité d'anatomie descriptive*, Tom. II, Paris: Adrien Delahaye.

Sartor K (1978) Detailed myelographic diagnosis: the spinal arteries in the Amipaque myelogram *ROFO* **129:** 575–808.

Sasaki Y, Wagner HN (1971) Measurement of the distribution of cardiac output in unanesthetized rats. *J Appl Physiol* **30:** 879–884.

Scaglietti O (1960) Surgical vascular crisis for the treatment of painful manifestations of arthrosis of the hip. *Sperimentale* **110:** 296–304.

Schenk R, Willeneger H (1964) Zur Histologie der primären Knochenheilung. *Langenbecks Arch Chir* **308:** 440–452.

Scheuermann HW (1920) Coxa valga caused by a separation of the epiphysis. *Acta Orthop Scand* **1:** 178.

Schiepers C (1993) Skeletal fluoride kinetics of 18F- and positron emission tomography (PET): *in vivo* estimation of regional bone blood flow and influx rate in humans. In: *Bone Circulation and Vascularization in Normal and Pathological Conditions* (eds A Schoutens, SPF Hughes, JWM Gardenieres), New York: Plenum, 95–100.

Schlatter C (1903) Verletzungen des schnabelförmigen Fort satzes der oberen Tibia-epiphyse. *Beitr Clin Chir* **36:** 874

Schmid K, McNair MB (1956) Characterization of the proteins of human synovial fluid in certain disease states. *J Clin Invest* **35:** 815–824.

Schmorl G (1929) Zur pathologischen Anatomie der Wirbelsaüle. *Klin Wochenschr* **8:** 1243–1249.

Schnitzer JE, McKinstry, Light TR, Ogden JA (1982) Quantification of regional chondro-osseous circulation in canine tibia and femur. *Am J Physiol* **242:** H365–H375.

Schoefl GI (1963) Studies on inflammation. III. Growing capillaries: their structure and permeability. *Virchows Arch Path Anat Physiol* **337:** 97–141.

Schoutens A, Bergmann P, Verhas M (1979) Bone blood flow measured by ^{85}Sr microspheres and bone seeking clearances in the rat. *Am J Physiol* **236:** H1–H6.
Schüller M (1889) Mittheillung über die kunstliche Steigerung des Knochenwachstums beim Menschen. *Berl Klin Wschr* **26:** 21–24, 50–54.
Schumacher S (1935) Zur Anordnung der Gefässkanäle in der Diaphyse langer Röhrenknochen des Menschen. *Z Mikrosk Anat Forsch* **38:** 145–160.
Schwalbe G (1876) Über die Ernährungskanäle der Knochen und das Knochenwachstum. *Z Anat EntwGesch* **1:** 307–352.
Schwann T (1839) *Mikroscopische Untersuchungen über der Übereinstimmung in der Struktur und dem Wachstum der Thiere und Pflanzen*, Berlin: Sander.
Schweigk H (1932) Untersuchungen über die Leberdurchblutung und den Pfortaderkreislauf. *Arch Exp Path Pharmak* **168:** 693–714.
Seliger WG (1970) Tissue fluid movement in compact bone. *Anat Rec* **166:** 247–255.
Selye H (1934) On the mechanism controlling the growth in length of the long bones. *J Anat* **68:** 289–292.
Semb H (1971) Bone marrow blood flow studies by iodoantipyrene clearance technique. *Surg Gynecol Obstet* **133:** 472–474.
Servelle M (1948) Stase veineuse et croissance osseuse. *Bull Acad Nat Med* **132:** 471–474.
Shamos MH, Levine LS, Shamos LI (1963) Piezoelectric effect in bone. *Nature* **197:** 81.
Sharpey W (1848) In: Quain J, *Elements of Anatomy* 5th edn (eds R Quain, W Sharpey), London: Taylor, Walton & Maberly.
Sharpey W, Ellis GV (1856) In: Quain J, *Elements of Anatomy* 6th edn (eds W Sharpey, GV Ellis), London: Walton & Maberly.
Shaw NE (1963) Observations on the intramedullary blood flow and marrow pressure in bone. *Clin Sci* **24:** 311–318.
Shaw NE (1966) The relation between blood flow in muscles and the circulation in bones. In: *Calcified Tissues, 1965* (eds H Fleisch, HJJ Blackwood, M Owen), Berlin: Springer.
Shaw NE, Harris NH (1960) Treatment of osteoarthritis of the hip by myelotomy: a preliminary report. *Proc R Soc Med* **53:** 949–950.
Shim SS (1963) *The Effects of Epinephrine on Bone Blood Flow in Dogs and Rabbits*, MSc Thesis, University of British Columbia.
Shim SS, Patterson FP (1966) A direct method of qualitative study of bone blood circulation. *Surg Gynecol Obstet* **125:** 261–268.
Shim SS, Copp DH, Patterson FP (1966) Bone blood flow in the limb following complete sciatic nerve section. *Surg Gynecol Obstet* **123:** 333–335.
Shim SS, Copp DH, Patterson FP (1968) Measurement of the rate and distribution of the nutrient and other arterial blood supply in long bones of the rabbit: a study of the relative contributions of the three arterial systems. *J Bone Joint Surg* **50B:** 178–183.
Shim SS, Hawk HE, Yu WY (1972) The relationship between blood flow and marrow cavity pressure of bone. *Surg Gynecol Obstet* **135:** 353–360.
Shulman SS (1959) Observations on the nutrient foramina of the human radius and ulna. *Anat Rec* **134:** 685–697.
Siffert RS (1956) The effect of staples and longitudinal wires on epiphyseal growth: an experimental study. *J Bone Joint Surg* **38A:** 1077–1088.
Sim FA, Kelly PJ (1970) Relationship of bone remodelling, oxygen consumption, and blood flow in bone. *J Bone Joint Surg* **52A:** 1377–1389.
Simpson ME, Asling CW, Evans HM (1950) Some endocrine influences on skeletal growth and differentiation. *Yale J Biol Med* **23:** 1–27.
Singh M, Brookes M (1971) Bone growth and blood flow after experimental venous ligation. *J Anat* **108:** 315–322.
Skawina A, Miaśkiewicz C (1982) Nutrient foramina in femoral tibial and fibular bones in human fetuses. *Folia Morphol (Warsz)* **41:** 469–481.
Skawina A, Wyczółkowski M (1987) Nutrient foramina of humerus, radius and ulna in human fetuses. *Folia Morphol (Warsz)* **46:** 17–24.
Skawina A, Litwin JA, Gorczyca J, Miodoński AJ (1994a) The vascular system of human fetal long bones: a scanning electron microscope study of corrosion casts. *J Anat* **185:** 369–376.
Skawina A, Litwin JA, Gorgczyca J, Miodoński AJ (1994b) Blood vessels in epiphyseal cartilage of human femoral bone: a scanning electron microscopic study of corrosion casts. *Anat Embryol* **189:** 457–462.
Smith JW (1960) Collagen fibre patterns in mammalian bone. *J Anat* **94:** 329–344.

Sœur R (1949) The synovial membrane of the knee in pathological conditions. *J Bone Joint Surg* **31A:** 317–340.
Somjen D, Binderman I, Berger E, Harrel A (1980) Bone remodelling induced by physical stress is prostaglandin mediated. *Biocheim Biophys Acta* **629:** 91–100.
Somogyi B (1964) Blood supply of the fetal spine. *Acta Morph Hung* **12:** 261–274.
Sorby H (1856) On slaty cleavage as exhibited in the Devonian limestone of Devonshire. *Phil Mag* **11:** 20.
Soulié A (1904) Sur les applications de la radiographie stérioscopique à l'étude des artères des os. *CR Assoc Anat* **6:** 172–174.
Spalteholz KW (1911) *Über das Durchsichtigmachen von menschlichen and tierischen Präparaten; etc.*, Leipzig: S Hirzel.
Spira E, Farin I, Karplus H (1963) The capillary conducting channels in the distal epiphyses of radius and ulna of the rabbit. *J Anat* **97:** 255–258.
Stanek KA, Smith TL, Murphy WR, Coleman TG (1983) Haemodynamic disturbances in the rat as a function of the number of microspheres injected. *Am J Physiol* **245:** H290–H293.
Stanley E (1849) *A Treatise on Diseases of Bone*, London.
Stein AH Jr, Morgan HC, Porras RF, Reynolds FC (1957) Variations in normal bone marrow pressures. *J Bone Joint Surg* **39A:** 1129–1134.
Stein AH Jr, Morgan HC, Porras RF (1958) The effect of pressor and depressor drugs on intramedullary bone marrow pressure. *J Bone Joint Surg* **40A:** 1103–1110.
Stein AH Jr, Morgan HC, Porras RF (1959) The effect of an arterio-venous fistula on intramedullary bone pressure. *Surg Gynecol Obstet* **109:** 287–290.
Steinbach HL, Jergeson F, Gilfillan RS, Petrakis NL (1957) Osseous phlebography. *Surg Gynecol Obstet* **40A:** 215–226.
Sterling K, Grey SJ (1950) Determination of the circulating red *cell volume* in man by radio-active chromium. *J Clin Invest* **29:** 1614–1619
Stilwell DL (1959) The vascular supply of vertebral structures. Gross anatomy: rabbit and monkey. *Anat Rec* **135:** 169–183.
Strangeways TSP (1920) Observations on the nutrition of articular cartilage. *Br Med J* **1:** 661–663.
Streeter GL (1949) Developmental horizons in human embryos (4th issue). A review of the histogenesis of cartilage and bone. *Contrib Embryol Carnegie Inst* **33:** 149–167.
Strehler BL (1962) *Time, Cells and Ageing*, London: Academic.
Studitsky AN (1936) Experimentalanalyse der Differrenzierungsfaktoren primäre Skelete. *Z Zellforsch mikrosk Anat* **24:** 269–302.
Stump CW (1925) The histogenesis of bone. *J Anat* **59:** 136–154.
Sugiura Y (1958) A morphological and physiological study of bone sensitivity. *Arch Jap Chir* **27:** 597–608.
Suzuki T, Kurokawa K, Okabe K, Ito K, Hatori T, Imai K, Yamanaka H (1991) Correlation between the prostatic vessels and vertebral venous system of the dog. *Jap J Urol* **82:** 1742–1747.
Suzuki T, Kurokawa K, Okabe K, Ito K, Yamanaka H (1992) Correlation between the prostatic vein and vertebral venous system under various conditions. *Prostate* **21:** 153–165.
Swiontkowski MF, Tepic S, Perren SM, Moor R, Ganz R, Rahn BA (1986) Laser Doppler flowmetry for bone blood flow measurement: correlation with microsphere estimates and evaluation of the effect of intracapsular pressure on femoral head blood flow. *J Orthop Res* **4:** 362–371.
Testut L (1880) *Vaisseaux et nerfs des tissus conjonctif fibreux, séreux et osseux: anatomie et physiologie*, Thèse d'agrégation, Paris: G Masson.
Testut L, Latarjet A (1948) *Traité d'Anatomie Humaine*, Tom I, Paris: G Doin.
Thiersch K (1865) Thiersch Graft. *Arch Mik Anat* 149.
Thomas HO (1886) *Contributions to Surgery and Medicine, Part VI. The principles of the treatment of fractures and dislocations*, London: Longman.
Thomas NR (1967) The tension theory of eruption. *J Anat* **102:** 143.
Thurston TJ (1982) Distribution of nerves in long bones as shown by silver impregnation. *J Anat* **143:** 719–728.
Tilling G (1958) The vascular anatomy of long bones: a radiological and histological study. *Acta Radiol Suppl* **161:** 1–107.
Tocantins LM, O'Neill JF (1941) Infusions of blood and other fluids into the general circulation via the bone marrow: technique and results. *Surg Gynecol Obstet* **73:** 281–287.
Tomes CS (1882) *A Manual of Dental Anatomy*, 2nd edn, London: Churchill.
Tomlin DH, Henry KM, Kon SK (1953) Autoradiographic study of growth and calcium metabolism in the long bones of the rat. *Br J Nutr* **7:** 235–252.

Tøndevold E (1983) Haemodynamics of long bones. *Acta Orthop Scand* **54:** suppl 205, 1–48
Tøndevold E, Eliasen P (1982) Regional vascular volumes and dynamic haematocrit compared to regional perfusion in canine cancellous and cortical bone. *Acta Orthop Scand* **53:** 197–203.
Töndury G (1958) *Entwicklungsgeschichte und Fehlbildungen der Wirbelsäule*. Stuttgart: Hippokrates.
Tonna EA, Cronkite EP (1962) Changes in the skeletal cell proliferative response to trauma concomitant with ageing. *J Bone Joint Surg* **44A:** 1557–1568.
Torreilles JFC (1962) *Contribution à l'étude de la vascularization interne de l'humérus du chien*, Thèse. Toulouse: Imprimerie Moderne.
Tothill P (1984) Bone blood flow measurement. *J Biomed Eng* **6:** 251–256.
Tothill P, McCormick J (1976) Bone blood flow in the rat determined by the uptake of radioactive particles. *Clin Sci Mol Med* **51:** 403–406.
Tothill P, Hooper G (1984) Invalidity of single passage measurements of the extraction of bone seeking tracers in rats and rabbits. *J Orthop Res* **2:** 75–79.
Tothill P, McPherson JN (1978) Post-mortem migration of bone seeking radionuclides in the rat and rabbit and its effect on estimates of bone uptake. *Clin Sci Mol Med* **55:** 221–223.
Tothill P, McPherson JN (1980) Limitations of radioactive microspheres as tracers for bone blood flow and extraction rate studies. *Calcif Tissue Int* **31:** 261–265.
Tothill P, McPherson JN (1986) The distribution of blood flow to the whole skeleton in dogs, rabbits and rats measured with microspheres. *Clin Phys Physiol Meas* **7:** 117–123.
Tothill P, Hooper G, McCarthy ID, Hughes SPF (1985) The variation with flow of the extraction of bone seeking tracers in recirculation experiments. *Calcif Tissue Int* **37:** 312–317.
Tothill P, Hooper G, Hughes SPF, McCarthy ID (1987) Bone blood flow measured with microspheres: the problem of non-entrapment. *Clin Phys Physiol Meas* **8:** 51–55.
Tower SS (1937a) Function and structure in the chronically isolated lumbo-sacral spinal cord of the dog. *J Comp Neurol* **67:** 109–131.
Tower SS (1937b) Trophic control of non-nervous tissues by the nervous system. *J Comp Neurol* **67:** 241–267.
Toynbee J (1841) Researches tending to prove the non-vascularity and the peculiar uniform mode of organization and nutrition of certain animal tissues. *Phil Trans R Soc* **131:** 159–192.
Treharne RW (1981) Review of Wolff's law and its proposed means of operation. *Orthop Rev* **10:** 35–47.
Trias A (1961) Effect of persistent pressure on the articular cartilage: an experimental study. *J Bone Joint Surg* **43B:** 376–386.
Trias A, Fery A (1979) Cortical circulation of long bones. *J Bone Joint Surg* **61A:** 1052–1059.
Triffit PD, Gregg PJ (1990) Measurement of blood flow to the tibial diaphysis using 11μm radioactive microspheres: a comparative study in the adult rabbit. *J Orthop Res* **8:** 642–645.
Trueta J (1953) Influence of the blood supply in controlling bone growth. *Bull Hosp Jt Dis NY* **14:** 147–157.
Trueta J (1954) Osteoarthritis of the hip. *Ann R Coll Surg* **15:** 174–192.
Trueta J (1957) The normal vascular anatomy of the human femoral head during growth. *J Bone Joint Surg* **39B:** 358–394.
Trueta J (1963) The role of the vessels in osteogenesis. *J Bone Joint Surg* **45B:** 402–418.
Trueta J (1968) *Studies of the Development and Decay of the Human Frame*, London: Heinemann.
Trueta J, Amato VP (1960) The vascular contribution to osteogenesis. 3. Changes in the growth cartilage caused by experimentally induced ischaemia. *J Bone Joint Surg* **42B:** 571–587.
Trueta J, Cavadias AX (1955) Vascular changes caused by the Küntscher type of nailing: an experimental study in the rabbit. *J Bone Joint Surg* **37B:** 492–505.
Trueta J, Harrison MHM (1953) The normal vascular anatomy of the femoral head in the adult man. *J Bone Joint Surg* **35B:** 442–461.
Trueta J, Morgan JD (1960) The vascular contribution to osteogenesis. I. Studies by the injection method. *J Bone Joint Surg* **42B:** 97–109.
Tucker FR (1949) Arterial supply to the femoral head and its clinical importance. *J Bone Joint Surg* **31B:** 82–93.
Trystrup N, Winkler K, Andreassen M (1962) Determination of the hepatic arterial blood flow and oxygen supply in man by clamping the hepatic artery during surgery. *J Clin Invest* **41:** 447–454.
Urist MR, McLean FC (1941) Calcification and ossification. I. Calcification in the callus in healing fractures in normal rats. *J Bone Joint Surg* **23A:** 1–16.
Urist MR, McLean FC (1952) Osteogenetic potency and new bone formation by induction in transplants to the anterior chamber of the eye. *J Bone Joint Surg* **34A:** 443–476.
Van Demark RE, Parke WW (1992) Avascular necrosis of the hamate – a case report with reference to the hamate blood supply. *J Hand Surg* **17A:** 1086–90.

Vanderhoeft P, de Marneffe R, Litvine J, van der Stricht J (1963) Mécanismes par lesquels une fistule artérioveneuse expérimentale modifie la croissance osseuse. Hypothèses. *Acta Chir Belg* **62:** 999–1012.
Vander Grend R, Deli PC, Glowczeskie F, Leslie B, Ruby LK (1994) Intraosseous blood supply of the capitate and its relation with aseptic necrosis. *J Hand Surg* **9A:** no 5, 677–683.
van der Stricht O (1892) Nouvelles recherches sur la genèse des globules rouges et des globules blancs du sang. *Arch Biol Paris* **12:** 199–344.
van Dyke D, Anger HO, Yano Y, Bozzini C (1965) Bone blood flow shown with F^{18} and the positron camera. *Am J Physiol* **209:** 65–70.
van Leeuwenhoek, Antonie (1674) Microscopical observations from M Leeuwenhoek concerning blood, milk, bones, the brain, spitle and cuticula etc. Letter to Royal Society dated 1 June. *Phil Trans R Soc* **9:** 121–128.
Vasciaveo F, Bartoli E (1961) Vascular channels and resorption cavities in the long bone cortex of the bovine bone. *Acta Anat* **47:** 1–33.
Vaubel E (1933) The form and function of synovial cells in tissue culture. II. The production of mucin. *J Exp Med* **58:** 85–95.
Veall N, Vetter H (1958) *Radioisotope Techniques in Clinical Research and Diagnosis*, London: Butterworths.
Venable CS, Stuck WG (1946) Muscle flap transplant for the relief of painful monoarticular osteoarthritis (aseptic necrosis) of the hip. *Ann Surg* **123:** 641–655.
Venturi JB (1797) *Recherches expérimentales sur le principe de la communication latérale du mouvement dans les fluides*, Paris: Houel & Ducros.
Verbout AJ (1974) *De vroeg-embryonale ontwikkeling van de wervelkolom van het schaap, met een kritische toetsing van de theorie der "Neugliederung"*, Thesis, University of Leiden.
Verbout AJ (1985) The development of the vertebral column. In: *Advances in Anatomy, Embryology & Cell Biology*, vol 90, Berlin: Springer.
Vesalius A (1555) *De Humani Corporis Fabrica*, Basel: Oporini.
Volkmann R (1863) Zur Histologie der Caries und Ostitis. *Arch Klin Chir* **4:** 437–474.
Von Bochmann G (1937) Die Entwicklung der Säugetierwirbel der hinteren Körperregionen. *Morph Jahrbuch* **79:** 1–53.
von Ebner V (1888) Urwirbel und Neugliederung der Wirbel-säule. *Sitzungsber Akad Wiss Wien III* **97:** 194–206.
von Eggeling H (1935) Gefässekanäle, Epiphysenkerne und Knochenwachstum. *Z Rassenk* **2:** 240–248.
von Friedländer F (1904) Beitrag zur Kenntnis der Architektur spongiöser Knochen. *Anat Hefte Abt 1* **23:** 235–282.
von Haller A (1743–56) *Iconum Anatomicorum Corporis Humani Fasciculi*, vol 5 (1752), Gottingae: Abram Vandenhoeck.
von Haller A (1763) *Experimentorum de Ossium Formatione. Opera Minora*, vol 2, Lausanne: Francisco Grasset.
von Roentgen WC (1895) Discovery of X Rays, for which he was awarded the Nobel Prize.
von Rustizky S (1872) Untersuchungen über Knochenmark. *Zentralbl Med Wiss* **10:** 56–564.
Vsevolodov GF (1959) Compact tissue veins of long cylindrical bones of extremities in man. *Arkh Anat Gistol Emb riol* **37:** 60–65.
Waine H (1958) Observations of osteoarthritis. *Arthritis Rheum* **1:** 454–461.
Waisbrod H, Treiman N (1980) Intraosseous venography in patellofemoral disorders: a preliminary report. *J Bone Joint Surg* **62B:** 454–456.
Walker RA (1985) *Ulex europeus* I – peroxidase as a marker of vascular endothelium: its application in routine histopathology. *J Pathol* **146:** 123–127.
Wardle EN (1964) Osteotomy of the tibia and fibula in the treatment of chronic osteoarthritis of the knee. *Postgrad Med J* **40:** 536–542.
Warren DJ, Ledingham JG (1974) Measurement of cardiac output distribution using microspheres; some theoretical and practical considerations. *Cardiovasc Res* **8:** 570–581.
Warwick R (1950) The relation of the direction of the mental foramen to the growth of the human mandible. *J Anat* **84:** 116–120.
Watermann R (1961) *Die Gefässkanäle der kniegelenksnahen Wachstumzonen*, Köln: Universitätverlag.
Watson-Jones Sir R (1952) *Fractures and Joint Injuries*, vol 1, 4th edn, London: Livingstone.
Weidenreich F (1923) Knochenstudien. I. Teil. Über Aufbau und Entwicklung des Knochens und den Charakter des Knochengewebes. *Z Anat EntwGesch* **69:** 382–466.
Weidenreich F (1930) Das Knochengewebe. In: *Handbuch der mikroskopischen Anatomie des Menschen*. W von Möllendorf, II/2, Berlin: Springer.

Weiland AJ, Berggren A (1981) Regional cortical blood flow measured by the hydrogen washout technique in composite canine rib grafts revascularized by microvascular anastomoses. *Int J Microsurg* **3:** 13–18.

Weiland M, Berggren A, Jones L (1982) The acute effects of blocking medullary blood supply on regional cortical blood flow in canine ribs as measured by the hydrogen washout technique. *Clin Orthop Rel Res* **165:** 265–272.

Weinmann DT, Kelly PJ, Owen CA, Orvis AL (1963) Skeletal clearance of C^{47} and Sr^{85} and skeletal blood flow in dogs. *Proc Staff Meet Mayo Clin* **38:** 559–570.

Weiss L (1959) The organization of the connective tissue elements in bone marrow. I. Fat cells. *Anat Rec* **133:** 439.

Weiss L (1960) The organization of the connective tissue elements in bone marrow. II. Reticular cells. *Anat Rec* **136:** 300.

Weiss L (1961) An electron microscopic study of the vascular sinuses of the bone marrow of the rabbit. *Bull Johns Hopkins Hosp* **108:** 171–178.

Weiss L, Root WS (1959) Innervation of the vessels of the marrow cavity of certain bones. *Am J Physiol* **197:** 1255–1257.

Welch RD, Johnston CE, Waldron MJ, Poteet B (1994) Bone changes associated with intraosseous hypertension in the caprine tibia. *J Bone Joint Surg* **75A:** 53–60.

White NB, Stein AH (1965) Observations on the rate of blood flow in the rabbit's tibia following ligation of the femoral vein. *Surg Gynecol Obstet* **121:** 1081–1084.

White NB, ter Pogossian M, Stein AH (1964) A method to determine the rate of blood flow in long bone and selected soft tissues. *Surg Gynecol Obstet* **119:** 535–540.

Whiteside LA (1984) Locomotor system: bones. Anatomy of blood circulation. In: *Blood Vessels and Lymphatics in Organ Systems* (eds DI Abramson, PD Dobrin), London: Academic, 674–697.

Whiteside LA, Lesker PA, Simmons DJ (1977a) Measurement of regional bone and bone marrow blood flow in rabbit using the hydrogen washout technique. *Clin Orthop Rel Res* **122:** 340–346.

Whiteside LA, Simmons, Lesker PA (1977b) Comparison of regional bone blood flow in areas with differing osteoblastic activity in the rabbit tibia. *Clin Orthop Rel Res* **124:** 267–270.

Wicker P, Tarazi RC (1982a) Coronary blood flow measurements with left atrial injection of microspheres in conscious rats. *Cardiovasc Res* **16:** 580–586.

Wicker P, Tarazi RC (1982b) Importance of injection site for coronary blood flow determinations by microspheres in rats. *Am J Physiol* **242** (Heart Circ Physiol 11): H94–H97.

Wiedman MP, Tuma RF, Mayrovitz HN (1981) *An Introduction to Microcirculation. Biophysics and Bioengineering Series*, vol 2, New York: Academic.

Wijeratne DE (1973) *Bone Growth and Vascularity in the Denervated Limb*, PhD Thesis of the University of London.

Wilkes CH, Visscher MB (1975) Some physiological aspects of bone marrow pressure. *J Bone Joint Surg* **57A:** 49–57.

Willans SM, McCarthy ID (1991) Heterogeneity of blood flow in tibial cortical bone: an experimental investigation using microspheres. *J Orthop Res* **9:** 168–173.

Williams MA (1985) Quantitative methods in biology: Stereological techniques. In: *Practical Methods in Electron Microscopy*, vol 6 (eds AM Glauert), Amsterdam: North Holland.

Willis TA (1949) Nutrient arteries of the vertebral bodies. *J Bone Joint Surg* **31A:** 538–540.

Willmer EN (1965) *Cells and Tissues in Culture*, vol I, London: Academic.

Wilson PD, Thompson TC (1939) Clinical consideration of methods equalizing leg length. *Ann Surg* **110:** 992–1015.

Winslow JB (1776) *An Anatomical Exposition of the Structure of the Human Body*, 5th edn (trans G Douglas), London: JF Rivington.

Wolff J (1868) Die Ossification des hyalinen Knorpels. *St Petersb Med Z* **14:** 1–11.

Wolff J (1870) Über die innere Architektur der Knochen und ihre Bedeutung für die Frage vom Knochenwachstum. *Virchows Arch Path Anat Physiol* **50:** 389–453.

Wolff J (1892) *Das Gesetz der Transformation der Knochen*, Berlin: Hirschwald (reprinted 1991, Stuttgart: Schattaeur).

Wollenberg GA (1909) Die Aetologie der Arthritis deformans im Lichte des Experimentes. *Arch Orthop Mech Unfallchir* **7:** 226.

Wood P (1959) *Diseases of the Heart and Circulation*, 3rd edn, London: Eyre & Spottiswoode.

Wood-Jones FW (1949) *The Principles of Anatomy as Seen in the Hand*, London: Baillière, Tindall & Cox.

Wootton R (1974) The single passage extraction of 18F in rabbit bone. *Clin Sci Mol Med* **47:** 73–77.

Wootton R (1988) Errors in bone blood flow measured with microspheres due to sample preparation technique. *Clin Phys Physiol Meas* **9:** 273–276.

Wootton R (1993) Measurement of bone blood flow in humans. In: *Bone Circulation and Vascularization in Normal and Pathological Conditions* (eds A Schoutens, SPF Hughes, JWM Gardenieres, J Arlet), New York: Plenum, 85–93.
Wootton R, Doré C (1986) The single passage extraction of ^{18}F in rabbit bone. *Clin Phys Physiol Meas* **7:** 333–343.
Wootton R, Reeve J, Veall N (1976) The clinical measurement of skeletal blood flow. *Clin Sci Mol Med* **50:** 261–268.
Wray JB, Lynch CJ (1959) The vascular response to fracture of the tibia in the rat. *J Bone Joint Surg* **41A:** 1143–1148.
Wu YK, Miltner LJ (1937) Procedure for stimulation of longitudinal growth of bone. Experimental study. *J Bone Joint Surg* **19:** 909–921.
Wyatt DG (1977) Theory, design, and use of electromagnetic flow meters. In: *Cardiovascular Dynamics and Measurements* (eds NH Hwang, NA Normann), Baltimore: University Park Press, chap 2.
Yasuda I (1953) Fundamental aspects of fracture treatment. *J Kyoto Med Soc* **4:** 395–406. (Translated and reprinted in *Clin Orthop* 1977; **124:** 5–8.)
Yeh C-K, Rodan GA (1984) Tensile forces enhance prostaglandin E synthesis in osteoblastic cells grown on collagen ribbons. *Calcif Tissue Int* **36:** S67–S71.
Yoffey JM (1962) A note on the thick-walled arteries of bone marrow. *J Anat* **96:** 425–426.
Yoffey JM, Hudson G, Osmond DG (1965) The lymphocyte in guinea-pig bone marrow. *J Anat* **99:** 841–860.
Young RW (1962) Cell proliferation and specialization during endochondral osteogenesis in young rats. *J Cell Biol* **14:** 357–370.
Zallone A, Teti A (1993) Animal models of bone physiology. *Curr Opin Rheumatol* **5:** 363–367.
Zamboni L, Pease DC (1961) The vascular bed of red bone marrow. *J Ultrastruct Res* **5:** 65–85.
Zawisch-Ossenitz C (1926) Histologische Untersuchungen über Gefässeinschluss und Gefässentwicklung im Knochen. *Z Mikrosk Anat Forsch* **6:** 76–161.
Zawisch-Ossenitz C (1927) Ueber Begriff und Bedeutung der durchbohrenden Knochenkanäle. *Z Mikrosk Anat Forsch* **9:** 585–606.
Zeirler KL (1965) Equations for measuring blood flow by external monitoring of radioisotopes. *Circ Res* **16:** 309–321.

Author Index

Roman numerals refer to pages in the text; *italic* numerals refer to pages in the Bibliography.

Subject Index

The items in this index are arranged alphabetically under the major subject headings shown in **bold** type. Some secondary and tertiary headings are shown in a natural, evolutionary order rather than alphabetically.

Zeitfracht Medien GmbH
Ferdinand-Jühlke-Straße 7
99095 Erfurt, Deutschland
produktsicherheit@kolibri360.de